Myasthenia Gravis
Disease Mechanism and Immunointervention

Other Books of Interest

Adaptation Biology and Medicine
(Vol 1. Subcellular Basis)
N.K. Ganguly and P.K. Singhal

Adaptation Biology and Medicine
(Vol. 2. Molecular Basis)
K.B. Pandolf et al

Advanced Histopathology
S.W.H. Stamp

Auditory Evoked Responses in Clinical Practice
A. Malhotra

Essentials of Clinical Toxicology
S.B. Lall

Diarrhoeal Diseases: Research Perspectives
N. Appaji Rao and N.K. Ganguly

Immunomodulation
S.N. Upadhyay

Immunopharmacology
S.N. Upadhyay

Introduction to Rational Use of Drugs
R.R. Chaudhary and C.D. Tripathi

Liver and Environmental Xenobiotics
S.V. Rana and K. Taketa

Multi-Drug Resistance in Emerging and Re-emerging Diseases
R.C. Mahajan and Amu Therwath

Neural Trauma and Brain Protection
V.K. Khosla and V.K. Kak

Radiobiological Concepts in Radiotherapy
D. Bhattacharjee and B.B. Singh

Rapid Eye Movement Sleep
B. Mallick and S. Inoué

Recombinant and Synthetic Vaccines
G.P. Talwar et al

Reproductive Immunology
Satish K. Gupta

Myasthenia Gravis

Disease Mechanism and Immunointervention

EDITOR
Premkumar Christadoss

Narosa Publishing House
New Delhi Chennai Mumbai Calcutta
London

EDITOR
Premkumar Christadoss
Professor
Department of Microbiology and Immunology
University of Texas Medical Branch
Galveston, Texas 77555-1070, USA

NAROSA PUBLISHING HOUSE
6 Community Centre, Panchsheel Park, New Delhi 110 017
22 Daryaganj, Prakash Deep, Delhi Medical Association Road, New Delhi 110 002
35–36 Greams Road, Thousand Lights, Chennai 600 006
306 Shiv Centre, D.B.C. Sector 17, K.U. Bazar P.O., New Mumbai 400 705
2F-2G Shivam Chambers, 53 Syed Amir Ali Avenue, Calcutta 700 019
3 Henrietta Street, Covent Garden, London WC2E 8LU, UK

ISBN 81-7319-294-4

Published by N.K. Mehra for Narosa Publishing House, 6 Community Centre, Panchsheel Park, New Delhi 110 017 and printed at Replika Press Pvt. Ltd., Delhi 110 040 (India).

Preface

Autoimmune myasthenia gravis (MG) is a classical autoimmune disease for which the target antigen, nicotinic acetylcholine receptor, has been cloned, sequenced and biochemically characterized. Antibodies to acetylcholine receptors destroy acetylcholine receptor at the neuromuscular junction, thus leading to defective neuromuscular transmission, muscle fatigue and weakness. Females of child-bearing age are more prone to develop MG, but after age 40, the incidence in both male and female are equivalent. The incidence is approximately 1 in 10,000 people. Target antigens have been characterized for only a very few other autoimmune diseases. Therefore, MG could serve as a prototype for other autoimmune diseases, especially antibody-mediated autoimmune diseases (e.g., Graves disease, SLE, hemolytic anemia, pemphigous vulgaries, etc.).

In the last few years, rapid advances have been made in unraveling the cellular and molecular mechanisms involved in the pathogenesis of MG, both in the animal model, experimental autoimmune MG (EAMG), and in human MG. Significant advances are being made in characterizing the cells and molecules involved in the autoimmune response to the acetylcholine receptor (AChR). These advances are leading to the development of specific methods of immunointervention in EAMG. Further understanding of the intricate involvement of the major histocompatibility complex (MHC) and non-MHC genes, T cell receptor (TCR), costimulator molecule, and specific cytokines in the afferent and efferent autoimmune response of AChR should pave the way to future antigen/clone-specific therapy of MG.

Every five years, the New York Academy of Sciences hosts an International Conference on MG and Related Disorders. It was felt that more frequent conferences on MG were necessary to address the rapid progress of MG research by disseminating current knowledge, and initiating future strategy through scientific interaction. In November 1998, an international MG workshop was held in Mysore, India, as a satellite Congress of the International Congress of Immunology, New Delhi, India. The theme was "Myasthenia Gravis: Disease Mechanisms and Immunointervention." The majority of the workshop's oral presentations were selected from leading current research. Scientists, clinicians, students and postdoctral fellows participated in this workshop. Day 1 was devoted to pathogenic mechanisms involving the thymus, MHC, T cell epitopes, and TCR genes in MG and EAMG. Day 2 was devoted to other pathogenic mechanisms involving non-MHC genetic polymorphism, costimulator molecules, cytokines, and hormones in MG and EAMG pathogenesis. Day 2 was also devoted to specific immunointervention in EAMG. The workshop was further complemented by poster presentations and tours of historic Mysore, which provided a friendly, interactive atmosphere.

Thus, this book is the outcome of the MG workshop proceedings in Mysore. The majority of the chapters in this book are contributed by world-renowned authors and their students. The book not only contains a timely review of specific topics, but also up-to-date findings. Scientists will find, in this volume, the latest in MG/EAMG cutting-edge research. Clinicians will be interested in the applications of the various immunointervention strategies into clinical trials in MG patients. Finally, students will not only be interested in reading the latest in EAMG/MG research, but also will find information to help them develop a future strategy to unravel the precise mechanism of disease.

To summarize, in this book, the readers should find up-to-date information related to immunological mechanisms involved in MG pathogenesis and various modalities for possible approaches to immunointervention to treat MG. I hope that the first International Workshop on MG and this book on the workshop proceedings will lay a foundation for future frequent workshops on MG, not only to promote research on the subject, but also to find a cure for this debilitating illness.

PREMKUMAR CHRISTADOSS

Acknowledgement

The following are the sponsors who provided funds to organize the MG workshop: The Department of Microbiology and Immunology, University to Texas Medical Branch, USA; Association Francaise Contre Les Myopathies, France; TEVA Pharmaceutical, Israel; and Crescent Healthcare, Inc., dba Ultracare Home Health, USA.

I would like to thank the organizing committee (Sonia Berrih-Aknin, Sanjeevi Carani, Marc H. Debaets, Sara Fuchs, Anthony Infante, Ann Kari Lefvert, Norman Talal, Socrates Tzartos and Hartmut Wekerle) who trusted in me and helped in the organization of the MG workshop. Special thanks goes to Octavious Bunshaw and Sumathi Hubert for coordinating the conference in "Southern Star", Mysore. My appreciation to Sam Baron and Stanley Lemon for their support, encouragement and suggestions during the organization of the workshop and in compiling this book for publication. Last, but not least, my gratitude to Mardelle Susman and Lyska Morrison, respectfully, for their excellent editorial and secretarial assistance.

List of Participants

Ahmed Ansar
Virginia-Maryland Regional College of Veterinary Medicine
Virginia Tech, 1410 Prices Fork Road
Blacksburg, VA 24061, USA
Phone: 540-231-7757 (7758)
Fax: 540-231-3426
E-mail: ansarahmd@vt.edu

Fulvio Baggi
Department of Neuromuscular Diseases
National Neurological Institute "Carlo Besta"
Via Celoria 11 - 20133, Milan, Italy
Phone: (39) 022394255
Fax: (39) 0270633874

Sonia Berrih-Aknin
Hopital Marie Lannelongue,
CNRS—Laboratorie de Physiologie Thymique
133, avenue de la Résistance
92350 Le Plessis-Robinson
Phone: 01.40.94.28.00 ext. 35.65
Fax 01.46.30.45.64
E-mail: berrih@pratique.fr

Ana Cardona
Laboratoire de Technologie Cellulaire
Institute Pasteur
28, rue de Doctcur Roux
75724 Paris cédex 15

Bianca M. Conti-Fine
Department of Biochemistry
Molecular Biology and Biophysics
University of Minnesota
1479 Gortner Ave.
St. Paul, MN 55108.
Phone: 612-624-6796
Fax: 612-625-5780
E-mail: conti@biosci. cbs.umn.edu

Premkumar Christadoss
Department of Microbiology and Immunology
University of Texas Medical Branch
3.142A Medical Research Building
Galveston TX. 77555-1070
Phone: (409) 772-5857
Fax: (409) 747-6869
Email: pchrista@utmb. edu

Sara Fuchs
Department of Immunology
Weizmann Institute of Science
Rehovot 76100, Israel
Tel: (+972)-8-9342618
Fax: (+972)-8-9344141
E-mail: lifuchs@weizmann.weizmann.ac.il

Stefanie Gutsche
Institute of Pathology
University of Würzburg
Josef-Schneider-Str.2
D-97080 Würzburg
Tel. 0931/201-3878:
Fax: 0931/201-3440

Viola Hoffacker
Institute of Pathology
University of Würzburg
Josef-Schneider-Str.2
D-97080 Würzburg
Tel. 0931/201-3790
Fax: 0931/201-3440

DeRen Huang
Karolinska Institute
Immunological Research Unit, CMM L8:03
Karolinska Hospital
Stockholm, S-171-76 Sweden
Phone: 46-8-51773447
Fax: 46-8-313147
E-mail: huang.de.ren@cmm.ki.se

Peter Karachunski
University of Minnesota
Dept. of Biochemistry, 140 Gortner Lab
1479 Gortner Avenue
St. Paul, MN 55108
Phone: 612-624-3790
Fax: 612-625-5780
E-mail: karachhun@biosci.cbs.umn.edu

Ann Kari Lefvert
Immunological Research Unit
CMM, L8/03
Karolinska Hospital
S-171 76 Stockholm
Sweden Phone: 46-8-51773084
Fax: 46-8-313147
e-mail: Ann.Kari.Lefvert@cmm.ki.se

Alexander Marx
Institute of Pathology
University of Würzburg
Josef-Schneider-Str.2
D-97080 Würzburg
Tel. 0931/201-5420
Fax: 0931/201-3440

Georg matell
Department of Neurology
Karolinska Institute
Stockholm, S-171 76 Sweden
Phone: 46-(0)-8-51772324
Fax: 46-(0)8-517-73757

Konstantinos Poulas
Hellenic Pasteur Institute
127 VAs. Sofias Avenue
Athens 115 21 Greece
Phone: 30-1-6430044
Fax: 30-1-6423498
E-mail: kpoulas@mail.pasteur.gr

Mathilde Poussin
University of Texas Medical Branch
Department of Microbiology and Immunology
11th and Mechanic, 142 MRB
Galveston, TX 77555-1070
Phone: 409-772-5857
Fax: 409-747-6869
E-mail: mapoussi@utmb.edu

Ioannis Roxanis
University of Oxford
Neurosciences Group
Institute of Molecular Medicine
John Radcliffe Hospital
Oxford 0X3 9DU United Kingdom
Phone: 0044-1865-222320

Berthold G.C. Schalke
Universitat Regensburg in Bezirksklinikum
Department of Neurology
Universitats Str 84
D-93053 Regensburg Germany
Phone: 0049-941-941-3010
Fax: 0049-941-941-3005

Fu-Dong Shi
Microbiology and Tumor Biology Center (MTC)
Karolinska Institute
Stockholm, S-171 77
Sweden
TEL: 46-8-728 63 02
Fax: 46-8-32 67 02.
E-mail: Fu-Dong.Shi@cnsf.ki.se

K. Sivakumar
Barrow Neurological Group
500 West Thomas Road, Suite 300
Phoenix, AZ 85013
Phone: 602-279-7300
Fax: 602-287-8076

Socrates Tzartos
Hellenic Pasteur Institute
127, Vas. Sofias Avenue
115 21 Athens Greece
Phone: 30-1-6457831
Fax: 30-1-6457831
E-mail: tzartos@mail.pasteur.gr

Carani B. Sanjeevi
Department of Molecular Medicine
Center for Molecular Medicine
L8:03, Karolinska Hospital
SE-171 76 Stockholm, Sweden
Telephone: 46-8-51776254
Fax: 46-8-51776179
E-mail: sanjeevi.carani@molmed.ki.se

Jian-ming-Wu Wu
Johns Hopkins Schools of Medicine
Baltimore, MD 21287
Phone: 410-614-4205
Fax: 410-955-1961
E-mail: wu@welchlink.welch.jhu.edu

Contents

II. Immunointervention 150–205

Myasthenia Gravis: Disease mechanisms and immunointervention
P. Christadoss (Ed)

1. Current Concepts on the Structure of Acetylcholine Receptor with Relevance to Myasthenia Gravis and Experimental Autoimmune Myasthenia Gravis Pathogenesis

Socrates Tzartos

Department of Biochemistry, Hellenic Pasteur Institute
127 Vas. Sofias Ave., Athens 11521, Greece

Introduction

Myasthenia gravis (MG) is an autoimmune disease caused by the destructive activity of antibodies to the acetylcholine receptor (AChR) of the neuromuscular junction. Our understanding of MG has been remarkably advanced compared to the level of understanding pertinent to AChR. However, an in-depth understanding of the structure and function of the AChR, and of its antigenic structure more specifically, is critical for complete comprehension of the disease and for the production of specific immunotherapeutic approaches.

AChR Structure and Function

The muscle-type nicotinic AChR (i.e. that of the neuromuscular junction and the electric organs of electric fish) is the best known member of the nicotinic AChR family, which also includes neuronal AChRs, and of the larger ligand-gated ion channel gene superfamily, which includes the receptors for $GABA_A$, serotonin ($5HT_3$) and glycine. The muscle-type AChR is a glycoprotein composed of five homologous subunits, present in the stoichiometry $\alpha_2\beta\gamma\delta$, and with a total molecular weight of about 290,000 kD; in adult muscle, the embryonic γ-subunit is replaced by the homologous ε-subunit. The neuronal nicotinic AChRs also have a pentameric structure, but are composed only of α and β subunits (α2-α9, β2-β4), which are homologous to the muscle-type subunits (reviewed in [1, 2]).

The amino acid sequences for all the AChR subunits from several species are known. The number of amino acids per muscle-type AChR subunit varies from 437 for the α-subunit to 495-501 (depending on the species) for the δ-subunit. Within a given species, the five subunits are approximately 40% homologous. Comparing AChRs from sources as different as *Torpedo* electric organ and human muscle, the α-subunits show about an 80% identity of residues and the other subunits about 55%. The N-terminus of each subunit is located extracellularly, but the location of the C-terminus is still a matter of debate (reviewed in [1, 2]).

Acetylcholine released from the nerve terminal binds to the AChR and causes the cation channel (an intrinsic part of the AChR) to open, thus allowing Na^+ to enter the muscle cell or electroplaque. Acetylcholine binds to two binding sites per AChR molecule, one on each α-subunit. Cysteine residues at α192 and α193 play a critical role in acetylcholine binding and function, while the residues Trp86, Tyr93, Trp149, Tyr151, Tyr190 and Tyr198 also seem to be implicated in acetylcholine binding. In addition, certain residues on the δ-(Trp57, Thr119, Asp180, Glu189) and γ-subunits (Trp55, Tyr117, Asp174, Glu183) contribute to the high- and low-affinity sites for acetylcholine, respectively. The binding sites for several acetylcholine agonists and antagonists have been extensively studied. Snake venom α-toxins, a group of small proteins of an approximate molecular weight of between 7,500–8,000 kD and include α-bungarotoxin from the banded krait *Bungarus multicinctus*, bind with high affinity (K_D approx. 2×10^{-11} M) to both α-subunits near the acetylcholine-binding sites, and competitively block AChR function. Peptides derived from the sequence α180-200 can bind α-bungarotoxin; the smallest peptide able to do so is α189-195 (reviewed in [1-3]).

Assembly of a fully functional AChR requires all four types of subunits. The subunits are organized around the channel in the order $\alpha\beta\alpha\gamma\delta$ or $\alpha\gamma\alpha\beta\delta$. The extracellular N-terminal half of each subunit (about 200 amino acid residues) is followed by four hydrophobic domains, M1-M4, with M1, M2 and M3 being separated by short sequences, while M3 and M4 are separated by a large cytoplasmic domain, the least conserved part of the molecule when comparing the different subunits. These four hydrophobic domains are thought to constitute a transmembrane and to form the ion channel. One of the two current models for the AChR predicts that M1-M4 form four hydrophobic α-helices, each of which crosses the membrane once. The M2 helices from each subunit line the cation channel. M1 may link the ligand binding site with M2 and also seems to contribute to the lining of the channel (reviewed in [1, 2]).

The structure and function of the cation channel have been extensively investigated, both by the use of non-competitive blockers of the AChR, which act directly on the channel, and by site-directed mutagenesis. These studies have demonstrated the presence of critical residues within the channel and identified their role in channel function. Three acidic amino acids at the ends of the M2 domain of each subunit form a negatively charged ring at the extracellular end of the pore and two negatively charged rings at the cytoplasmic end that act as selectivity filters, while rings of hydrophobic residues in the interior of the channel also play a crucial role [1, 2].

Electron microscopy of tubular crystals of *Torpedo* post-synaptic membranes has been used to reconstruct the three-dimensional structure of the AChR at both the closed and open channel configurations of the AChR at 9 Å resolution [4]. The AChR is a cylinder, 110–120 Å in length and 80 Å wide, extending out from both sides of the membrane and with a pseudo-five-fold symmetry axis running down the center of the molecule and lying approximately perpendicular to the plane of the membrane. The extracellular part of the molecule has an irregular outer surface, while its inner surface is smooth and forms a wall lining the synaptic entrance of the channel, which is a tube with a diameter at the entrance well of 25 Å, narrowing to about 7-8 Å at the transbilayer region. The synaptic domain of each subunit contains three intertwined rods (α-helices); in the α-subunits, these helices form a cavity approximately 30 Å above the bilayer surface that may constitute the ACh-binding site. The membrane-spanning region shows a high degree of rotational symmetry. The central pore is lined by five helices, but is surrounded by a continuous rim corresponding to a β-barrel. Thus, in contrast to the four transmembrane α-helix model, these data suggest that each subunit may contain only one transmembrane α-helix, apparently the M2 domain, while two or three of the M1, M3, M4 domains of each subunit possibly form the surrounding β-barrel. The transmembrane M2 helices appear to bend or kink, and to be oriented in such a way that their close approach occludes the central pore, forming a barrier to ion permeation. The binding of ACh induces a small degree of rotation of the subunits in the extracellular domain that triggers a change in the conformation of the kinked α-helices lining the membrane-spanning pore, thus increasing the diameter of the pore at the level of the kink [4].

MG and Experimental Autoimmune MG

Mainly because of the well-characterized autoantigen involved, i.e. the skeletal muscle AChR, the autoimmune disease MG has been extensively studied. It is characterized by weakness and fatigability of the skeletal muscles. Symptoms usually begin with drooping of the eyelids and double vision, followed, in most cases, by impairment of speech and swallowing. During later stages, the muscles of the limbs and trunk are usually affected, and respiration may eventually be impaired. The disease occurs in about one in 10,000–20,000 individuals, with a higher incidence in women of child-bearing age. Young onset MG is associated with the HLA antigens A1, B8 and DR3, whereas old onset MG is associated with the HLA antigens A3, B7 and DR2 (reviewed in [5-10]).

The new era in the study of MG started in 1973 with two seminal publications, when Patrick and Lindstrom reported that rabbits immunized with *Electrophorus electricus* AChR developed symptoms of MG and Fambrough and collaborators observed that muscle biopsies of MG patients had a reduced content of α-bungarotoxin binding sites compared with biopsies from healthy controls. Two years later, it was shown that MG symptoms could be passively transferred to mice using the IgG fraction from human MG sera (reviewed in [5, 10]).

The detection and measurement of anti-AChR antibodies in the sera of suspected MG patients constitutes the most objective and quantitative diagnosis of the disease [5]. Antibodies against the human AChR can be detected in the sera of about 85% of MG patients, but are essentially absent in healthy humans. Anti-AChR antibody production is controlled by autoimmune AChR-specific helper T-cells (reviewed in [7]).

Autoantibodies against other (non-AChR) muscle or non-muscle body constituents are also frequent in MG and the incidence of other autoimmune diseases in MG patients is elevated [8]. These observations suggest a major autoimmune abnormality in MG patients, but, most probably, it is primarily the action of the anti-AChR antibodies that causes the MG symptoms.

For a given patient, variations in serum anti-AChR antibody titer correlate well with clinical improvement. In contrast, studies of populations of MG patients show only a weak correlation between total anti-AChR antibody concentration and disease severity, and it is still unclear whether this is due to certain antibody subpopulations being more potent than others in causing impairment of neuromuscular transmission or to other factors [5].

MG patients have decreased numbers of AChR molecules at their neuromuscular junctions, resulting in impaired neuromuscular transmission. This decrease is caused by the anti-AChR antibodies and seems to be the main effect of these antibodies. At least two antibody-mediated mechanisms account for the observed loss: (1) Bivalent and polyvalent antibodies crosslink membrane-bound AChRs, resulting in an increased rate of internalization and degradation (antigenic modulation). (2) The bound AChR antibodies bind and activate complement, causing lysis of the membrane (reviewed in (5, 10)). In addition to the AChR loss, direct block of the function of the remaining AChRs by antibodies against the acetylcholine binding site may be a significant factor in impairing neuromuscular transmission [11, 12].

Several models have contributed dramatically to our understanding of human MG:

(A) Experimental autoimmune MG has been induced in all species tested (rats, mice, rabbits, chicken, monkeys and sheep) by injection with purified heterologous or homologous AChR, AChR subunits or their fragments, or by passive transfer of polyclonal or monoclonal anti-AChR antibodies (reviewed in [5]).

(B) In addition to human MG, idiopathic autoimmune MG also occurs in dogs; the anti-AChR antibody specificity pattern in canine MG is very similar to that seen in human MG, suggesting a similar mechanism of induction [5].

(C) A small percentage of rheumatoid arthritis or Wilson's disease patients who receive D-penicillamine develop symptoms of MG and their sera contain anti-AChR antibodies [13]; both the symptoms and antibodies disappear when the drug is withdrawn. The anti-AChR antibody specificity patterns in these patients seem to be similar to those in idiopathic MG patients [3] and it appears that the drug may mimic the unknown trigger of idiopathic MG.

(D) Approximately 10–15% of infants having mothers with MG develop myasthenic symptoms for a few weeks after birth, due to the transferred anti-AChR antibodies (neonatal MG) [14].

Although the mechanism involved is not yet understood, the thymus undoubtedly plays a crucial role in MG. Most MG patients have thymic hyperplasia, while about 10% have thymomas. Thymic lymphocytes from MG patients spontaneously produce anti-AChR antibodies and stimulate antibody production by peripheral blood cells. AChR present on the surface of myoid cells of the thymus is a possible candidate for the trigger of the autoimmune response in human MG [15]. Several AChR subunits are also present in thymic epithelial cells and may also play an important triggering role [16]. Other proteins, detected in epitheliomas of MG thymomas, but not in those of non-MG thymomas, appear to share certain epitope(s) with the AChR and may be involved in the initiation of the immune response against the AChR [8].

Current treatments for MG are relatively efficient, but generally incomplete and non-specific. Nevertheless, using established treatments, the majority of patients can now live a tolerable life, and deaths from MG no longer occur with frequency [10]. The most commonly used treatments are: (a) Anticholinesterase drugs, which inhibit the hydrolysis of acetylcholine released at the neuromuscular junction, resulting in a prolonged action on the remaining AChRs. (b) Thymectomy, which often results either in remission (in about one-third of thymectomized patients) or in improvement (in another one-third). (c) Immunosuppressive drugs (e.g. corticosteroids and azathioprine) are given to those patients who do not respond to the above treatments; however, such drugs have serious side effects that limit their use. (d) Plasmapheresis results in an immediate decrease in antibody titer which is accompanied by clinical improvement. (e) The intravenous infusion of high doses of normal human immunoglobulin is as effective as plasmapheresis in MG exacerbation and has a lower risk [17], but its mechanism of action is unclear. Various approaches to specific immunotherapy are currently being investigated, but are still at the experimental stage (reviewed in [10]).

Several informative reviews and books on various aspects of MG have been published recently [5-10].

Antigenic Structure of AChR

The AChR is a very potent immunogen. Various species of animals immunized with intact or fragmented AChR respond by the production of antibodies to various sites on the molecule. Generally, when the intact AChR is used as an immunogen, most of the antibodies are directed against extracellular regions of the AChR, while injection of denatured AChR subunits usually results in antibodies directed against cytoplasmic regions of the molecule (reviewed in [3, 5]).

The majority of antibodies (both polyclonal and monoclonal) against intact solubilized AChR from fish electric organs or mammalian muscle compete with each other for binding to a specific region on the α-subunit, the main immunogenic region (MIR) [3]. The MIR seems to be mainly restricted to a small region, but is clearly not a single epitope. Antibodies to other extracellular regions on each of the AChR subunits have also been produced. The epitopes for many of these mAbs have been identified using several approaches.

Antibody competition experiments suggest that the antibody repertoire in MG patients is similar to that in experimental rats immunized with intact AChR. The anti-MIR fraction also seems to dominate the antibody repertoire in human MG, although certain arguments against this notion have been proposed [18], and we await direct proof for the occurrence and role of anti-MIR antibodies in human MG. More direct experiments on human MG have shown the predominance of anti-α-subunit antibodies, although antibodies to other subunits clearly do exist. Antibodies binding to, or near, the acetylcholine and α-bungarotoxin binding sites also occur in MG, as do antibodies capable of displacing bound α-bungarotoxin, although the extent of their contribution to symptoms in the average MG patient is uncertain.

T cell epitopes on the AChR have been studied using recombinant proteins or synthetic peptides, and peripheral blood lymphocytes or T cell lines and clones from AChR-injected animals and MG patients. In certain species, such as the Lewis rat, there appears to be a major T cell epitope, present on the α-subunit and distinct from the MIR, whereas in other animal species and in MG patients, the response appears to be much more heterogeneous and can involve other AChR subunits. Current knowledge of the T cell epitope repertoire in experimental and human MG has been presented in detail in recent reviews [7, 19] and it is also presented in this volume by Conti-Fine and collaborators.

The in-depth understanding of the antigenic structure of the AChR at both the B and T cell epitope levels is a prerequisite for a complete understanding of the disease and for the production of specific immunotherapeutic approaches.

Main Immunogenic Region (MIR)

Identification of MIR

As mentioned above, a large fraction of the antibodies derived from rats immunized with intact AChR are directed against the MIR on the extracellular region of each α-subunit (reviewed in [3]).

Although the binding of anti-MIR antibodies is basically conformation-dependent, the weak binding of certain anti-MIR mAbs to denatured AChR subunits and to peptides made it possible to localize the MIR. Several anti-MIR mAbs were found to bind to the AChR α-subunit, indicating that the MIR is on the α-subunit. Using α-subunit proteolytic peptides, recombinant α-subunit segments and many synthetic peptides, the MIR was finally localized between α67-76 of human (WNPDDYGGVK) and *Torpedo* (WNPADYGGIK) AChR [3, 20]. The contribution of this region to the MIR was confirmed by the use of site-directed AChR mutants [21]. The antigenic role of each residue within the sequence α67-76 was tested using single residue substitutions of α67-76, and region α68-71 was found to be the most critical segment of the MIR [22, 23].

The conformation of *Torpedo* α67-76 and several of its analogues has been studied by two-dimensional NMR spectroscopy. In DMSO, α67-76 assumes a folded conformation, stabilized essentially by three interactions involving the D71, G74 and K76 amide protons. Any Ala substitution, except that on α75, significantly alters the conformation of the decapeptide. In the presence of anti-MIR mAb6, these peptides acquire a folded conformation, even in aqueous solutions. Molecular dynamics simulations, using NMR geometrical constrains, have been carried out for the free *Torpedo* peptide in DMSO, and for the more active [Ala] MIR analogue in the mAb6-bound state. It was observed that the β-folded structure of the N-terminal N68-P-A-D71 sequence was required for mAb6 recognition. It seems that the type I β-turn found in the free peptide is slightly modified into a type III β-turn in the mAb6-bound peptide. The C-terminal sequence is folded in two different ways according to the free or bound state of the peptides: two overlapping β/β or β/α turns result in a short helical sequence in the free *Torpedo* peptide, whereas the bound analogue is folded by an uncommon hydrogen bond closing an 11-membered cycle. Only the N-terminal part of the natural *Torpedo* peptide is bound to the mAb6, and the rigidly folded C-terminal part remains unbound. On the contrary, the rather flexible C-terminal part of the [Ala] MIR analogue is fashioned by mAb6, in such a way that the entire molecule is bound to the antibody. In this structure, the three hydrophobic side chains are oriented on the same side of the peptide backbone and are probably directly involved in peptide-antibody recognition [24].

Several approaches have been used to determine the epitope specificities of antibodies in MG sera. Although synthetic peptides have been used in some studies for MG antibody mapping, we believe that, since the binding of most anti-AChR antibodies is conformation-dependent, the outcome of such mapping may be misleading. We have tested human MG sera using competition experiments between anti-MIR mAbs and MG sera for binding to the intact AChR. In these studies, the proportion of MG serum antibodies prevented from binding by the anti-MIR mAbs varied from patient to patient, but, overall, approximately 65-70% of the human anti-AChR antibodies were inhibited from binding by either whole anti-MIR mAbs or their Fab fragments. This suggests that about two-thirds of MG antibodies may be directed against the MIR [3]. However, the determination of the actual epitopes for these antibodies requires the use of direct approaches. The use of AChR hybrids and mutants should offer such a direct mapping approach. As a first step, *Torpedo*-mouse and *Torpedo*-human AChR hybrids were used to confirm the immunodominance of the α-subunit in MG sera [25], and at least 50% of MG antibodies were found to bind to the α-subunit, whereas few antibodies seemed to bind to other subunits.

The MIR is clearly not a single epitope, but rather a small distinct region [3]. This fact has been stressed since the beginning, yet some confusion still exists [18]. Even among those mAbs which bind to α67-76, the various amino acid residues in the site contribute differently to the binding of each mAb [23], and the reactivity with different AChRs from various species varies considerably among these mAbs. Furthermore, the binding of other anti-MIR mAbs is entirely conformation-dependent, i.e. they do not bind, to an appreciable extent, to any synthetic peptide, yet mutation analysis shows that the epitope of at least one (mAb 35) includes the residues α68 and α71 [21]. They belong to various Ig subclasses, and anti-idiotypic antibodies show only a weak, if any, cross-reaction between anti-MIR mAbs. Finally, the nucleotide and amino acid sequences of their variable domains differ significantly [26–28]. The actual epitopes for the anti-MIR antibody fraction of human MG sera are not known. Steric hindrance is very likely to play an important role; however, this possibility does not negate the notion of, and significance of, a MIR in human MG.

The three-dimensional location of the MIR on the intact AChR (at 17 Å resolution) has been determined by electron crystallography of AChR tubes labeled with Fab or Fv fragments of mAb 35 [29], which were found to bind to the extreme synaptic ends of the two a-subunits and extend from the MIR away from the axis of the AChR towards the synaptic cleft (Fig. 1). No other subunits seemed to be directly involved in the MIR site. These extreme ends of the α-subunits are the most accessible parts of the AChR, and this accessibility may be relevant to the high immunogenicity of the MIR. Such antibodies, which extend from the MIR away from the AChR axis and into the synaptic cleft, do not need to penetrate between the closely-packed postsynaptic AChRs, and thus bind with a minimum of steric interference. Finally, in agreement with earlier biochemical observations, the orientation of the antibody fragments is such that it does not normally allow an intact antibody to cross-link two α-subunits on the same AChR molecule, and thus, anti-MIR antibodies cross-link different AChR molecules and are, therefore, particularly effective at enhancing the AChR degradation rate and the binding of complement.

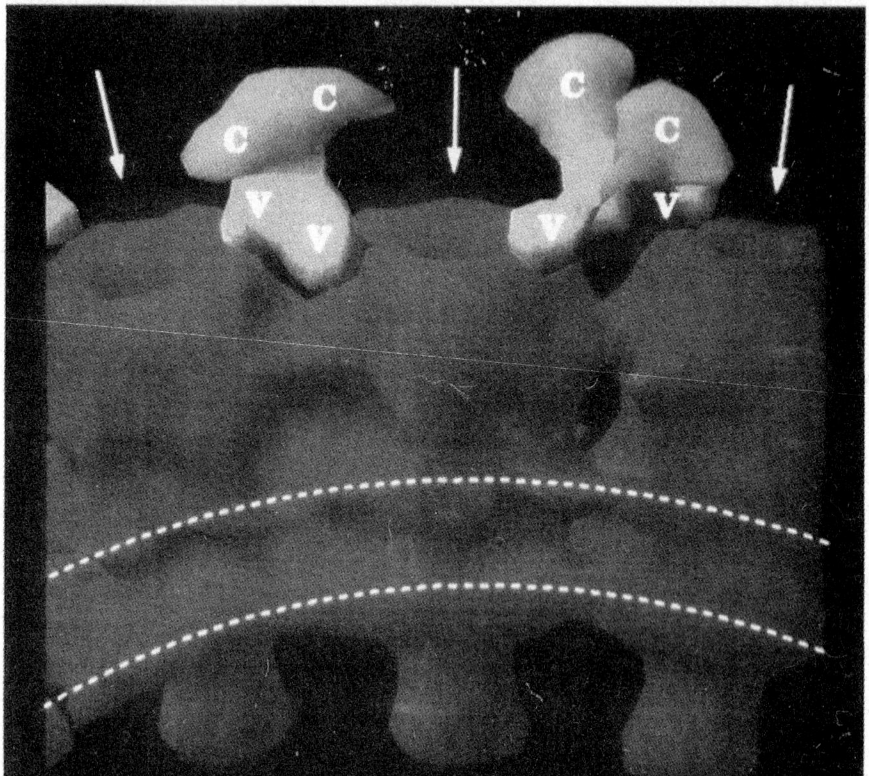

Fig. 1. Three-dimensional localization of the MIR by electron crystallography. Side view of the binding of 4 Fab fragments of anti-MIR mAb 35 to the MIR of the AChR. Variable and constant domains of Fab are marked as V and C, respectively. Pairs of Fab (V+C) binding to adjacent AChR molecules do not resolve and appear as if fused together (from [29], by permission).

Pathogenicity of anti-MIR antibodies

The potential functional roles of anti-MIR mAbs have been studied both in experimental animals and in muscle-cell cultures. Seven separate anti-MIR mAbs were found to induce MG symptoms in experimental animals within 1–3 days. Most of the animals showed severe MG symptoms and lost approximately one-half of their muscle AChR [3, 30] (Papanastasiou et al. unpublished). Similarly, animals injected with two apparently anti-MIR mAbs [18, 31] also exhibited MG symptoms and loss of muscle AChR. In contrast, four mAbs to non-MIR sites did not cause either MG symptoms or AChR loss [3]. Experiments on mice with a new set of anti-AChR mAbs have confirmed the above data: four out of five anti-MIR mAbs tested induced experimental MG, whereas none of three extracellular, but non-MIR, mAbs induced MG symptoms or AChR loss [32]. Several other mAbs capable of passively transferring MG are known to be directed against the α-subunit and, although for most of these the actual binding site has not been clearly localized, the most extensively studied mAb in this group, mAb 132A, was found to be anti-MIR [33].

The ability of anti-MIR mAbs to cause AChR loss via antigenic modulation has been studied in various animal and human muscle cell cultures [30, 34]. Almost all anti-MIR mAbs tested produced a 2–3 fold increase in the AChR degradation rate, as compared with its degradation rate in the absence of antibody, i.e., they produced an effect very similar to that of MG serum antibodies. mAbs directed against sites near the MIR also induced AChR degradation, whereas five non-MIR mAbs had no effect. In addition, bivalent $F(ab)_2$ fragments of an anti-MIR mAb, when injected into rats, were capable of causing AChR loss and MG symptoms. Since these antibody fragments lack the Fc portion which fixes complement, it can be concluded that AChR antigenic modulation alone induced by anti-MIR antibodies is capable of causing MG [30].

The effect on the AChR of anti-MIR antibodies from MG sera has only been tested indirectly, as this antibody fraction cannot yet be isolated quantitatively. The approach used was to shield the MIR of AChRs in cell culture with a univalent antibody fragment (Fab or Fv) of an anti-AChR mAb. (Univalent antibody fragments do not cross-link the AChRs and thus do not cause antigenic modulation.) Then we added the MG serum to measure its ability to downregulate the protected AChR. Using this approach, it was found that the AChR in cell cultures was efficiently protected by anti-MIR mAb fragments (by 60-80%) against the antigenic modulation induced by human MG sera [26, 34], indicating that the MIR may be the major pathogenic region of the AChR.

The above protective ability of the anti-MIR univalent Fab against AChR-loss in cell cultures, suggests a possible therapeutic approach to MG by the use of protecting univalent anti-MIR fragments. Recently we are investigating the efficacy of this approach in rats against passive transfer of MG by an anti-MIR mAb. We showed that rats were efficiently protected against the pathogenic activity of intact anti-MIR mAbs by the use of high-affinity Fab fragments from an anti-MIR mAb (Papanastasiou and col., unpublished), implying that a scheme for the efficient protection of the MIR in human MG patients may provide a useful therapeutic approach. However, the application of such an approach would require a number of modifications to the available anti-MIR recombinant antibody fragments [26], i.e., their humanization and the enhancement of their affinity for the AChR [35].

Towards this aim, we have engineered single-chain Fv fragments from three anti-MIR mAbs which exhibit moderate to high affinity for human AChR (K_D from 80 to 0.6 nM) [26, 28]. A humanized, single-chain Fv, consisting of the six

CDRs of one anti-MIR Fv (mAb 198) and the framework regions of a human immunoglobulin, was subsequently engineered. When expressed in *E. coli*, the humanized fragment exhibited a very low affinity for *Torpedo* AChR and undetectable affinity for human AChR. However, by substituting four residues in the VH framework regions (selected by molecular modelling) with those of the original rat VH, a dramatic recovery of binding affinity for both *Torpedo* and human AChRs was obtained that was only four times lower than that of the original Fv [35]. Nevertheless, the binding affinity of these fragments must be further increased in order for them to be of therapeutic use.

Immunogenicity of the cholinergic ligand binding site

Antibodies to the ligand-binding sites can be induced in experimental animals and are present in some MG patients. Usually such antibodies are detected simply by their ability to block a-bungarotoxin binding to the AChR. However, antibodies that block α-bungarotoxin binding do not necessarily block ACh binding and channel function.

Immunization of mice with intact AChR has occasionally produced mAbs directed against the α-bungarotoxin- and acetylcholine-binding sites [36–41]. mAb WF6 completely blocks toxin binding but it blocks only one-half of the ACh binding sites and does not block the binding of any small antagonists tested, suggesting the presence of separate binding sites for the different agonists and antagonists [36]. Interestingly, this mAb also blocks ACh-induced channel openings [36, 42], while, in the absence of agonist, itself acts as an agonist and activates mouse muscle AChR ion channels [42]. WF6 was shown to bind to α181-200 and, to a lesser extent, to α55-74 and α134-153 [40]; similarly, α-bungarotoxin bound to α181-200 and, to a lesser extent, to α55-74, whereas two other mAbs, the binding of which was inhibited by all cholinergic ligands, bound predominantly to α55-74 and to a lesser extent to α181-200. These results suggest that the cholinergic binding site is formed by two or more discontinuous sequence segments of the α-subunit [40].

Richman et al. ([41], and references therein) identified rat anti-AChR mAbs which blocked agonist-induced ion fluxes through *Torpedo* membrane vesicles. Some of these were characterized as directed against the a-subunit and the binding site of one that competes with agonists and antagonists was mapped to residues α187-205, i.e. the sequence which contains the major parts of the ligand binding site(s).

Monoclonal antibodies directed against the cholinergic binding site have proven to be unusually efficient inducers of experimental MG. Since the tested mAbs did not bind well to mammalian AChR, they were tested in chicken hatchlings [37] and found to induce hyperacute experimental MG within about one hour of injection without signs of postsynaptic membrane destruction, followed by death within a few hours. Apparently the antibodies directly block ACh binding, thus inhibiting ion channel opening [41].

In human MG, antibodies that inhibit ACh binding and/or function could be powerful mediators of the disease, although the actual contribution of such antibodies to the overall pathogenicity of MG antibodies is still uncertain. Several laboratories have proved that such antibodies exist in MG sera. The reported frequency of seropositive MG sera containing antibodies that block a-bungarotoxin binding to the AChR varies from 7 to 98%, depending on the type and specificity of the assay [11, 12, 18]. Drachman and collaborators detected blocking antibodies in 88% of MG sera tested, and noted a significant correlation between the degree of block and clinical status [11]. Vernet-der Garabedian et al. [12], using a novel assay detected blocking antibodies in 97% of the sera, but no significant correlation was found between the titers of blocking antibodies and clinical status. However, in neonatal MG, the occurrence of maternal blocking antibodies and their ability to cross the placenta seem to play a role in the efficiency of disease transfer. It has been shown that the sera of those MG mothers who transfer disease contain 5 times more blocking antibody than those of mothers who do not transfer disease. In addition, higher percentages of blocking antibodies crossed the placenta in affected neonates compared with non-affected ones.

Antibodies from some MG patients are capable of blocking or opening the AChR ion channel. The IgG fraction and $F(ab)_2$ fragments from an MG serum acted as an inhibitor of agonist-induced mouse AChR ion channels and as an activator of the same channels in the absence of ligand; this activation, as in the case of mAb WF6 described above, was blocked by the antagonist tubocurarine [42]. Thus, it seems that the ability of mAb WK6 to activate AChR channels is not a rare event, and such events may play a role at the neuromuscular junction in certain patients.

Other extracellular immunogenic regions

Antibodies to non-MIR extracellular sites on the α-and non-α-subunits can be produced in experimental animals and are found in MG sera. Such antibodies have been identified mainly by the use of antibody competition experiments, interspecies AChR hybrid molecules and AChR fragments. A number of mAbs directed to β, γ, δ, ε subunits have been obtained and characterized [43, 4]. Their precise epitope localization has not been able yet to be determined. Antibodies to various recombinant fragments or synthetic peptides have also been produced.

In competition experiments between anti-AChR mAbs and MG sera, antibodies to the β- and γ-subunits, as well as to a non-MIR region on the α-subunit, were detected in human sera [45]. Using *Torpedo*-mammalian hybrid AChR molecules (*Torpedo* α/mouse $\beta\gamma\delta$, mouse α/*Torpedo* $\beta\gamma$, human α/*Torpedo* $\beta\gamma\delta$ and *Torpedo* $\alpha\beta(\gamma)$/ human δ [25] and Loutrari & Tzartos, unpublished results), the subunit specificities of MG antibodies were partially, but directly, revealed. About 48% of the antibodies from 50 MG sera bound to the human α/*Torpedo* $\beta\gamma\delta$ hybrid and were thus identified as anti-α-subunit (and mostly anti-MIR); therefore some, or all, of the remaining 52% of antibodies could be directed against other subunits, but it is equally possible that the binding of some α-subunit-specific antibodies may have been impaired due to the hybrid AChRs assuming a different conformation from those of the native molecule. Direct proof of the presence of large percentages of antibodies to non-α-subunits was provided in two out of ten MG sera in which about 40 and 25% of the antibodies bound to the *Torpedo* α/mouse $\beta\gamma\delta$ hybrid and by at least two out of 50 MG sera in which about 34 and 20% of the antibodies bound to the *Torpedo* $\alpha\beta(\gamma)$/human δ hybrid (Loutrari and Tzartos, unpublished results). Unfortunately, the available hybrids did not allow the binding site of the antibodies to be localized to a single subunit. Human monoclonal Fab fragments have been produced using phage-display technology, and at least two out of 26 Fab were identified as being anti-γ-subunit [46].

An interesting issue is the question of whether MG antibodies are specific for adult and/or embryonic AChRs, which differ by one subunit (γ in the embryo; ε in the adult). Most of our mAbs bind to both AChRs, and this is consistent with the notion of the MIR and of the prevalence of anti-α-subunit antibodies. Some MG sera bind preferentially to one or other type of AChR, and this seems to be relevant to the transfer of neonatal MG and to fetal arthrogryposis. Vernet-der Garabedian et al. [14] detected a strong correlation between the occurrence of neonatal MG and the anti-embryonic/anti-adult AChR ratio, suggesting that antibodies to embryonic AChR may play a critical role in the pathogenesis of neonatal MG. Arthrogryposis multiplex congenita is a rare fetal condition that results from lack of fetal movement and occasionally complicates pregnancy in MG mothers. It has been shown that sera from mothers with a history of this disease specifically inhibit the function of fetal, but not adult, AChR [47]. The relative occurrence and pathogenic role of antibodies to the γ- and ε-subunits in disease states require further investigation.

Antigenic Structure of the Cytoplasmically-Located Region of AChR

In general, when intact AChR is used to immunize experimental animals, most of the antibodies are directed against extracellular parts of the AChR. This also seems to be the case in human MG. In contrast, when sodium dodecyl sulfate-denatured AChR, or its isolated subunits, are used, most of the antibodies are directed against cytoplasmic sites of the molecule (reviewed in [3]).

Cytoplasmic epitopes have been detected and studied by several groups. Lindstrom and colleagues (reviewed in [5]) found that most antibodies from sera of rats immunized with *Torpedo* AChR α-subunit bound to α338-366 or α150-165. Palace et al. [48] immunized four inbred strains of mice with almost full-length human recombinant α-subunit (α37-429) and studied the epitopes of the antibodies produced by their binding to smaller recombinant fragments and synthetic peptides; they found that the majority of the antibodies bound within the cytoplasmic region α325-368 and also reacted with intact human AChR. Antibodies to the cytoplasmic region can also be produced following immunization with intact solubilized AChR. When rats were immunized with intact *Torpedo* AChR, the majority of those antibodies that were able to bind to synthetic peptides bound to α330-410 [5], but this does not exclude the possibility that a large proportion of the total antibody population was incapable of binding to any synthetic peptide.

The epitopes for over 40 mAbs that bind to the cytoplasmic regions of the α, β, γ and δ-subunits have been precisely determined by the use of several hundred synthetic peptides, mimicking parts of the subunit sequences [49-51] (Fig. 2).

Most mAbs bind to restricted areas within the large cytoplasmic loop between M3 and M4 (at α341-382, β338-376, γ364-398 and δ350-396) of each subunit. Epitopes, with sizes ranging from 4 to 11 amino acids, have been identified. Comparison of the peptide mapping data with earlier mappings of the same mAbs using competitive binding experiments with the intact AChR as antigen showed the antibody competition approach to be both highly sensitive and very reliable. For example, mAbs specific for epitopes separated only by 6-7 residues showed very little cross-competition [49-51].

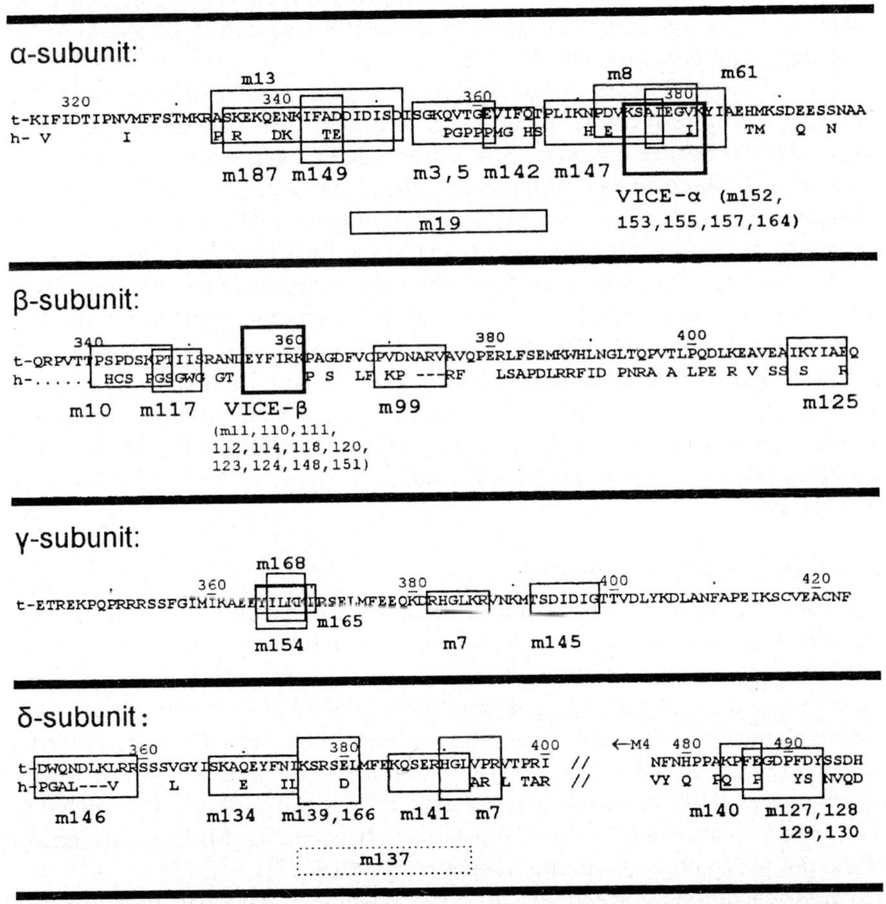

Fig. 2. Monoclonal antibody epitopes on the α, β, γ and δ-subunits of AChR. The relevant part of amino acid sequence of each subunit of the *Torpedo* AChR (t-) is shown, with non-conserved amino acid residues of the corresponding human subunit (except the γ-subunit) indicated below (h-). mAbs were tested mainly on Torpedo peptides. Epitopes for various mAbs are represented by rectangles. m187, m149 etc. represent mAb code numbers. Only the essential parts of epitopes are shown, except for anti-α-subunit mAbs 13, 187, 19 and anti-δ-subunit mAb 137 whose epitopes may be smaller than those of the identified peptides. Epitope for mAb 137 was determined indirectly from antibody competition experiments. Bold rectangles correspond to VICE-α and VICE-β. Based on results from [49–51].

Among the many cytoplasmic epitopes localized on all four subunits, two highly immunogenic cytoplasmic epitopes (VICE-α at α373–380 and VICE-β at β352–359) were identified on the α- and β-subunits; five and eleven mAbs, respectively, bound to each epitope [49, 50]. VICE-α is potentially a crucial pathogenic site, since the mAbs which bind to it also bind to a non-AChR protein (recently identified as a neurofilament NF-M protein) present in thymomas from MG patients, but absent in thymomas from non-MG individuals [8].

Certain mAbs bind to AChR tyrosine phosphorylation sites on the β- (VICE-β), γ- and δ-subunit, and some of these mAbs are capable of blocking the ligand-activated ion channel, suggesting a functional role for each single AChR tyrosine phosphorylation site [50, 51].

Anti-AChR antibodies in human MG sera bind mainly to conformational epitopes; therefore the determination of their specificities requires the use of native AChR. Earlier antibody competition studies suggested that most MG antibodies are directed against the extracellular part of the AChR. To determine whether even small quantities of such antibodies exist in MG sera, we performed competition experiments based on the inhibition by MG sera of the binding of mAb to the human AChR, rather than inhibition by mAbs of the binding of MG sera performed earlier [52]. When mAbs directed against two cytoplasmic epitopes on the α- or β-subunits (α373-380 and β354-360) were used as test mAbs, 17% or 9% of MG sera inhibited the binding of the anti-α- or anti-β-subunit mAbs, respectively, by $\geq$ 50% (Fig. 3). These results suggest the presence, in several MG sera, of antibodies directed against cytoplasmic regions of the AChR. Their possible role in the autoimmune mechanism involved in MG, remains to be determined.

Cross-Reactive Antibodies

Some anti-AChR antibodies seem to cross-react with other molecules. Molecular mimicry mechanisms involving AChR-like epitopes on non-AChR exogenous and endogenous molecules have been suggested to contribute to the induction of MG. Reported cross-reactivities of anti-AChR antibodies or epitope homologies with exogenous molecules include epitope sharing between AChR and bacterial proteins [53], between AChR α157-170 and a homologous domain of herpes simplex virus (HSV) glycoprotein D [10], between the MIR and U1 snRNP (a marker of two other autoimmune diseases) or between the MIR and a segment of the pol polyprotein of several human retroviruses [7].

Cross-reactivities with endogenous body constituents have also been observed and implicated in MG pathogenetic mechanisms. Mohan et al. [54] detected cross-reactivity of MG antibodies with an enzymatically important region in the head of the myosin heavy chain and the MIR of the AChR, and the presence of anti-myosin antibodies correlated significantly with disease severity. As mentioned earlier, mAbs to VICE-α (located between residues at 373-380 of the AChR α-subunit) bind also to a neurofilament protein (NF-M, p153), present in MG thymomas but not in non-MG thymomas, as well as to muscle fast troponin I [8]. These intriguing cross-reactivities may underlie molecular mimicry mechanisms which trigger the initial steps of the autoimmune response in MG.

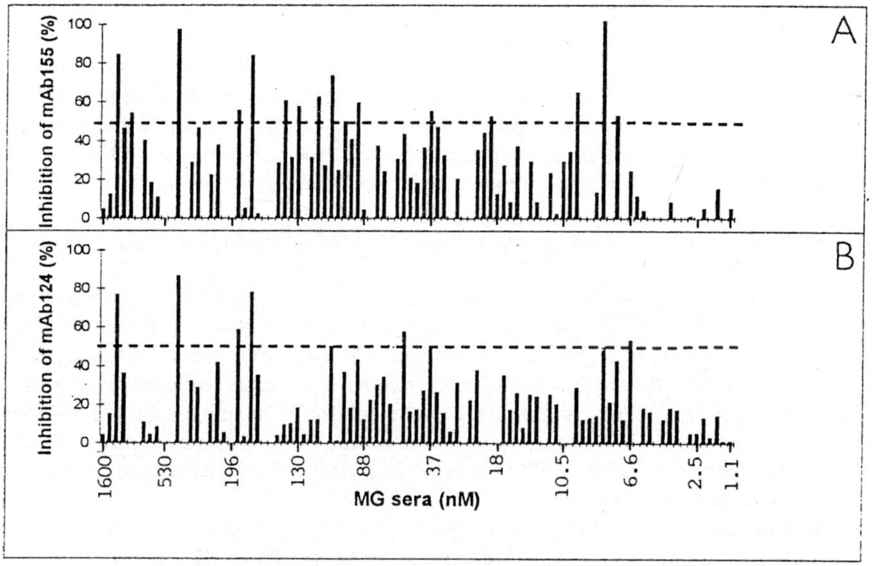

Fig. 3. Indirect detection of MG serum antibodies to two cytoplasmic regions of human AchR. Toxin-labeled AChR was incubated with Fab fragments of one of 95 sera, then mAb 155 (A—directed against the cytoplasmic epitope VICE-α) or mAb 124 (B—directed against the cytoplasmic epitope VICE-β) was added. Subsequently, mAb-bound labeled AChR was selectively immuno-precipitated. Sera are arranged in order of decreasing titer and the titers, in nM, of the 10th, 20th etc. sera (plus the first and last) are indicated. 50% cut-off of inhibition is shown by horizontal lines. Based on [52].

Conclusion

Our understanding of the antigenic structure of muscle AChR is steadily advancing. However, two major difficulties make progress slower than would be expected from the amount of efforts devoted. These are to-date the lack of diffraction quality crystals of the AChR for high resolution structural studies and the non-continuous, conformational nature of the majority of the epitopes for anti-AChR antibodies of MG patients. Yet, these obstacles are partially overcome by various laborious approaches, like electron cryo-microscopy of 2D crystals, use of AChR hybrid molecules, antibody-competition experiments, or phage-display human antibodies.

Acknowledgements

Supported by grants from the Greek General Secretariat of Research and Technology, the Association Francaise Contre Les Myopathies and the contract BIO4-CT98-0110 of the Biotechnology program of EC.

References

1. Galzi, J.L. and J.P. Changeux. 1994. Neurotransmitter-gated ion channels as unconventional allosteric proteins. *Curr. Opin. Struct. Biol.* 4: 554.

2. Karlin, A. and M.H. Akabas. 1995. Towards a structural basis for the function of nicotinic acetylcholine receptors and their cousins. *Neuron* 15: 1231.
3. Tzartos, S.J., T. Barkas, M.T. Cung, A. Mamalaki, M. Marraud, P. Orlewski, D. Papanastasiou, C. Sakarellos, M. Sakarellos-Daitsiotis, P. Tsantili and V. Tsikaris. 1998. Anatomy of the antigenic structure of a large membrane autoantigen, the muscle-type nicotinic acetylcholine receptor. *Immunol. Rev.* 163: 89.
4. Unwin, N. 1995. Acetylcholine receptor channel imaged in the open state. *Nature* 373: 37.
5. Lindstrom, J., D. Shelton, and Y. Fugii. 1988. Myasthenia Gravis. *Adv. Immunol.* 42: 233.
6. Tournier-Lasserve, E. and J.F. Bach. 1993. The immunogenetics of myasthenia gravis, multiple sclerosis and their animal models. *J. Neuroimmunol.* 47: 103.
7. Conti-Fine, B., M.P. Protti, M. Bellone and F.M. Howard Jr. (eds) 1997. *Myasthenia Gravis: The Immunobiology of an Autoimmune Disease*. Springer, New York,
8. Marx, A., A. Wilisch, A. Schultz, S. Gattenlohner, R. Nenninger and H.K. Muller-Hermelink. 1997. Pathogenesis of myasthenia gravis. *Virchows Archiv.* 430: 355.
9. Richman, D.P. (ed.). 1998. Myasthenia gravis and related diseases. *Ann.N.Y. Acad. Sci.* Vol. 841.
10. Drachman, D.B. 1998. Myasthenia gravis. In *The Autoimmune Diseases* (ed. N.R. Rose & I.R. Mackay) 3rd edition, Academic Press, San Diego. p. 637.
11. Drachman, D.B., R.N. Adams, L.F. Josifek and S.G. Self. 1982. Functional activities of autoantibodies to acetylcholine receptors and the clinical severity of myasthenia gravis. *N. Engl., J. Med.* 307: 769.
12. Vernet-der Garabedian, B., E. Morel and J.F. Bach. 1986. Heterogeneity of antibodies directed against the alpha-bungarotoxin binding site on human acetylcholine receptor and severity of myasthenia gravis. *J. Neuroimmunol.* 12: 65.
13. Russell, A.S. and J.M. Lindstrom. 1978. Penicillamine-induced myasthenia gravis associated with antibodies to acetylcholine receptor. *Neurology.* 28: 847.
14. Vernet-der Garabedian, B., M. Lacokova, B. Eymard, E. Morel, M. Faltin, J. Zajac, O. Sadovsky, M. Dommergues, P. Tripon and J.F. Bach. 1994. Association of neonatal myasthenia gravis with antibodies against the fetal acetylcholine receptor. *J. Clin. Invest.* 94: 555.
15. Wekerle, H., U.-P. Ketelsen, A.D. Zurn and B.W. Fulpius. 1978. Intrathymic pathogenesis of myasthenia gravis: transient expression of acetylcholine receptor on thymus-derived myogenic cells. *Eur. J. Immunol.* 8: 579.
16. Wakkach, A., T. Guyon, C. Bruand, S. Tzartos, S. Cohen-Kaminsky and S. Berrih-Aknin. 1996. Expression of acetylcholine receptor genes in human thymic epithelial cells-Implications for myasthenia gravis. *J. Immunol.* 157: 3752.
17. Koffman, B.M. and M.C. Dalakas. 1997. Effect of high-dose intravenous immunoglobulin on serum chemistry, hematology, and lymphocyte subpopulations: Assessments based on controlled treatment trials in patients with neurological diseases. *Muscle Nerve* 20: 1102.
18. Lennon, V.A. and G.E. Griesmann. 1989. Evidence against acetylcholine receptor having a main immunogenic region as target for autoantibodies in myasthenia gravis. *Neurology.* 39: 1069.
19. Willcox, N. 1993. Myasthenia Gravis. *Curr. Opin. Immunol.* 5: 910.
20. Tzartos, S.J., A. Kokla, S. Walgrave and B. Conti-Tronconi. 1988. Localization of the main immunogenic region of human muscle acetylcholine receptor to residues 67-76 of the α-subunit. *Proc. Natl. Acad. Sci. USA* 85: 2899.
21. Saedi, M.S., R. Anand, W.G. Conroy and J. Lindstrom. 1990. Determination of amino acids critical to the main immunogenic region of intact acetylcholine receptors by *in vitro* mutagenesis. *FEBS Lett.* 267: 55.

22. Bellone, M., F. Tang, R. Milius and B.M. Conti-Tronconi. 1989. The main immunogenic region of the nicotinic acetylcholine receptor - identification of amino acid residues interacting with different antibodies. *J. Immunol.* 143: 3568.
23. Papadouli, I., C. Sakarellos, and S.J. Tzartos. 1993. High-resolution epitope mapping and fine antigenic characterization of the main immunogenic region of the acetylcholine receptor. Improving the binding activity of synthetic analogues of the region. *Eur. J. Biochem.* 211: 227.
24. Orlewski, P., M. Marraud, M.T. Cung, V. Tsikaris, M. Sakarellos-Daitsiotis, C. Sakarellos, E. Vatzaki and S.J. Tzartos. 1996. Compared structures of the free nicotinic acetylcholine receptor main immunogenic region (MIR) decapeptide and the antibody-bound [A(76)]MIR analogue: A molecular dynamics simulation from two-dimensional NMR data. *Biopolymers* 40: 419.
25. Loutrari, H., A. Kokla, N. Trakas and S.J. Tzartos. 1997. Expression of human-Torpedo hybrid acetylcholine receptor for analysing the subunit specificity of antibodies in sera from patients with myasthenia gravis. *Clin. Exp. Immunol.* 109: 538.
26. Mamalaki, A., N. Trakas and S.J. Tzartos. 1993. Bacterial expression of a single-chain Fv fragment which efficiently protects the acetylcholine receptor against antigenic modulation caused by myasthenic antibodies. *Eur. J. Immunol.* 23: 1839.
27. Graus, Y.F., M.H. DeBaets, P.W.H.I. Parren, S. Berrih Aknin, J. Wokke, P.J.V. Vriesman and D.R. Burton. 1997. Human anti-nicotinic acetylcholine receptor recombinant Fab fragments isolated from thymus-derived phage display libraries from myasthenia gravis patients reflect predominant specificities in serum and block the action of pathogenic serum antibodies. *J. Immunol.* 158: 1919.
28. Tsantili, P., S.J. Tzartos and A. Mamalaki. 1999. High affinity scFv antibody fragments protecting the human nicotinic acetylcholine receptor. *J. Neuroimmunol.* (In Press)
29. Beroukhim, R. and N. Unwin. 1995. Three-dimensional location of the main immunogenic region of the acetylcholine receptor. *Neuron* 15: 323.
30. Loutrari, H., A. Kokla and S.J. Tzartos. 1992. Passive transfer of experimental myasthenia gravis via antigenic modulation of acetylcholine receptor. *Eur. J. Immunol.* 22: 2449.
31. Lennon, V.A. and E.H. Lambert. 1980. Myasthenia gravis induced by monoclonal antibodies to acetylcholine receptors. *Nature* 285: 238.
32. Graus, Y., F. Meng., A. Vincent, P. van Breda Vriesman and M. de Baets. 1995. Sequence analysis of anti-AChR antibodies in experimental autoimmune myasthenia gravis. *J. Immunol.* 154: 6382.
33. Agius, M.A., G.M. Twaddle and R.H. Fairclough. 1998. Epitope spreading in experimental autoimmune myasthenia gravis. *Ann. N. Y. Acad. Sci.* 841: 365.
34. Tzartos, S.J., D. Sophianos, and A. Efthimiadis. 1985. Role of the main immunogenic region of acetylcholine receptor in myasthenia gravis. An Fab monoclonal antibody protects against antigenic modulation by human sera. *J. Immunol.* 134: 2343.
35. Papanastasiou, D., A. Mamalaki, E. Eliopoulos, K. Poulas, C. Liolitsas and S.J. Tzartos. 1999. Construction and characterization of a humanized single chain Fv antibody fragment against the main immunogenic region of the acetylcholine receptor. *J Neuroimmunol.* (In Press)
36. Fels, G., R. Plumer-Wilk, M. Schreiber and A. Maelicke. 1986. A monoclonal antibody interfering with binding and response of the acetylcholine receptor. *J. Biol. Chem.* 261: 15746.
37. Souroujon, M.C., A.R. Pachner and S. Fuchs. 1986. The treatment of passively

transferred experimental myasthenia with anti-idiotypic antibodies. *Neurology.* 36: 622.

38. Dowding, A.J. and Z.W. Hall. 1987. Monoclonal antibodies specific for each of the two toxin-binding sites of Torpedo acetylcholine receptor. *Biochemistry.* 26: 6372.
39. Heidenreich, F., A. Vincent, A. Roberts and J. Newsom-Davis. 1988. Epitopes on human acetylcholine receptor defined by monoclonal antibodies and myasthenia gravis sera. *Autoimmunity* 1: 285.
40. Conti Tronconi, B.M., F. Tang, B.M. Diethelm, S.R. Spencer, S. Reinhardt Maelicke and A. Maelicke. 1990. Mapping of a cholinergic binding site by means of synthetic peptides, monoclonal antibodies and alpha-bungarotoxin. *Biochemistry* 29: 6221.
41. Mihovilovic, M., D. Donnelly-Roberts, D.P. Richman and M. Martinez-Carrion. 1994. Pathogenesis of hyperacute experimental autoimmune myasthenia gravis. *J. Immunol.* 152: 5997.
42. Bufler, J., S. Kahlert, S. Tzartos, K.V. Toyka, A. Maelicke and C. Franke. 1996. Activation and blockade of mouse muscle nicotinic channels by antibodies directed against the binding site of the acetylcholine receptor. *J. Physiol-London.* 492: 107.
43. Tzartos, S.J., L. Langeberg, S. Hochschwender, L. Swanson and J. Lindstrom. 1986. Characteristics of monoclonal antibodies to denatured Torpedo and to native calf acetylcholine receptors: species, subunit and region specificity. *J. Neuroimmunol.* 10: 235.
44. Jacobson, L., D. Beeson, S. Tzartos and A. Vincent. 1999. Monoclonal antibodies raised-globulin human acetylcholine receptor bind to all five subunits of the fetal isoform. Submitted.
45. Tzartos, S.J., M. Seybold and J. Lindstrom. 1982. Specificities of antibodies to acetylcholine receptors in sera from myasthenia gravis patients measured by monoclonal antibodies. *Proc. Natl. Acad. Sci. USA* 79: 188.
46. Matthews, I., S. Farrar, S.M. Mclachlan, B. Rapoport, N. Willcox, A. Vincent and J. Newsom-Davis. 1998. Production of Fab fragments against the human acetylcholine receptor from myasthenia gravis thymus lambda and kappa phage libraries. *Ann. N.Y. Acad. Sci.* 841: 418.
47. Riemersma, S., A. Vincent, D. Beeson, C. Newland, S. Hawke, B. Vernet-der Garabedian, B. Eymard and J. Newsom-Davis. 1996. Association of arthrogryposis multiplex congenita with maternal antibodies inhibiting fetal acetylcholine receptor function. *J. Clin. Invest.* 98: 2358.
48. Palace, J., A. Vincent, D. Beeson and J. Newsom-Davis. 1994. Immunogenicity of human recombinant acetylcholine receptor alpha subunit: Cytoplasmic epitopes dominate the antibody response in four mouse strains. *Autoimmunity.* 18: 113.
49. Tzartos, S.J. and M.S. Remoundos. 1992. Precise epitope mapping of monoclonal antibodies to the cytoplasmic side of the acetylcholine receptor alpha subunit-dissecting a potentially myasthenogenic epitope. *Eur. J. Biochem.* 207: 915.
50. Tzartos, S.J., C. Valcana, R. Kouvatsou and A. Kokla. 1993. The tyrosine phosphorylation site of the acetylcholine receptor beta-subunit Is located in a highly immunogenic epitope implicated in channel function. Antibody probes for beta-subunit phosphorylation and function. *EMBO. J.* 12: 5141.
51. Tzartos, S.J., E. Tzartos and J.S. Tzartos. 1995. Monoclonal antibodies against the acetylcholine receptor gamma-subunit as site specific probes for receptor tyrosine phosphorylation. *FEBS Lett.* 363: 195.
52. Tzartos, S.J. and M.S. Remoundos. 1999. Detection of antibodies directed against

the cytoplasmic region of the human acetylcholine receptor in sera from myasthenia gravis patients. *Clin. Exp. Immunol.* (In Press).

53. Stefansson, K., M.E. Dieperink, D.P. Richman, C.M. Gomez and L.S. Marton. 1985. Sharing of antigenic determinants between the nicotinic acetylcholine receptor and proteins in Escherichia coli, Proteus vulgaris, and Klebsiella pneumoniae. *N. Engl. J. Med.* 312: 221.
54. Mohan, S., R.J. Barohn, C.E. Jackson and K.A. Krolick. 1994. Evaluation of myosin-reactive antibodies from a panel of myasthenia gravis patients. *Clin. Immunol. Immunopathol.* 70: 266.

Myasthenia Gravis: Disease mechanisms and immunointervention
P. Christadoss (Ed)

2. Tolerance of a Transgenic Self Antigen Expressed in the Thymus: Implication for Myasthenia gravis

Anne-Marie Salmon[1], Corinne Bruand[2], Ana Cardona[3], Jean-Pierre Changeux[1] and Sonia Berrih-Aknin[2]

[1]Unité de Neurobiologie moléculaire, CNRS URA-1284, Institut Pasteur, 28 rue du Docteur Roux, 75015 Paris

[2]Laboratoire de Physiologie Thymique, CNRS ESA-8078, Hôpital Marie Lannelongue, 133, avenue de la Résistance, 92350 Le Plessis-Robinson

[3]Laboratoire de Technologie Cellulaire, Institut Pasteur, 28, rue du Docteur Roux, 75724 Paris cédex 15

Introduction

The thymus plays a central and probably a primary role in MG, as thymectomy is an effective therapy for many patients [1]. Further, thymic abnormalities (hyperplasia or thymoma) are found histologically in 70 to 80% of MG patients [2]. The presence of an autoantigen in the thymus has been suggested by several studies, but its low expression has made it difficult to detect, except in very rare myoid cells [3]. Other cell types have also been reported to contain antigens that cross-react with antibodies to AChR [4], namely epithelial cells from thymomas [5]. By molecular biology approaches, murine epithelial cell lines from the thymic cortex and medulla, as well as human thymic epithelial cells in culture, were shown to express the α-subunit AChR mRNA [6, 7].

To determine whether the AChR, or cross-reactive antigens, are expressed in the thymus, we studied mice transgenic for the α subunit gene promoter linked to the β-galactosidase (LacZ reporter) gene, and investigated to what extent the α subunit gene promoter enhanced LacZ gene expression. We used two models of transgenic mice expressing the nlsLacZ gene (with nuclear localisation sequence) under the control of α AChR promoter sequences; the first, Tg1, was constructed with an 842-bp fragment and the second, Tg2, with a 3300-bp fragment of the α AChR promoter.

Results and Discussion

1. Characteristics of the Transgenic Mouse Lineages

As described by Klarsfeld et al [8] and Salmon and Changeux [9], the α842 promoter sequence confers a spatio-temporal β-gal expression which closely parallels that of the endogeneous embryonic gene. Other lines were established with a transgene containing a longer promoter sequence of the α-subunit gene (3300 bp) derived from the chicken α subunit gene cloned by Klarsfeld et al [10]. Two founder mice, selected by DNA PCR and β-gal expression in tail muscle at birth, showed stable integration of the α3300nlsLacZ transgene and are referred to as Tg2 mice. The copy number of the transgene was roughly the same (about 3 copies) in α842NLZ2-8 (Tg1) and α3300NLZ4-14 (Tg2) mice. β-gal was mainly expressed in muscle and appeared similar in embryonic muscles in the Tg2 and Tg1 lines. Muscle staining intensity fell after birth, but β-gal expression, analyzed in leg muscles and diaphragm, remained positive until adulthood in Tg2, but not in Tg1 mice. These observations suggest that the distribution of β-gal expression in the muscle was closer to endogeneous α expression in Tg2 than in Tg1 mice.

2. The α AChR Promoter Confers Intrathymic Expression in Transgenic Mice

2.1 Nature of the expressing cell and localisation

Contradictory data have been published on AChR expression in the thymus. Since the discovery of α-bungarotoxin binding sites in the thymus [11], there has been a vigorous debate as to whether or not the thymus expresses an authentic AChR or rather an AChR-like protein, and where such a protein might be located. Myoid cells and epithelial cells have been reported to express AChR-like molecules [4-7, 11-14]. For example, Marx et al observed immunoreactivity with a monoclonal antibody directed against the cytoplasmic portion of the AChR both in myasthenic thymomas and in cortical epithelial cell lines derived from them [14]; it was subsequently shown to be due to a non-AChR cross-reactive 153 kD protein [15]. Expression of AChR genes in the thymus has been investigated by means of molecular biology. Geuder et al did not detect AChR mRNA by northern blot analysis [16], but Wheatley et al, using reverse transcription followed by the polymerase chain reaction (RT-PCR) detected the AChR α subunit mRNA in SV40-immortalized murine cortical and medullar epithelial cell lines [6]. By the same method, Kaminsky et al [17] demonstrated the presence of α and other subunits of the muscle AChR in whole thymus preparations. More recently, the different subunits of the adult AChR were detected at the mRNA level in human TEC [7].

In Tg1 mice, β-gal-positive cells were labelled with an anti-desmin antibody, demonstrating their myoid nature, while controls (fluorescent antibodies) were consistently negative. In Tg2 mice, in addition to myoid cells, numerous cells were stained which were located mainly in the cortical area. Double staining with anti-keratin antibodies showed that most β-gal-positive cells displayed the epithelial phenotype. In the medulla, some epithelial cells also express the β-gal antigen. Thus, both the thymic cortex and medulla of Tg2 mice expressed β-gal [18]. Therefore, by using transgenic mice expressing the LacZ gene under the control of the α AChR promoter, we obtained strong evidence that the AChR is present in two types of thymic cells: myoid cells, which are rare, dispersed throughout the thymus and show a high level of expression; and epithelial cells, which are numerous and predominantly located in the outer cortex [18]. This expression is consistent with data from Wheatley et al. reporting α-AChR mRNA expression in a cortical epithelial cell line [6].

This study shows that thymic expression of the transgene differed in the two mouse lines. In the Tg1 model, the 842-bp promoter fragment conferred exclusive transgene expression in myoid cells, while in the Tg2 model the longer promoter fragment (3300 bp) also led to expression in thymic epithelial cells. Differences in the number of gene copies or the site of transgene insertion could not explain these observations, since the number of copies was 3 to 4 in both mouse lines, and two distinct lines were raised for each construct and yielded similar results, thus ruling out the difference in the insertion site. The different thymic expression is more likely due to the length of the promoter. In Tg1 mice, 842 bp was sufficient for the expression in myoid cells, in keeping with the expression of the transgene in skeletal muscle of this transgenic line [8]. The expression in other cell types (TEC) in Tg2 mice would require DNA elements present upstream in the 3.3-Kb fragment, which are probably activated by factors present in TEC.

Table 1. Expression of β-gal in the thymus of Tg1 and Tg2 mice

	Transgenic mice[a]	
	Tg1[a]	Tg2[a]
Promoter	850 pb	3300 pb
Expression of β-gal cell type	myoid	myoid and epithelial
Level of expression in the thymus (pg/ml)	56	975

[a]In Tg1 mice, cells expressing β-gal are myoid cells and the level of expression evaluated in ELISA is 56 pg/ml at day 4 post natal. In Tg2 mice epithelial cells and myoid cells express β-galactosidase and the expression is about 20 times higher than in Tg1 mice.

2.2 Quantification of β-galactosidase

To measure total β-gal protein expression in the thymus and peripheral lymphoid organs of Tg1 and Tg2 mice, we extracted total protein and applied a β-gal ELISA method. As shown in Table 1, we confirmed that the thymus expressed β-gal. Secondary lymphoid organs (lymph nodes and spleen) and serum were consistently negative (data not shown). At day 4, post-natal thymic expression was about 20 times lower in Tg1 than in Tg2 mice. Expression was much higher in neonates than in adult mice. At 8 weeks, β-gal could not be detected in the thymus of Tg1 mice, but was still faintly detected in Tg2 mice (not shown).

3. Anti β-Gal Response in Tg Mice

Studies of the interaction of T cells with major histocompatibility antigens showed that the thymus is the primary site of self-tolerance induction, and that mechanisms, including programmed cell death and functional inactivation, eliminate self-reactive T lymphocytes [19]. Tolerance induction occurs in the thymus when immature thymocytes are selected to move into the mature thymocyte pool via interactions with self-antigens [20, 21]. Intrathymic antigen injection led to unresponsiveness to the same antigen in several experimental models [22, 23]. In this study we examined T cell proliferation and antibody production in response to β-gal as a self-antigen.

3.1 Antibody response

The anti β-gal antibody response was investigated after immunizing Tg1 and Tg2 mice with β-gal, by comparison with non transgenic control mice. Serum was collected from the day of immunization until 120 days post immunization. The ability to produce specific anti-β-gal antibodies was assessed by an ELISA method. Tg1 mice showed a significant specific response to β-gal, which was significantly weaker than that of non-transgenic control mice ($p < 0.0001$, ANOVA). By contrast, the response was clearly impaired in Tg2 mice ($p < 0.0001$ compared to Tg1 and non transgenic control mice, ANOVA). The mean maximal responses were 874, 35 and 1187 μg/ml in Tg1, Tg2 and control mice, respectively (Table 2). In Tg2 mice the mean anti-β-galactosidase antibody titer was, therefore, 34 times lower than in the control group. *Torpedo* AChR was used as a control antigen, and anti-AChR antibodies were analysed by radioimmunoassay. The three mouse lines responded very similarly, indicating that these mouse lines present the same ability to produce antibodies upon immunization (Table 2).

Table 2. Anti β-gal and anti-AChR antibody production in Tg1 and Tg2 after challenge with β-gal and -AChR, respectively

	Mice		
	Controls	Tg1	Tg2
anti-β-gal antibodies (μg/ml)[a]	1187 ± 121	874 ± 110	35.4 ± 30
anti-AChR antibodies (nM)[a]	325 ± 151	275 ± 58	332 ± 170

[a]Results are expressed as mean ± SD of the maximum level of antibodies for 3 or 4 mice. This level is obtained between day 50 and 60 for β-gal antibodies and between days 40 to 50 for anti-AChR antibodies. β-gal antibodies were titrated by ELISA and AChR antibodies were detected by radioimmunoprecipitation.

3.2 Anti β-Gal Proliferation Assay and Cytokine Profile

The ability of T cells from immunized mice to proliferate in response to β-gal is shown in Table 3. Cultured lymph node cells from Tg1 and Tg2 mice showed lower β-gal-dependent proliferation than controls ($p < 0.0001$ for both transgenic lines, ANOVA). The results obtained in Tg1 mice suggested that the β-gal proliferative response was much more sensitive to tolerance induction than was anti-β-gal antibody production, as the antibody reponse was reduced by about 30% relative to the mean control value, while antigen-specific proliferation fell by about 90%.

In order to further explore the Th1/Th2 response in the transgenic mice, Tg1, Tg2 and control mice were immunized with β-gal. Eight days later, lymph node cells were cultured in the presence of β-gal, and supernatants were titrated for their contents in IL-4 and IFN-γ (Table 3). Compared to cells from non-transgenic control mice, cells from Tg1 mice produced comparable levels of IL-4, but much lower levels of IFN-γ, while cells from Tg2 mice produced low levels of IFN-γ and undetectable levels of IL-4. The calculated ratio IL-4/IFN-γ was 0.5, 2.6 and 0 for control, Tg1 and Tg2 mice, respectively, underlining an imbalance in favor of the Th2 cell type in Tg1 mice (Table 3).

Table 3. β-galactosidase T cell proliferation

	Mice		
	Controls	Tg1	Tg2
β-gal proliferation (cpm)[a]	28728 ± 9220	1213 ± 1389	369 ± 588
IL4 / IFNγ ratio[a]	0,46	2,63	0,05

[a]Mice were challenged with β-galactosidase and proliferation towards β-gal were measured in the lymph node cells. Cell proliferation results are expressed as the mean ± SD for 3 or 4 mice. IL-4 and IFNγ were titrated in the supernatant of the cultures by ELISA.

These data raise the question of why tolerance towards a T cell-dependent self-antigen fails in Tg1 mice, even though they express a significant level of β-galactosidase in their thymus. Several mutually compatible explanations can be forwarded: (1) myoid cells may not be able to present the antigen to developing T cells, or co-stimulatory signals may be lacking. This is unlikely, as these mice were virtually unresponsive in the T cell proliferation assay. (2) The localisation of expressing cells could be important. Indeed, in the Tg1 line, the expression was limited to some isolated cells essentially in the medulla, while in the Tg2 line, expressing cells were found mainly in the cortex and faintly in the medulla. (3) The kinetics of antigen expression may be important. Self tolerance is achieved mainly by the deletion and inactivation of autoreactive T cells during thymic development [19-21]. In the Tg1 model, β-gal expression decreases after birth, whereas β-gal expression increases after birth and is still present in adulthood in Tg2 mice. Thus it is possible that the significant decrease of β-gal expressing cells in Tg1 mice after birth is responsible for the incomplete tolerance in these mice. (4) Finally, the self-antigen is not sufficiently abundant in Tg1 mice to induce full tolerance. Differences in the frequency, duration and intensity of contacts between T cells and the tolerating tissue are probably crucial. Limiting levels of expression of self antigen influence the efficiency of negative selection, enabling potentially self-reactive T cells to escape tolerance induction [24, 25]. In Tg1 mice we found that total expression of β-gal was about 20 times lower than in Tg2 mice. Thus, expression in Tg1 mice may be just sufficient for T cell proliferation unresponsiveness, but too low to induce tolerance in terms of antibody production. A Th1 > Th2 > B cell gradient of sensitivity to tolerance induction has been forwarded (26). The level of β-gal expression could thus be sufficient for tolerance induction of Th1 cells but not Th2 cells in Tg1 mice, while both Th1 and Th2 populations are tolerized in Tg2 mice. This is supported by the cytokine profile analysis.

In myasthenia gravis, an antibody response to the AChR is raised, thus indicating that thymic AChR expression levels are too low to induce tolerance. Several arguments support this hypothesis: (1) immunization of mice with affinity-purified mouse AChR induces not only anti-AChR antibody responses but also myasthenic symptoms in some animals, even when AChR is injected without adjuvants [27]; (2) AChR-reactive T and B cells have been reported not only in MG patients but also in controls [28]. (3) The level of AChR protein has been examined in a previous report [29] that indicates that the number of AChR molecules is around 0.9 fmole/mg of tissue, that is about 8 (adult age) and 80 (neonatal) times less than the β-galactosidase expression detected in the Tg2 mice. Thus, even if the distribution of β-gal in Tg2 mice looks similar to that of the endogeneous gene, a major difference in the amount of the antigen expressed could explain why an anti-β-gal response did not take place in Tg2 mice, while an anti-AChR reponse was obtained. Environmental antigens may activate T cells which cross-react with the autoantigen, thereby initiating autoimmunity. Thus, as in other models, autoimmunity in MG is not necessarily due to a break-down of self tolerance. Indeed, in transgenic mice expressing the glycoprotein of lymphocytic choriomeningitis virus (LCMV-GP) under the control of the rat insulin promoter, viral glycoprotein on islet β cells is ignored by the immune system. However, in appropriate priming conditions, an immune reaction against this antigen can be mounted and can induce autoimmunity [30].

Conclusion

Our results show that the tolerance of developing T cells in the thymus is dependent on the level of expression of the self antigen. Similar observations have been recently reported in other models of autoimmunity. In the human insulin-dependent diabetes mellitus (IDDM) that results from the autoimmune destruction of the insulin-producing pancreatic β-cells, the susceptibility to diabetes is higher in patients with lower insulin thymic expression, indicating that high thymic expression might prevent β-cell destruction by promoting the deletion in the thymus of insulin-reactive, diabetogenic T cells [31, 32]. In the experimental model of autoimmune uveoretinitis, a correlation between constitutive expression of ocular autoantigens in the thymus and resistance to autoimmunity was evidenced [33].

The two transgenic mice lines described in this study are powerful tools not only for characterizing the cells potentially expressing AChR but also for exploring the mechanisms of tolerance towards an antigen differentially expressed in the thymus. Furthermore, as the self antigen is transiently expressed in the thymus, these models could also contribute to our understanding of how self tolerance is maintained during aging.

Acknowledgments

This work was supported by grants from CNRS (Centre National de la Recherche Scientifique), CNAMTS (Caisse Nationale d'Assurance Maladie des Travailleurs Salariés), AFM (Association Française contre les Myopathies) and Pasteur Institute.

References

1. Le Brigand, H., P. Levasseur, A.R. Miranda, C. Gaud and I. Wojakowski. 1980. Surgical treatment of myasthenia gravis by thymectomy: A report on 248 cases. *Ann. Chir.* 34: 169–172.
2. Berrih-Aknin, S., E. Morel, F. Raimond, D. Safar, C. Gaud, J.P. Binet, P. Levasseur and J.F. Bach. 1987. The role of the thymus in myasthenia gravis: Immunohistological and immunological studies in 115 cases. *Ann. N.Y. Acad. Sci.* 505: 50–70.
3. Schluep, M., N. Willcox, A. Vincent, G.K. Dhoot and J. Newsom-Davis. 1987. Acetylcholine receptors in human thymic myoid cells *in situ*: an immunohistological study. *Ann. Neurol.* 22: 212–222.
4. Marx, A., T. Kirchner, F. Hoppe, R. O'Conner, B. Schalke, S. Tzartos and H.K. Muller-Hermelink. 1989. Proteins with epitopes of the acetylcholine receptor in epithelial cell cultures of thymomas in myasthenia gravis. *Am. J. Pathol.* 134: 865–877.
5. Hara, Y., S. Ueno, T. Uemichi, N. Takahashi, S. Yorifuji, Y. Fujii and S. Tarui. 1991. Neoplastic epithelial cells express α-subunit of muscle nicotinic acetylcholine receptor in thymomas from patients with myasthenia gravis. *FEBS Lett.* 279: 137–140.
6. Wheatley, L.M., D. Urso, K. Tumas, J. Maltzman, E. Loh and A.I. Levinson. 1992. Molecular evidence for the expression of nicotinic acetylcholine receptor alpha-chain in mouse thymus. *J. Immunol.* 148: 3105–3109.
7. Wakkach, A., T. Guyon, C. Bruand, S. Tzartos, S. Cohen-Kaminsky and S. Berrih-Aknin. 1996. Expression of acetylcholine receptor genes in human thymic epithelial cells. Implications for Myasthenia Gravis. *J Immunol* 157: 3752–3760.
8. Klarsfeld, A., J.L. Bessereau, A.M. Salmon, A. Triller, C. Babinet and J.P. Changeux. 1991. An acetylcholine receptor α-subunit promoter conferring preferential synaptic expression in muscle of transgenic mice. *EMBO J.* 10: 625–632.
9. Salmon, A.M. and J.P. Changeux. 1992. Regulation of an acetylcholine receptor LacZ transgene by muscle innervation. *Neuro Report* 3: 973–976.
10. Klarsfeld, A. and J.P Changeux. 1985. Activity regulates the levels of acetylcholine receptor α-subunit mRNA in cultured chicken myotubes. *Proc. Natl. Acad. Sci.* 82: 4558–4562.
11. Engel, W.K., J.L. Trotter, D.E. McFarlin and C.L. McIntosh. 1977. Thymic epithelial cell contains acetylcholine receptor. *Lancet* 1: 1310–1311.
12. Kao, I. and D.B. Drachman. 1978. Thymic muscle cells bear acetylcholine receptors: possible relation to myasthenia gravis. *Science* 195: 74–75.
13. Wekerle, H., U.P. Ketelson, A.D. Zurn and B.W. Fulpius. 1978. Intrathymic pathogenesis of myasthenia gravis: transient expression of acetylcholine receptors on thymus-derived myogenic cells. *Eur. J. Immunol.* 8: 579–582.
14. Marx, A., T. Kirchner, F. Hoppe, R. O'Conner, B. Schalke, S. Tzartos and H.K. Müller-Hermelink. 1989. Proteins with epitopes of the acetylcholine receptor in epithelial cell cultures of thymomas in myasthenia gravis. *Am. J. Pathol.* 134: 865–877.
15. Marx, A., R. O'Connor, K.I. Geuder, F. Hoppe, B. Schalke, S. Tzartos, I. Kalies, T. Kirchner and H.K. Muller-Hermelink. 1990. Characterization of a protein with an acetylcholine receptor epitope from myasthenia gravis-associated thymomas. *Lab. Invest.* 62: 279–286.
16. Geuder, K.I.R., R. Schoepfer, T. Kirchner, A. Marx and H.K. Muller-Hermelink. 1989. The gene of the α-subunit of the acetylcholine receptor: molecular

organization and transcription in myasthenia-associated thymomas. *Thymus* 14: 179–186.

17. Kaminski, H.J., R.A.F. Fenstermaker, W. Abdul-Karim, J. Clayman and R.L. Ruff. 1993. Acetylcholine receptor subunit gene expression in thymic tissue. *Muscle Nerve* 16: 1332–1337.
18. Salmon A.M., C. Bruand, A.Cardona, J.P. Changeux and S. Berrih-Aknin. 1998. An acetylcholine receptor α subunit promoter confers intrathymic expression in transgenic mice. Implications for tolerance of a transgenic self antigen and for autoreactivity in myasthenia gravis. *J. Clin. Invest.* 101: 2340–2350.
19. Nossal, G.J.V. 1994. Negative selection of lymphocytes. *Cell* 76: 229–239.
20. Kappler, J.W., N. Roehm and P. Marrack. 1987. T cell tolerance by clonal elimination in the thymus. *Cell* 49: 273–280.
21. Kisielow, P., H. Blüthmann, U.D. Staerz, M. Steinmetz and H. Von Boehmer. 1988. Tolerance in T-cell-receptor transgenic mice involves deletion of nonmature CD4+8+ thymocytes. *Nature* 333: 742–746.
22. Posselt, A.M., C.F. Barker, J.E. Tomaszewski, J.F. Markmann, M.A. Choti, A. Naji. 1990. Induction of donor-specific unresponsiveness by intrathymic islet transplantation. *Science* 249: 1293–1295.
23. Remuzzi, G., M. Rossini, O. Imberti and N. Perico. 1991. Kidney graft survival in rats without immunusuppressants after intrathymic glomerular transplantation. *Lancet* 337: 750–752.
24. Oehen S.U., P.S. Ohashi, K. Bürki, H. Hengartner, R.M. Zinkernagel and P. Aichele. 1994. Escape of thymocytes and mature T cells from clonal deletion due to limiting tolerogen expression levels. *Cell. Immunol.* 158: 342–352.
25. Iwabuchi, K., K.I. Nakayama, R.L. McCoy, F. Wang, T. Nishimura, S. Habu, K.M. Murphy and D.Y. Loh. 1992. Cellular and peptide requirements for *in vitro* clconal deletion of immature thymocytes. *Proc. Natl. Acad. Sci.* 9000–9004.
26. Husby, S., J. Mestecky, Z. Moldoneanu, S. Holland and C.O. Elson. 1994. Oral tolerance in humans. T cell but not B cell tolerance after antigen feeding. *J. Immunol.* 152: 4663.
27. Jermy, A., D. Beeson and A. Vincent. 1993. Pathogenic autoimmunity to affinity-purified mouse acetylcholine receptor induced without adjuvant in BALB/c mice. *Eur. J. Immunol.* 23: 973–976.
28. Link, H., O. Olsson, J. Sun, W.Z. Wang, G. Andersson, H.P. Ekre, T. Brenner, O. Abramsky and T. Olsson. 1991. Acetylcholine receptor-reactive T and B cells in myasthenia gravis and controls. *J. Clin. Invest.* 87: 2191–2195.
29. Ohshima F., K. Kondo and T. Tsubaki. 1978. Binding of iodine 125 a-bungarotoxin to the thymus of mice. *Arch Neurol* 35: 31–32.
30. Ohashi, P.S., S. Oehen, K. Buerki, H. Pircher, C.T. Ohashi, B. Odermatt, B. Malissen, R.M. Zinkernagel and H. Hengartner. 1991. Ablation of tolerance and induction of diabetes by virus infection in viral antigen transgenic mice. *Cell* 65: 304–317.
31. Vafiadis P., S.T. Bennett, J.A. Todd, J. Nadeau, R. Grabs, C.G. Goodyer, S. Wickramasinghe, E. Colle and C. Polychronakos. 1997. Insulin expression in human thymus is modulated by *INS* VNTR alleles at the *IDDM2* locus. *Nature genetics* 15: 289–292.
32. Pugliese A., M. Zeller, A. Fernandez, L.J. Zalcberg, R.J. Bartlett, C. Ricordi, M. Pietropaolo, G.S. Eisenbarth, S.T. Bennett and D.D. Patel. 1997. The insulin gene is transcribed in the human thymus and transcription levels correlate with allelic variation at the *INS* VNTR-*IDDM2* susceptibility locus for type 1 diabetes. *Nature genetics* 15: 293–297.
33. Egwuagu C.E., P. Charukamnoetkanok and I. Gery. 1997. Thymic expression of autoantigens correlates with resistance to autoimmune disease. *J. Immunol.* 159: 3109–3112.

Myasthenia Gravis: Disease mechanisms and immunointervention
P. Christadoss (Ed)

3. Low Levels of Acetylcholine Receptor Delta-Subunit Message and Protein in Human Thymus Suggests the Occurrence of 'Triplet Receptors' in Thymic Myoid Cells

Alexander Marx[1], Annette Wilisch[1], Stefanie Gutsche[1], Viola Hoffacker[1], Anja Schultz[1], Socrates Tzartos[2], Wilfried Nix[3], Berthold Schalke[4], Christiane Schneider[5] and Hans-Konrad Müller-Hermelink[1]

[1]Institute of Pathology, University of Würzburg, Germany

[2]Hellenic Pasteur Institute, Athens, Greece

[3]Department of Neurology, University of Mainz, Germany

[4]Department of Neurology, University of Regensburg, Germany

[5]Department of Neurology, University of Würzburg, Germany

Introduction

Myasthenia gravis (MG) is an autoimmune disease caused by autoantibodies against the acetylcholine receptor (AChR) at the neuromuscular junction [1]. The muscular AChR has been extensively characterized [2], but whether the muscular AChR plays a role during the initiation of MG is unknown [3]. The muscular AChR is a pentameric ion channel composed of 4 different subunits [2, 4]. The fetal AChR expressed during intrauterine life and after denervation of adult muscle exhibits an $\alpha_2\beta\delta\gamma$ composition, while the adult AChR expressed after birth in innervated muscle exhibits an $\alpha_2\beta\delta\varepsilon$ composition [4]. The α-subunit contains the main epitopes recognized by MG autoantibodies [2]. The human muscle AChR α-subunit exists as two isoforms, P3A$^-$ and P3A$^+$ [5]. The P3A$^+$ isoform does not bind α-bungarotoxin or monoclonal antibodies against the AChR main immunogenic region and is not integrated into functional AChR [6]. Studies on the expression of the various AChR subunits in thymus and thymoma are reported by Gutsche et al [16].

The pathogenetic relevance of thymic pathology for the development of MG is undisputed [3, 7], but whether it is involved in the triggering of MG is unknown [8]. Seventy percent of MG patients have thymitis. In these patients autoantibody production occurs inside the thymus, and autosensitization probably takes place via exposure of antigen presenting cells and autoreactive T cells to muscular AChR expressed on thymic myoid cells [9, 10, 11]. Ten percent of MG patients have a thymic epithelial tumor (thymoma). Most thymomas appear to contribute to the pathogenesis of paraneoplastic MG by abnormal (non-tolerogenic) intratumorous generation of mature T cells from immature precursors, but whether muscular AChR drives the autoimmune process as assumed in thymitis is not known [16, 17]. In screening thymomas and thymuses for expression of message for the various AChR subunits, we realized that the δ-subunit message was by far the least abundant or even undetectable. In agreement with these findings no δ-subunit protein could be detected in thymic myoid cells, while α-subunit protein was readily identified. These findings imply that there may occur "triplet AChR" on thymic myoid devoid of δ-subunits with the presumed composition $\alpha_2\beta\gamma_2$.

Material and Methods

Tissues

Thirty-five thymomas, 7 hyperplastic thymuses, 3 normal thymuses and 2 tumor biopsies of rhabdomyosarcoma patients were studied by RT-PCR using tissue snap-frozen within four hours after surgery. Thymomas were classified according to Müller-Hermelink and co-workers [12]: 12 cortical thymomas (CT), 4 "well differentiated thymic carcinoma" (WDTC), 17 mixed thymomas (MXT), and 2 medullary thymomas (MDT). Normal thymuses ($n = 3$, age range 3 d to 51 y, sex ratio (f/m) = 1/2) were obtained from patients without immunological disorders undergoing thoracic surgery. Thymuses with typical lymphofollicular thymitis (THY, $n = 7$, age range 11 to 61 y only women) and two different ex vivo rhabdomyosarcoma biopsies were tested. MG was diagnosed in all THY ($n = 7$), MDT ($n = 2$) and WDTC ($n = 4$) cases and in 9 of the 17 MXT and 7 of the 12 CT cases. For PCR based detection of muscular AChR gene expression, the embryonal and alveolar rhabdomyosarcoma cell lines TE 671 and RD, respectively, were used as positive controls.

Reverse Transcriptase Polymerase Chain Reaction (RT-PCR)

Total RNA was prepared from 0.1 g snap-frozen tissue or from 10^6 cultured cells using Trizol reagent (Gibco Life Technologies, Eggenstein, Germany). After cDNA synthesis with oligo-dT specific primers and MMLV reverse transcriptase, 1/20 of each reaction mixture was amplified using Taq polymerase and sequence specific primers. The oligonucleotide primers were derived from published sequences. Amplification was performed applying the following parameters. By denaturation for 30 sec at 94°C, annealing for 30 sec at a primer specific temperature and amplification for 30 sec at 72°C. An RT-PCR with GAPDH-specific primers and ethidium staining of rRNA was performed to confirm the integrity of the RNA.

One-fourth of the amplified cDNA was electrophoretically separated on a 2% agarose gel, stained with ethidium bromide and a picture was taken using a videoprinter. The picture was digitized, saved on disk and used for final picture processing. Ethidium bromide staining of the AChR amplification products revealed bands of expected molecular size and subsequent sequencing of the PCR products confirmed that the cDNA fragments were identical to the published AChR sequences. Primer sequences, annealing temperatures and number of cycles are available on request. For the nested PCR analysis of the AChR δ-subunit a second pair of primers was chosen, which are located within the cDNA sequence which was amplified using the first pair of primers (δ1). Instead of cDNA the amplification product of the first round of PCR was used for nested PCR.

Immunofluorescence

For double labeling of myoid cells in frozen tissue sections the histological slides were incubated first with the respective AChR specific antibody (Table 1) and second with a biotin-SP-conjugated donkey anti-rat serum (Dianova, Hamburg, Germany, dilution 1:1,000). Subsequently, the slides were incubated with Cy^{TM3}-conjugated streptavidin (Dianova, Hamburg, Germany, dilution 1:1,000). To label the second antibody, slides were then incubated with an anti-Desmin antibody (Immunotech, Hamburg, Germany, undiluted), followed by a FITC (Fluorescein thiocyanate)-labeled goat anti-mouse serum (Dianova, Hamburg, Germany, dilution 1:1,000). Each incubation step was for 30 minutes and followed by washing with Tris buffer, pH 7.4. As controls, the respective first antibodies were omitted, excluding cross-reactivities of the biotin- or FITC-labeled sera. Specimens were investigated under a Zeiss axiophot microscope.

Table 1. Antibodies used for immunofluorescence

Monoclonal antibody	Subunit, region and epitope specificity	Dilution	Animal	Reference
Mab 195 (IgG1)	α 67-74, MIRa	1:40	rat	38
Mab 198 (IgG2a)	α 67-74, MIR	1:20	rat	38
Mab 61 (IgG2a)	α 375-389	1:40	rat	39
Mab 7 (IgG1)	δ 389-396, cytoplasmic	undiluted[b]	rat	40
Mab 137 (IgM)	δ 376-392, cytoplasmic	undiluted	rat	39
Mab 141 (IgG2a)	δ 385-392, cytoplasmic	1:10	rat	39

[a]MIR: main immunogenic region of the muscular AChR α subunit (extracellular).
[b]Undiluted: Cell culture supernatant.

Results

The AChR δ-subunit was investigated using two different PCR primer pairs: one specific for a sequence located more 3′ and another specific for a sequence located more 5′ in the AChR δ-cDNA. This subunit gene was always strongly expressed in different muscles and rhabdomyosarcomas, but not in any of the thymic tissues (normal thymus, thymitis or thymoma) investigated (Fig. 1). To increase the sensitivity, we performed a nested PCR. In this type of experiment the δ-subunit could be detected in 24 out of 31 cases (Fig. 1). No expression after the second PCR round was detected in two THY, one MXT, two CT and two WDTC cases. This indicates that the δ-subunit mRNA is present in thymic tissue, albeit in very low concentrations.

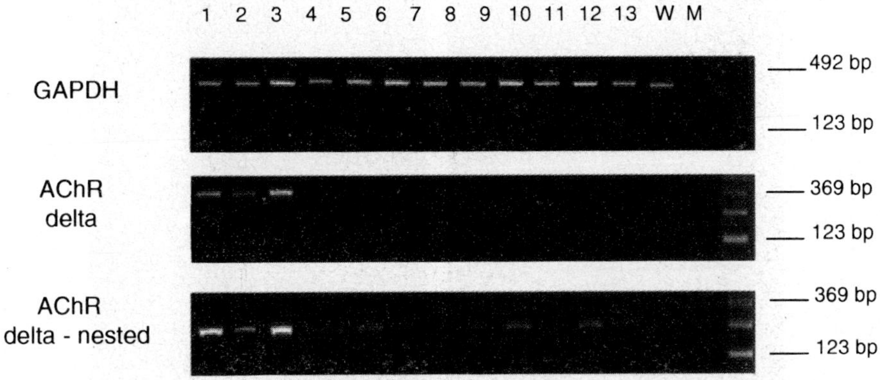

Fig. 1. Detection of AChR δ-subunit RNA by RT-PCR. In thymus and thymoma the δ-subunit could only be detected using nested PCR in about two-thirds of the cases whereas in normal muscle, *ex vivo* rhabdomyosarcoma tissue and in rhabdomyosarcoma cell line TE671 a signal was seen after the first round of PCR. Shown here are the results with δ1 primers. 1: TE 671; 2: normal muscle tissue; 3: *ex vivo* rhabdomyosarcoma tissue; 4: normal thymus; 5-7: thymitis; 8-10: mixed thymoma; 11-13: cortical thymoma; W: negative control (water); M: marker of a 123bp ladder

To check these results we also performed immunohistochemistry and immunofluorescence experiments. In thymoma, previous investigations could not detect α-subunit protein by immunohistochemistry [11]. This finding was confirmed here (not shown). In addition, δ-subunit expression could neither be found in thymomas, nor in non-neoplastic thymuses (not shown), although α-subunit expression was detectable on thymic myoid cells as reported previously [9, 11]. This surprising finding was further studied by double immunofluorescence (Fig. 2). The AChR α-subunit could be detected with different antibodies (Mabs 61, 195, 198, Table 1) both in three normal thymuses and in embryonal rhabdomyosarcoma at the cell surface of thymic myoid cells and neoplastic muscle cells, respectively. By contrast the δ-subunit (Mabs 7, 137, 141, Table 1) could only be detected in the rhabdomyosarcoma.

Conclusion

The lack or extreme reduction of δ-subunit message and protein in thymomas and non-neoplastic thymuses alike, distinguishing them from normal muscle and rhabdomyosarcomas. Since AChR α- and γ-subunits were detected on the myoid cell surface in a previous study [13] and confirmed here for the α-subunit (Fig. 2), we conclude that AChRs devoid of δ-subunits are inserted into the myoid cell membrane. Such receptors have not been described under physiological conditions. However, transfection experiments showed, that in the absence of δ-subunit message "triplet AchR" composed of α, β and γ subunits form pentameric channels ($\alpha_2\beta\gamma_2$) that are inserted into the cell membrane [4, 13]. The occurrence

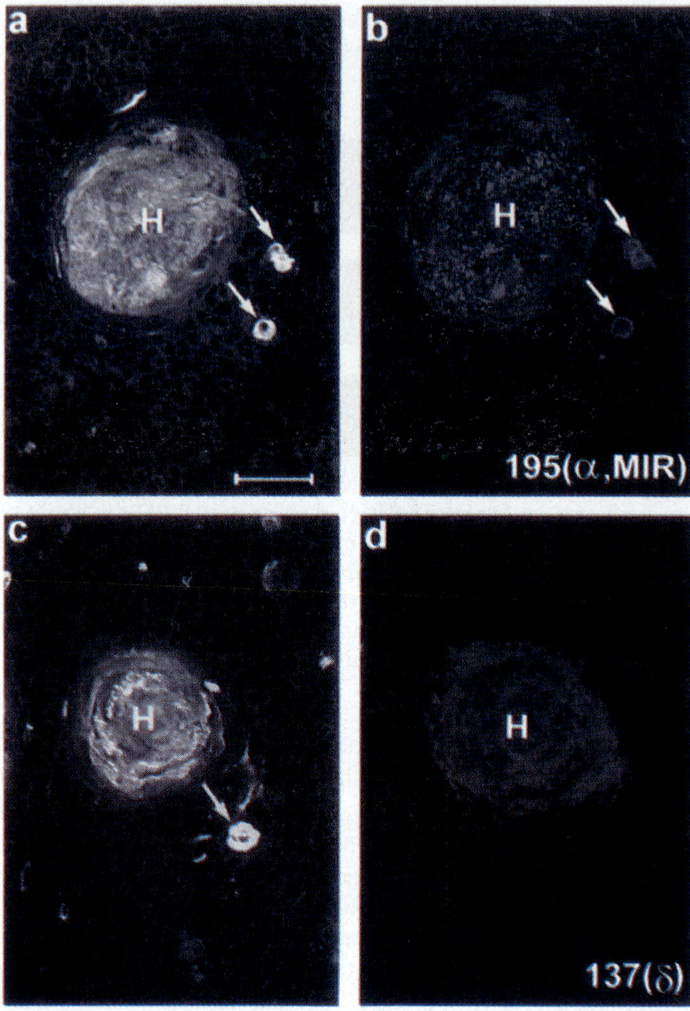

Fig. 2. Detection of muscular AChR α- but not δ-subunit in thymic myoid cells (normal thymus) by immunofluorescence. Arrows indicate thymic myoid cells, which stain positive with anti-desmin (a,c) and anti-AChR α Mab195 against the MIR of AChR α-subunit (b) (MIR: main immunogenic region, α67-74). No reactivity of myoid cells was seen with anti-AChR δ antibody Mab137 (d). Respective positive and negative results were also obtained with anti-MIR AChR α antibody Mab198 and anti-δ antibodies Mab7 and Mab141 (not shown here). Identical results were obtained with two other normal thymuses (Magnification × 250, indicated scale: 0.05 mm, H: Hassall's corpuscle).

of such "triplet AChRs" on myoid cells might reflect specific thymic microenvironmental properties (to be defined) or the unique regulation of the AChR δ-subunit gene by myogenic factors that differentially activate or repress its transcription in myotubes and myoblasts, respectively [14]. To address the thus far unresolved question, whether thymic myoid cells play a role for the shaping of the normal T cell repertoire (perhaps by providing dendritic cells in the thymic medulla with tolerogenic AChR peptides), it might be interesting on the basis of our findings to study the frequency of δ-specific versus α-, β- and γ-specific T cells in the normal T cell repertoire. Finally, our results offer a possibility to test the hypothesis that myoid cells are involved in the pathogenesis of thymitis-associated MG by providing AChR as immunogen [10]. This hypothesis has been supported by demonstrating that thymic tissue with thymitis (expressing γ-positive AChR) is enriched for γ-subunit specific B and T cells (reviewed in [15]) If this scenario is correct, the lack of intrathymic δ-subunit protein (Fig. 2) predicts that δ-subunit specific T cells should be rare among intrathymic anti-AChR autoreactive T cells.

Acknowledgements

We thank E. Oswald, C. Kohaut and E. Schmitt for technical assistance. This work was supported by the DFG-grant Ma 1484/2-2 and the BIOMED (BMH1-CT93-1100) grant.

References

1. Lindstrom J., D. Shelton and Y. Fujii (1988). Myasthenia gravis. *Adv. Immunol.* 42: 233–284.
2. Tzartos S.J., T. Barkas, M.T. Cung et al. (1998). Anatomy of the antigenic structure of a large membrane autoantigen, the muscle-type nicotinic acetylcholine receptor. *Immunol. Rev.* 163: 89–120: 89–120.
3. Vincent A. (1994). Aetiological factors in development of myasthenia gravis. *Adv. Neuroimmunol.* 4: 355–371.
4. Sumikawa K. and R. Miledi. (1989). Assembly and insertion of a multi-subunit nicotinic acetylcholine receptor into plasma membranes. In: Molecular biology of neuroreceptors and ion channels, Maelicke A. (ed) Springer-Verlag Berlin, Heidelberg, New York, London, Tokio: 451–467.
5. Beeson D., A. Morris, A. Vincent and J. Newsom Davis (1990). The human muscle nicotinic acetylcholine receptor alpha-subunit exist as two isoforms: a novel exon. *EMBO J* 9: 2101–2106.
6. Newland C.F., D. Beeson A. Vincent and J. Newsom-Davis (1995). Functional and non-functional isoforms of the human muscle acetylcholine receptor. *J. Physiol* (Lond) 489: 767–778.
7. Willcox N (1993). Myasthenia gravis. *Curr. Opin. Immunol.* 5: 910–917.
8. Sommer N, G.C. Harcourt, N. Willcox, D. Beeson and J. Newsom Davis (1991). Acetylcholine receptor-reactive T lymphocytes from healthy subjects and myasthenia gravis patients. *Neurology* 41: 1270–1276.
9. Schluep M., N. Willcox, A. Vincent, G.K. Dhoot and J. Newsom-Davis (1987). Acetylcholine receptors in human thymic myoid cells in situ: an immunohistological study. *Ann. Neurol.* 22: 212–222.
10. Wekerle H. and U.P. Ketelsen. (1977). Intrathymic pathogenesis and dual genetic control of myasthenia gravis. *Lancet* 1: 678–680.
11. Kirchner T., S. Tzartos, F. Hoppe, B. Schalke, H. Wekerle and H.K. Müller-Hermelink (1988). Pathogenesis of myasthenia gravis. Acetylcholine receptor-related antigenic determinants in tumor-free thymuses and thymic epithelial tumors. *Am. J. Pathol.* 130: 268–280.

12. Müller-Hermelink H. K., A. Marx and T. Kirchner (1994). Advances in the diagnosis and classification of thymic epithelial tumors. *In*: Recent Advances in Histopathology, Anthony, P and MacSween, R, (eds). Edinburgh, Churchill Livingstone, 49–63.
13. Sine S.M. and T. Claudio (1991). Gamma- and delta-subunits regulate the affinity and the cooperativity of ligand binding to the acetylcholine receptor. *J. Biol. Chem.* 266: 19369–19377.
14. Simon A. M. and S.J. Burden (1993). An E box mediates activation and repression of the acetylcholine receptor delta-subunit gene during myogenesis. *Mol. Cell Biol.* 13: 5133–5140.
15. Marx A., A. Wilisch, A. Schultz, S. Gattenlöhner, R. Nenninger and H.K. Müller-Hermelink (1997). Pathogenesis of myasthenia gravis. *Virchows Arch.* 430: 355–364.
16. S. Gutsche, A. Wilisch, V. Hoffacker, A. Schultz, S. Tzartos, W. Nix, B. Schalke, C. Schneider, H.-K. Muller-Hermelink and A. Marx (1999). Expression of the Acetylcholine Receptor a Subunit Gene is Associated with Paraneoplastic Myasthenia Gravis in Mixed Thymoma. *In*: Myasthenia Gravis: Disease Mechanism and Immunointervention, P. Christadoss (Ed), Narosa Publishing House, New Delhi, 42–50.
17. V. Hoffacker, A. Schultz, R. Nenninger, S. Tzartos, H.-K. Müller-Hermelink and A. Marx (1999). Abnormal Thymocyte Development and Neurofilament-Reactive Thymocytes in Thymoma. *In*: Myasthenia Gravis: Disease Mechanism and Immunointervention, P. Christadoss (Ed), Narosa Publishing House, New Delhi, 51–57.

Myasthenia Gravis: Disease mechanisms and immunointervention
P. Christadoss (Ed)

4. Aberrant Encounter of Acetylcholine Receptor-Expressing Cells with the Lymphoid Infiltrates in the Thymus of Myasthenia Gravis Patients

Ioannis Roxanis, John Newsom-Davis and Nick Willcox

Neurosciences Group, Institute of Molecular Medicine,
John Radcliffe Hospital, University of Oxford

Introduction

The muscle weakness in myasthenia gravis (MG) is clearly mediated by autoantibodies to the acetylcholine receptor (AChR). Their production depends on helper T cells, the induction of which must be a crucial step in autosensitization [1]. MG patients with onset of the disease before 40 years of age (early onset MG-EOMG) typically show a characteristic thymic hyperplasia (reviewed in [1]). This is largely due to invasion of the extraparenchymal perivascular spaces by lymphoid infiltrates with germinal centers (GC) and T cell areas [2-4]. In parallel, the true thymic parenchyma also shows alterations, with rearrangement of the medullary epithelium into bands (medullary epithelial bands-MEB) [3, 4]. In normal thymus, the two compartments are separated by a laminin$^+$ basement membrane. By contrast, in the EOMG thymus, this barrier is frequently fenestrated [3, 4], and thymic epithelial cells (TEC) are occasionally seen protruding toward the lymphoid infiltrates. Such TEC are intermingled with abundant deposits of extracellular matrix (ECM) proteins (e.g. laminin) that are continuous with an analogous network in T cell areas. Furthermore, they express high levels of ECM protein receptors (integrins) and epidermal growth factor receptor (EGFR) [5], which could synergize in leading to TEC proliferation and migration. As a result, in the EOMG thymus, a considerable proportion of TEC is aberrantly exposed to the lymphoid infiltrates. Interestingly, it has been previously noticed that GC are frequently localized at sites of basement membrane fenestrations [3, 4]. There is also recent evidence that TEC express AChR subunits [6], though not whole AChR.

Myoid cells are rare, muscle-like cells found in the medulla of both the normal and EOMG thymus, including MEB [7]. As they express complete functional AChR [7, 8], they have been implicated as possible *agents provocateurs* in the initiation of the autoimmune response in EOMG [8-10].

In this study we tried to quantify the associations between basement membrane fenestrations and GC, and to assess whether myoid cells were localized at such sites. Using immunohistochemical techniques (3; Fig. 1 legend), we compared the thymuses of 36 EOMG patients (with detectable anti-AChR serum antibodies-'seropositives'), 4 patients who had undetectable anti-AChR antibodies at the time of thymectomy but later became marginally seropositive ('seroconverters'), and 8 consistently 'seronegative' MG patients.

Results and Discussion

Associations Between Basement Membrane Fenestrations and GC

Overall, the frequency of GC within the extraparenchymal lymphoid infiltrates ('extraparenchymal' GC), although characteristically variable between patients, was significantly higher in seropositives than in seroconverters, and especially seronegatives in whom they were extremely rare. The same was largely true for basement membrane fenestrations, but was not quantified.

In each patient subgroup, laminin fenestrations were seen near practically all of the extraparenchymal GC, creating aberrant contacts with the TEC (Fig. 1); these 'exposed' TEC are typically hyperplastic [5]. Furthermore, the GC borders frequently followed the edges of exposed MEB and lost contact only at sites where the basement membrane barrier was intact.

Therefore, extraparenchymal GC showed a preferential localization near exposed TEC, instead of a random one within the occasionally extremely large lymphoid infiltrates. This 'affinity' of GC for TEC implies a causal relationship between them. Since many fenestrations lacked a nearby GC (30–50%), whereas the opposite was extremely uncommon (0–10%), it seems likely that TEC hyperplasia provokes laminin breakdown and GC formation rather than the reverse. Since TEC apparently express AChR subunits [7], they may be well placed to initiate T cell autoreactivity. In addition, they have been shown to produce IL-1 and IL-6, both *in vitro* [11, 12] and *in situ* [13]. These two cytokines are known to play a role both in the earlier stages of B cell activation, proliferation and differentiation, and in the induction of their terminal differentiation [14]. Furthermore, they are known to synergize, increasing IL-2 production and proliferation of peripheral T cells [15]. Therefore, consistently with our findings, 'exposed' TEC might create a favorable microenvironment for T cell activation, B cell differentiation and GC formation.

Localization of Myoid Cells in Different Compartments of the EOMG Thymus

In all three subgroups of MG patients, we estimated the number of myoid cells in 3 different medullary compartments (Fig. 2): (a) relatively 'normal' medullary areas and intact MEB, (b) fenestrated MEB and (c) at the borders of fenestrated MEB or within the lymphoid infiltrates (partially or entirely 'extraparenchymal' myoid cells).

As shown in Fig. 2, a surprisingly high proportion of myoid cells was seen within the lymphoid infiltrates (Fig. 1, IV-arrows). This proportion, although

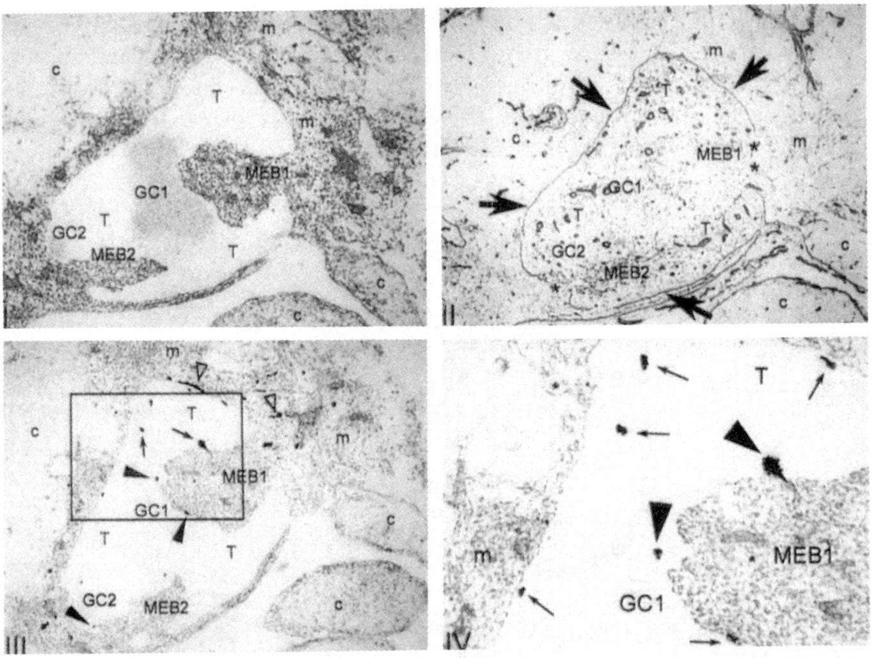

Fig. 1. Location of myoid cells relative to medullary epithelial bands (MEB) and germinal centers (GC) in a 'seroconverter' female MG patient (age 19 y; anti-AChR was undetectable before the thymectomy and showed a low positive titer after the operation; single fiber EMG was indicative of generalized MG). Adjacent sections were stained for: I—keratin (dark labeling; monoclonal antibody-mAb-LP34, DAKO, Glostrup, Denmark) and GC (pale; mAbs RFB4 and RFB6 against B cells and follicular dendritic cells, kind gifts of Prof. G. Janossy, London), II—laminin (polyclonal rabbit antibody, Sigma, Pool, UK), III—keratin (pale) and myoid cells (dark; mAb 42/25 against troponin I, Courtesy: Dr G.K. Dhoot, London) and IV—enlargement of the area marked in III. Two MEB (MEB1 and MEB2) are seen protruding towards a T cell area (T) through fenestrations (* in II) of the laminin$^+$ basement membrane which is intact elsewhere (arrows in II). The two GC (GC1 and GC2) are in contact with the exposed epithelium with no intervening laminin. 'Extraparenchymal' myoid cells in association with these GC are indicated with arrowheads in III. Other 'extraparenchymal' myoid cells are indicated with arrows in III and, in higher magnification, in IV, whereas myoid cells in relatively 'normal' medullary areas (m) are indicated with open arrowheads. c: cortex.

Method: Thymus samples were embedded in OCT (Bright, Huntingdon, UK), snap-frozen in isopentane (BDH, Poole, UK), cooled in liquid nitrogen and stored at −70°C. Five-μm cryostat sections were air-dried overnight, fixed in acetone (BDH) for 10 min and stored at −20°C.

For double immunoperoxidase staining, each successive indirect labeling procedure ended with a different chromogen. Sections were initially rehydrated in PBS, and then incubated with the first primary mAb (LP34 or 42/25) optimally diluted, followed by the appropriate secondary antibody (goat anti-mouse IgG, DAKO) diluted 1:50; finally, they were stained with diaminobenzidine tetrahydrochloride (DAB) and nickel chloride (black product). Sections were washed with PBS for 10 min between the incubations and for 20-30 min after the last one. Then the second primary antibodies (RFB4 plus RFB6 or LP34) were applied as above, before 3-amino-9-ethylcarbazole (AEC) was added, giving a clearly distinguishable red color.

variable between patients, was significantly higher in seropositives and seroconverters than seronegatives. Furthermore, in seropositives, the proportion of 'extraparenchymal' myoid cells was significantly correlated with the pre-operative duration of symptoms. Finally, myoid cells were occasionally seen even in contact with follicular dendritic cells of GC.

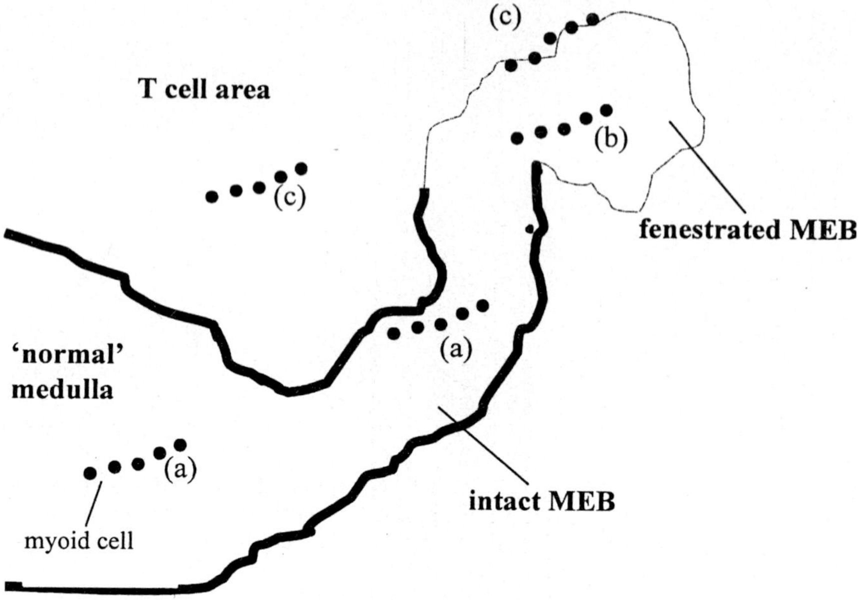

	Seronegatives	Seroconverters	Seropositives
Normal medulla/ Intact MEB (a)	**96** (79-100)%*	**76.5** (55-86)%	**36** (0-88)%
Fenestrated MEB (b)	**0** (0-8)%	**6**(0-8)%	**26** (0-67)%
'Extraparenchymal' sites (c)	**6** (0-13)%	**19** (12-37)%	**34** (0-63)%
Total myoid cells counted	951	668	2462

*median (range)

Fig. 2 Distribution of myoid cells in different microenvironments in the thymus of MG patients. MEB: medullary epithelial band.

Therefore, as with TEC, a considerable number of myoid cells were seen in aberrant encounter with the lymphoid infiltrates. The gradual increase of this number from seronegatives to seroconverters to seropositives and, finally, to seropositives with long duration of symptoms, might reflect a continuous process in which myoid cells play an active role.

Associations Between Basement Membrane Fenestrations, GC and Myoid Cells

Since only a proportion of fenestrations was associated with adjacent GC and, a considerable proportion of myoid cells were seen within the lymphoid infiltrates, we looked for associations between these components in the three subgroups of MG patients.

Interestingly, the co-occurrence of an 'extraparenchymal' myoid cell at a site of fenestration significantly increased the likelihood of a nearby GC, both in seropositives and seroconverters (Fig. 1 and 3). Further to their mere presence within the lymphoid infiltrates, this implies that myoid cells may play an active role in the GC formation and autoantibody synthesis in these subgroups of MG patients.

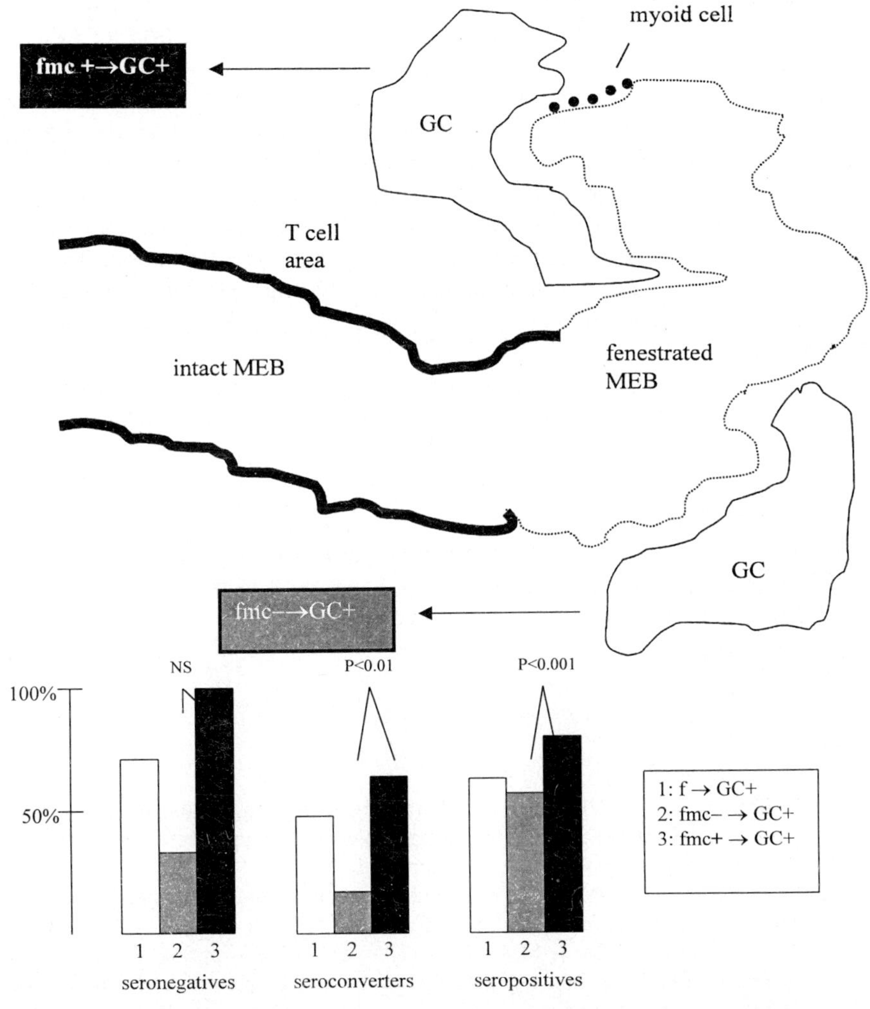

Fig. 3 The co-occurrence of an 'extraparenchymal' myoid cell at a site of fenestration (fmc+) significantly increased the likelihood of a nearby germinal centre (fmc+ → GC+).

Conclusions

Our main findings demonstrated that in the myasthenic thymus, whereas practically all GC or their coronas were in basement membrane-free contact with TEC, only a proportion of fenestrations had an adjacent GC. Myoid cells were frequently seen within the lymphoid infiltrates, especially in seropositives, and their co-occurrence at sites of fenestrations significantly increased the likelihood of a nearby GC.

The thymus has long been implicated as the site of anti-AChR autosensitization in MG [1, 2, 8-10]. Interestingly, despite the intrathymic presence of AChR on TEC and myoid cells, tolerance against all its epitopes is not complete [16]. Therefore, potentially autoreactive, AChR-specific T cells are present even in healthy individuals [17]. Such cells may well recirculate via high endothelial venules of T cell areas and aberrantly encounter TEC and myoid cells. The hypothesis that they might be sensitized by them is strongly supported by the significant co-occurrence of GC with 'exposed' TEC and myoid cells.

It is possible that epithelial hyperplasia is a primary event leading to autoimmunization of helper and/or cytotoxic T cells (either directly or via professional antigen-presenting cells) and early antibody formation. The co-localizing myoid cells might then induce antibody synthesis against the native AChR conformation, determinant spreading to fetal AChR epitopes and enhanced GC formation.

In order to assess their antigen-presenting potential, we are currently investigating the MHC and accessory molecule profile of TEC and myoid cells in different microenvironments of the EOMG thymus.

Acknowledgements

This work has been supported by the State Scholarships Foundation of Greece and the Human Capital and Mobility program of the European Union. We are grateful to Dr. K. Micklem for his kind advice on illustrations, and to many colleagues for mAbs.

References

1. Willcox N. and A. Vincent. 1988. Myasthenia gravis as an example of organ-specific autoimmune disease. *In* B lymphocytes in human disease. A.G. Bird and J.E. Calvert, eds. Oxford University Press, Oxford, pp. 469–506.
2. Levine G.D. and J. Rosai. 1978. Thymic hyperplasia and neoplasia: A review of current concepts. *Hum. Pathol.* 9: 495.
3. Schluep M., N. Willcox, M.A. Ritter, J. Newsom-Davis and A.N. Larche M., Brown. 1988. Myasthenia gravis thymus: Clinical, histological and culture correlations. *J. Autoimmun.* 1: 445.
4. Bofill M., G. Janossy, N. Willcox, M. Chilosi, L.K. Trejdosiewicz and J. Newsom-Davis. 1985. Microenvironments in the normal thymus and the thymus in myasthenia gravis. *Am. J. Pathol.* 119: 462.
5. Beeson D., A.P. Bond, L. Corlett, S.J. Curnow, M.E. Hill, L.W. Jacobson, C. MacLennan, A. Meager, A.-M. Moody, P. Moss, N. Nagvekar, J. Newsom-Davis,

N. Pantic, I. Roxanis, E.G. Spack, A. Vincent and N. Willcox. 1998. Thymus, thymoma and specific T cells in Myasthenia Gravis. *Ann. N.Y. Acad. Sci.* 841: 371.

6. Wakkach A., T. Guyon, C. Bruand, S. Tzartos, S. Cohen-Kaminsky and S. Berrih-Aknin. 1996. Expression of acetylcholine receptor genes in human thymic epithelial cells. Implications for myasthenia gravis. *J. Immunol.* 157: 3753.
7. Schluep M., N. Willcox, A. Vincent, G.K. Dhoot and J. Newsom-Davis. 1987. Acetylcholine receptors in human thymic myoid cells in situ: an immunohistological study. *Ann. Neurol.* 22: 212.
8. Kao I. and D.B. Drachman. 1976. Thymic muscle cells bear acetylcholine receptors: possible relation to myasthenia gravis. *Science.* 195: 74.
9. van de Velde R.L. and N.B. Friedman. 1970. Thymic myoid cells and myasthenia gravis. *Am. J. Pathol. 59:347.*
10. Wekerle H. and U.-P. Ketelsen. 1976. Intrathymic pathogenesis and dual genetic control of myasthenia gravis. *Lancet.* i: 678.
11. Le P.T., D.T. Tuck, C.A. Dinarello, B.F. Haynes and K.H. Singer. 1987. Human thymic epithelial cells produce interleukin 1. *J. Immunol.* 138: 2520.
12. Le P.T., S. Lazorick, L.P. Whichard, Y.-C. Yang, S.C. Clark, B.F. Haynes and K.H. Singer. 1990. Human thymic epithelial cells produce IL-6, Granulocyte-Monocyte-CSF and leukemia inhibitory factor. *J. Immunol.* 145: 3310.
13. Emilie D., O. Devergne, S. Cohen-Kaminsky, S. Berrih-Aknin and P. Galanaud. 1993. *In situ* production of interleukins in hyperplastic thymus from myasthenia gravis patients. *Ann. N. Y. Acad. Sci.* 681: 97.
14. Kishimoto T. 1989. The biology of interleukin-6. *Blood.* 74: 1.
15. Holsti M. A. and D. H. Raulet. 1989. IL-6 and IL-1 synergize to stimulate IL-2 production and proliferation of peripheral T cells. *J. Immunol.* 143: 2514.
16. Jermy A., D. Beeson and A. Vincent. 1993. Pathogenic autoimunity to affinity purified mouse acetylcholine receptor induced without adjuvant in BALB/c mice. *Eur. J. Immunol.* 23: 973.
17. Sommer N., G.C. Harcourt, N. Willcox, D. Beeson and J. Newsom-Davis. 1991. Acetylcholine receptor-reactive T lymphocytes from healthy subjects and myasthenia gravis patients. *Neurology.* 41: 1270.

Myasthenia Gravis: Disease mechanisms and immunointervention
P. Christadoss (Ed)

5. Expression of the Acetylcholine Receptor α-Subunit Gene is Associated with Paraneoplastic Myasthenia Gravis in Mixed Thymoma

Stefanie Gutsche[1], Annette Wilisch[1], Viola Hoffacker[1], Anja Schultz[1], Socrates Tzartos[2], Wilfried Nix[3], Berthold Schalke[4], Christiane Schneider[5], Hans-Konrad Müller-Hermelink[1] and Alexander Marx[1]

[1]Institute of Pathology, University of Würzburg, Germany

[2]Hellenic Pasteur Institute, Athens, Greece

[3]Department of Neurology, University of Mainz, Germany

[4]Department of Neurology, University of Regensburg, Germany

[5]Department of Neurology, University of Würzburg, Germany

Introduction

Myasthenia gravis (MG) is an autoimmune disease caused by autoantibodies against the acetylcholine receptor (AChR) at the neuromuscular junction [1]. The muscular AChR has been extensively characterized [2], but the etiology of MG is still obscure. Whether the muscular AChR or another (auto)antigen plays a role during the initiation of MG is unknown [3]. The muscular AChR is a pentameric ion channel composed of four different subunits. The α-subunit contains the acetylcholine binding site and the main epitopes recognized by MG autoantibodies [2]. The human muscle AChR α-subunit exists as two isoforms, P3A$^-$ and P3A$^+$ [4]. This is a result of alternative splicing of the P3A exon located between exons three and four. The P3A$^+$ isoform does not bind α-bungarotoxin or monoclonal antibodies against the AChR main immunogenic region and is not integrated into functional AChR [5]. The muscular AChR belongs to the family of nicotinic AChRs as do neuronal AChRs. Since muscular and neuronal AChRs share significant molecular homology [6], neuronal AChRs have been considered as candidate autoantigens able to elicit autoimmunity against the muscular AChR by molecular mimicry [7].

Thymic pathology is so specific and frequent in MG patients that its relevance for the pathogenesis of MG is undisputed [3, 8], but whether it is involved in the triggering of MG, i.e. its etiology, is unknown [9, 10]. Seventy per cent of MG patients have thymitis. In these patients autoantibody production occurs inside the thymus and autosensitization probably takes place via exposure of antigen presenting cells and autoreactive T cells to muscular AChR expressed on thymic myoid cells [11, 12]. Ten per cent of MG patients have a thymoma, which is an epithelial tumor that shares as a unique function the intratumorous thymus-like generation of mature T cells from immature precursors [13]. Based on histological, clinical and functional properties, medullary, mixed, and cortical thymoma and "well differentiated thymic carcinoma" are distinguished [13, 14]. In contrast to thymitis, there is no autoantibody production in thymomas, myoid cells are rare [15, 16] and epithelial AChR protein expression has not been detected [17, 18]. Nevertheless, expression of mRNA of muscular and neuronal AChR has been reported in thymomas, though not correlated with the occurrence of MG [7, 16]. Therefore, autosensitization in paraneoplastic versus thymitis-associated MG probably has a different pathogenesis [8].

The aim of this study was to investigate whether autoimmunity against the AChR is associated with the gene expression of muscular or neuronal AChR subunits in thymomas. We found that transcription only of the muscular AChR P3A$^-$ α-subunit gene exhibited a correlation with the presence or absence of MG in mixed but not cortical thymomas.

Material and Methods

Tissues and Cell Culture

Thirtyfive thymic epithelial tumors (TET), seven hyperplastic thymuses, three normal thymuses and two tumor biopsies of rhabdomyosarcoma patients were studied by RT-PCR using tissue snap-frozen within four hours after surgery. TETs were classified according to Müller-Hermelink and co-workers [15, 19]. Cortical thymoma (CT) and "well differentiated thymic carcinoma" (WDTC), though morphologically different, are so closely related in clinical, histogenetic and functional terms [13, 15] that they were considered as one tumor group here. CT and WDTC were compared with mixed thymomas (MXT), which are the second most frequent MG-associated tumors [15, 19]. In addition two medullary thymomas (MDT) were studied. Invasiveness of tumors was staged according to the proposal of Masaoka [20]. Normal thymuses were obtained from patients without immunological disorders undergoing thoracic surgery. Thymuses with thymitis (THY) and two different ex vivo rhabdomyosarcoma biopsies were tested. The tumor stage [20] ranged from I to II in MDT and MXT and from II to IVa in CT and WDTC. The clinical diagnosis of MG was routinely confirmed electromyographically and by the detection of anti-AChR autoantibodies by a radioimmunoassay using human muscle-derived, ^{125}J-labeled AChR. All thymitis cases corresponded to the typical lymphofollicular thymitis as reported by Kirchner and co-workers [21].

For PCR-based detection of muscular AChR gene expression the embryonal and alveolar rhabdomyosarcoma cell lines TE 671 and RD, respectively, were used as positive controls. The neuroblastoma cell line IMR 32 was used as positive control for neuronal AChR gene expression. All cell lines were cultured in DMEM supplemented with 10% heat inactivated fetal calf serum (Gibco, Eggenstein, Germany), 2mM L-Glutamine, 100 U/ml penicillin and 100 mg/ml streptomycin at 37°C and 5% CO_2.

Reverse Transcriptase Polymerase Chain Reaction (RT-PCR)
Total RNA was prepared from 0.1 g snap-frozen tissue cut into 7 µm sections on a cryostat or from 10^6 cultured cells using Trizol reagent (Gibco Life Technologies, Eggenstein, Germany) according to the manufacturer's instructions. After cDNA synthesis with oligo-dT specific primers and MMLV reverse trancriptase, 1/20 of each reaction mixture was amplified using Taq polymerase and sequence specific primers. The oligonucleotide primers were derived from published sequences.

Amplification of muscular ($\alpha, \beta, \gamma, \delta, \varepsilon$) and neuronal ($\alpha 3, \beta 4$) AChR subunit cDNA was performed applying the following parameters: denaturation for 30 sec at 94°C, annealing for 30 sec at a primer specific temperature and amplification for 30 sec at 72°C. A RT-PCR with GAPDH specific primers and ethidium staining of rRNA was performed to confirm the integrity of the RNA.

One-fourth of the amplified cDNA was electrophoretically separated on a 2% agarose gel, stained with ethidium bromide and a picture was taken using a videoprinter. The picture was digitalized, saved on disk and used for final picture processing. Ethidium bromide staining of the AChR amplification products revealed bands of expected molecular size and subsequent sequencing of the PCR products confirmed that the cDNA fragments were identical to the published AChR sequences. Primer sequences, annealing temperatures and number of cycles are available on request.

Statistical Analysis
The improved χ^2 test was used for statistical analysis of our data.

Results

Muscular AChR Subunits are Differently Expressed in Thymus and Thymoma

As shown in Table 1, a consistently combined expression of the α, β, γ and ε-subunit genes of the muscular AChR was detected in all normal thymuses, in all thymuses of patients with thymitis and in all positive controls (normal muscle, *ex vivo* rhabdomyosarcoma samples and rhabdomyosarcoma cell lines). Likewise, transcripts of the α, β, γ and ε-subunit genes of the muscular AChR could be amplified from thymoma cDNA. The AChR δ-subunit message was consistently undetectable in all thymuses and thymomas by conventional RT-PCR (see Marx et al., this volume). However, in 50% of all thymomas investigated, expression of one or two of the muscular subunit genes was missing, suggesting an incomplete expression of AChR proteins in these thymomas. The expression pattern of

Table 1. Expression of muscular and neuronal AChR subunits in non-neoplastic thymuses, thymomas, control tissues and cell lines given as the percentage of positive PCR-reactions (Upper lines, bold numbers). Numbers of investigated cases are given in brackets

Type of tissue/MG status[1]	Muscular AChR α^{11} P3A⁻/P3A⁺	Muscular AChRβ	Muscular AChRγ	Muscular AChRδ	Muscular AChRε	Neuronal AChR $\alpha 3$	Neuronal AChR $\beta 4$
NT[2]/	**100/100**	**100**	**100**	**0**	**100**	**50**	**100**
MG⁻	(3)/(3)	(3)	(3)	(3)	(3)	(2)	(2)
THY[3]/	**100/67**	**100**	**100**	**0**	**100**	**86**	**86**
MG+	(7)/(6)	(7)	(6)	(6)	(7)	(7)	(7)
MDT[4]/	**100/0**	**100**	**100**	**0**	**100**	**50**	**100**
MG+	(2)/(2)	(2)	(2)	(2)	(2)	(2)	(2)
MXT[5]/	**100/0**	**67**	**88**	**0**	**89**	**78**	**89**
MG+	(9)/(8)	(9)	(8)	(9)	(9)	(9)	(9)
MXT/	**25/0**	**100**	**60**	**0**	**100**	**80**	**80**
MG–	(8)/(8)	(5)	(5)	(8)	(5)	(5)	(5)
CT[6]/	**86/14**	**71**	**100**	**0**	**86**	**57**	**86**
MG+	(7)/(7)	(7)	(7)	(7)	(7)	(7)	(7)
CT/	**80/60**	**100**	**100**	**0**	**100**	**100**	**100**
MG–	(5)/(5)	(2)	(2)	(5)	(2)	(2)	(2)
WDTC[7]/	**50/0**	**50**	**100**	**0**	**75**	**25**	**75**
MG–	(4)/(4)	(4)	(4)	(4)	(4)	(4)	(4)
Rhabdo, RD and TE671[8]	**100/100**	**100**	**100**	**100**	**100**	**n.i.**[12]	**n.i.**
	(4)/(4)	(4)	(4)	(4)	(4)		
IMR 32[9]	**n.i.**	**n.i.**	**n.i.**	**n.i.**	**n.i.**	**100**	**100**
muscles[10]	**100/100**	**100**	**100**	**100**	**100**	**n.i.**	**n.i.**
	(3)	(3)	(3)	(3)	(3)		

[1]MG: Myasthenia gravis; [2]NT: normal thymus; [3]THY: thymitis; [4]MDT: medullary thymoma; [5]MXT: mixed thymoma; [6]CT: cortical thymoma; [7]WDTC: well differentiated thymic carcinoma;[8] Rhabdo: rhabdomyosarcoma; TE 671 and RD: rhabdomyosarcoma cell lines; [9]IMR 32: neuroblastoma cell line; [10]Muscles: 3 cases of muscle biopsies obtained from three different adults within 45 min. after surgery or autopsy; [11]P3A⁻, P3A⁺: isoforms of the muscular AChR a subunit; [12]n.i.: not investigated.

All RT-PCR experiments were carried out 2 to 4 times. In case of a negative signal, this result was confirmed in at least three repetitions.

AChR subunits did not correlate with specific thymoma subtypes. In addition, there was no correlation with AChR antibody titer or immunosuppressive treatment. For the muscular AChR subunit α, a statistically significant difference was seen in mixed thymomas. All 9 MXT patients with MG expressed the P3A$^-$ mRNA whereas only two out of eight MXT patients without MG expressed this subunit mRNA (Table 1). This indicates the predominant expression of the α-subunit in mixed thymomas associated with MG (χ^2 = 9.82 with α < 0.01) (Fig. 1). No such difference was found for patients with a cortical thymoma (χ^2 = 0.06).

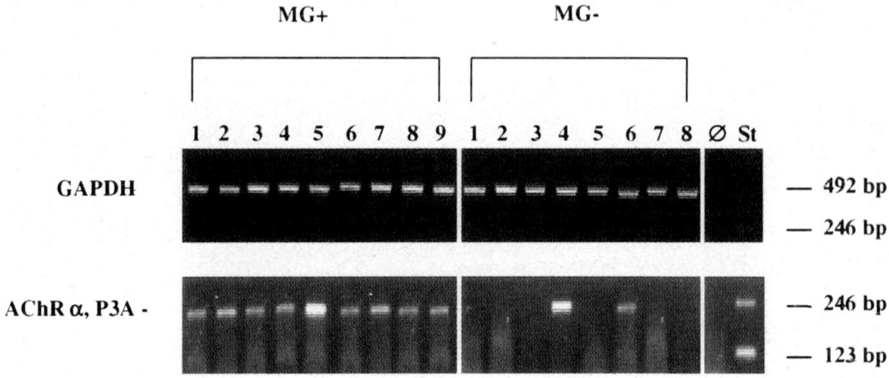

Fig. 1. The mRNA-Expression of the muscular AChR α-subunit P3A$^-$ is significantly correlated with myasthenia gravis in patients with mixed thymoma. χ^2 = 9.82 with α < 0.01. Ø : Negative control (water); St: Marker of a 123 bp ladder.

The expression levels of the muscular AChR α P3A$^-$ subunit in MXT with paraneoplastic MG were quite low. Therefore, it is not clear how such low levels might contribute to the pathogenesis of paraneoplastic MG in MXTs particularly since the respective proteins have not been detected in thymoma [17, 18]. However, the latter investigations [17, 18] do not exclude the intratumorous expression of extremely low levels of AChR protein. The low AChR α-subunit expression might be important, since even very low levels of intrathymic protein have profound effects on the T cell selection processes in the thymus [22, 23], and this might also be true for thymomas [13]. In this respect another autoimmune disease, insulin-dependent diabetes mellitus (IDDM), is instructive, since different numbers of repeats within a minisatellite upstream of the insulin gene seem to influence the amount of insulin mRNA in the thymus and the risk of IDDM [24, 25]. The studies suggest that large amounts of insulin in the thymus may more efficiently induce negative selection of insulin-specific T-lymphocytes (and protect from IDDM) while low amounts of insulin may favor positive selection and an increased IDDM risk [24, 25]. Therefore, antigen expression in the normal thymus seems to have an effect on tolerance induction that is just opposite to antigen expression in the abnormal microenviroment of MXTs.

Expression of the α Isoforms of Muscular AChR

Recently, the expression of two isoforms (P3A$^-$ and P3A$^+$) of the α-subunit of muscular AChR was described in muscle [4, 26] and thymic tissue [27]. In all normal thymuses and in four out of six thymuses from patients with thymitis both isoforms were detected (Table 1). In contrast, in all MXTs positive for the α-subunit (n = 11) only the P3A$^-$ isoform was expressed. In the group of CTs and WDTC (n = 15) the expression of the P3A$^+$ exon could be detected in only four CTs (Table 1). The difference between MXTs and CTs was not significant. We found the α-subunit isoform P3A$^+$ preferentially in non-neoplastic thymuses but not in MXTs and in only a minority of CTs. The latter result contradicts a recent study (27), which failed to detect P3A$^+$ expression in thymomas at all. Nevertheless the difference between thymomas and thymuses with respect to the expression of the P3A$^+$ isoform detected in our studies was statistically significant (Table 1). The investigation by Andreetta and co-workers (27) also describes a much lower expression of the P3A$^+$ isoform in comparison to the P3A$^-$ isoform in normal thymus and hyperplastic thymuses, which is confirmed by our results (Fig. 2), but contradicts an earlier report [28].

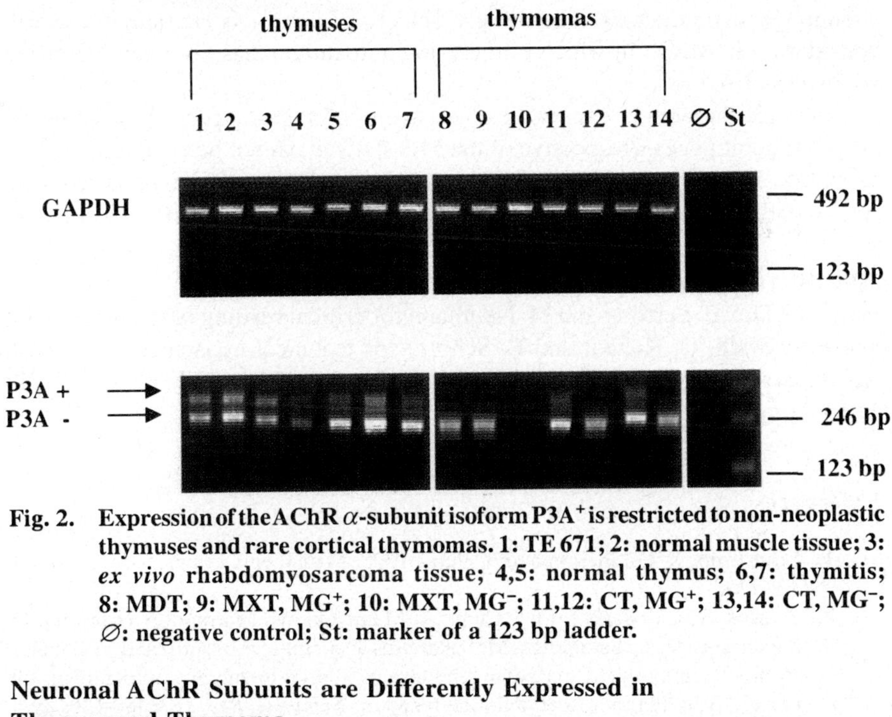

Fig. 2. Expression of the AChR α-subunit isoform P3A$^+$ is restricted to non-neoplastic thymuses and rare cortical thymomas. 1: TE 671; 2: normal muscle tissue; 3: *ex vivo* rhabdomyosarcoma tissue; 4,5: normal thymus; 6,7: thymitis; 8: MDT; 9: MXT, MG$^+$; 10: MXT, MG$^-$; 11,12: CT, MG$^+$; 13,14: CT, MG$^-$; Ø: negative control; St: marker of a 123 bp ladder.

Neuronal AChR Subunits are Differently Expressed in Thymus and Thymoma.

The α3 and β4-subunit genes of the neuronal AChR have been described to be expressed in a limited number of thymoma cases [7], but a statistical correlation concerning the MG status has not been reported. Both subunits were expressed in six out of nine thymuses and 18 out of 28 thymomas as well as in the positive control. In 11 cases (three thymuses and eight thymomas) either the α3 or the β4-subunit could be detected, and in two thymomas both subunits were missing (Table 1). The expression of the neuronal AChR subunits was neither correlated with a thymoma subtype nor with the presence or absence of MG, and no significant difference between thymuses and thymomas was detected.

Conclusions

From the highly significant correlation ($\alpha < 0.01$) between the expression of muscular AChR α-subunit (P3A⁻) message in MXTs and the occurrence of paraneoplastic MG in the patients with these tumors, we conclude that the gene encoding the α-subunit might play a role in the pathogenesis of paraneoplastic MG in MXTs. Since the levels of the AChR α-subunit message are very low in MXTs one may speculate that low-dose expression of $P3A^-$ AChR α-subunit protein in MG-associated mixed thymomas is optimal for intratumorous positive selection of AChR reactive T cells but too low to trigger negative selection. This scenario would explain why MG associated thymomas are selectively enriched in AChR-reactive T cells [29] that are not apparently activated in situ [14]. By contrast, the complete absence of AChR α-subunit protein in mixed thymomas might essentially preclude the positive selection of AChR reactive T cells, and negative selection may simply not be required to maintain tolerance in MG-negative MXTs. Such an immunological mechanism involving the AChR α-subunit gene product as a positively selecting protein is particularly worth considering in MXTs in which a triggering autoantigen has not been identified so far [13, 30].

Since all thymomas expressed at least one of the muscular and neutronal AChR subunit genes irrespective of the MG status it cannot be excluded that the expressed AChR subunit genes might be a necessary but not sufficient prerequisite for the pathogenesis of paraneoplastic MG irrespective of the thymoma subtype.

Acknowledgement

We thank Drs. E. Serfling and M. Neumann for critical reading of the manuscript and E. Oswald, C. Kohaut and E. Schmitt for technical assistance. This work was supported by the DFG-grant Ma 1484/2-2 and the BIOMED (BMH1-CT93-1100) grant.

References

1. Lindstrom, J., D. Shelton and Y. Fujii. 1988. Myasthenia gravis. *Adv. Immunol.* 42: 233.
2. Tzartos, S.J., T. Barkas, M.T. Cung, A. Mamalaki, M. Marraud, P. Orlewski, D. Papanastasiou, C. Sakarellos, M. Sakarellos-Daitsiotis, P. Tsantili and V. Tsikaris. 1998. Anatomy of the antigenic structure of a large membrane autoantigen, the muscle-type nicotinic acetylcholine receptor. *Immunol. Rev.* 163: 89–120: 89.
3. Vincent, A. 1994. Aetiological factors in development of myasthenia gravis. *Adv. Neuroimmunol.* 4: 355.
4. Beeson, D., A. Morris, A. Vincent and J. Newsom Davis. 1990. The human muscle nicotinic acetylcholine receptor alpha-subunit exist as two isoforms: a novel exon. *EMBO.* J. 9: 2101.
5. Newland, C.F., D. Beeson, A. Vincent and J. Newsom-Davis. 1995. Functional and non-functional isoforms of the human muscle acetylcholine receptor. *J. Physiol. (Lond).* 489: 767.
6. Lindstrom, J. 1996. Neuronal nicotinic acetylcholine receptors. In *Ion channels.* T. Narahashi, ed. Plenum Press, New York, p. 377.

7. Mihovilovic, M. and A.D. Roses. 1993. Expression of alpha-3, alpha-5 and beta-4 neuronal acetylcholine receptor subunit transcripts in normal and myasthenia gravis thymus. Identification of thymocytes expressing the alpha-3 transcripts. *J. Immunol.* 151: 6517.
8. Willcox, N. 1993. Myasthenia gravis. *Curr. Opin. Immunol.* 5: 910.
9. Sommer, N., G.C. Harcourt, N. Willcox, D. Beeson and J. Newsom Davis. 1991. Acetylcholine receptor-reactive T lymphocytes from healthy subjects and myasthenia gravis patients. *Neurology* 41: 1270.
10. Meinl, E., W.E. Klinkert and H. Wekerle. 1991. The thymus in myasthenia gravis. Changes typical for the human disease are absent in experimental autoimmune myasthenia gravis of the Lewis rat. *Am. J. Pathol.* 139: 995.
11. Schluep, M., N. Willcox, A. Vincent, G.K. Dhoot and J. Newsom-Davis. 1987. Acetylcholine receptors in human thymic myoid cells in situ: an immunohistological study. *Ann. Neurol.* 22: 212.
12. Wekerle, H. and U. P. Ketelsen. 1977. Intrathymic pathogenesis and dual genetic control of myasthenia gravis. *Lancet.* 1: 678.
13. Müller-Hermelink, H.K., A. Wilisch, A. Schultz and A. Marx. 1997. Characterization of the human thymic microenvironment: Lymphoepithelial interaction in normal thymus and thymoma. *Arch. of Hist. and Cyt.* 60: 9.
14. Nenninger, R., A. Schultz, V. Hoffacker, M. Helmreich, A. Wilisch, B. Vandekerckhove, T. Hunig, B. Schalke, C. Schneider, S. Tzartos, H. Kalbacher, H.K. Müller-Hermelink and A. Marx. 1998. Abnormal thymocyte development and generation of autoreactive T cells in mixed and cortical thymomas. *Lab. Invest.* 78: 743.
15. Kirchner, T., B. Schalke, J. Buchwald, M. Ritter, A. Marx and H.K. Müller-Hermelink. 1992. Well-differentiated thymic carcinoma. An organotypical low-grade carcinoma with relationship to cortical thymoma. *Am. J. Surg. Pathol.* 16: 1153.
16. Kornstein, M.J., O. Asher, and S. Fuchs. 1995. Acetylcholine receptor alpha-subunit and myogenin mRNAs in thymus and thymomas. *Am. J. Pathol.* 146: 1320.
17. Kirchner, T., S. Tzartos, F. Hoppe, B. Schalke, H. Wekerle and H.K. Müller-Hermelink. 1988. Pathogenesis of myasthenia gravis. Acetylcholine receptor-related antigenic determinants in tumor-free thymuses and thymic epithelial tumors. *Am. J. Pathol.* 130: 268.
18. Marx, A., R. O'Connor, K.I. Geuder, F. Hoppe, B. Schalke, S. Tzartos, I. Kalies, T. Kirchner and H.K. Müller-Hermelink. 1990. Characterization of a protein with an acetylcholine receptor epitope from myasthenia gravis-associated thymomas. *Lab. Invest.* 62: 279.
19. Müller-Hermelink, H.K., A. Marx and T. Kirchner. 1994. Advances in the diagnosis and classification of thymic epithelial tumors. In *Recent Advances in Histopathology.* P. Anthony and R. MacSween, eds. Edinburgh, Churchill Livingstone, p. 49.
20. Masaoka, A., Y. Monden, K. Nakahara and T. Tanioka. 1981. Follow-up study of thymomas with special reference to their clinical stages. *Cancer.* 48: 2485.
21. Kirchner, T., B. Schalke, A. Melms, T. von Kugelgen and H.K. Müller-Hermelink. 1986. Immunohistological patterns of non-neoplastic changes in the thymus in Myasthenia gravis. *Virchows. Arch. B. Cell. Pathol. Incl. Mol. Pathol.* 52: 237.
22. Hämmerling, G., G. Schonrich, F. Momburg, N. Auphan, B. Malissen, A.M. Schmitt-Verhults and B. Arnold. 1991. Non-deletional mechanisms of peripheral and central tolerance: studies with transgenic mice with tissue-specific expression of a foreign MHC class I antigen. *Immunol. Rev.* 122: 47.

23. Naujokas, M.F., L.S. Arneson, B. Fineschi, M.E. Peterson, S. Sitterding, A.T. Hammond, C. Reilly, D. Lo and J. Miller. 1995. Potent effects of low levels of MHC class II-associated invariant chain on CD4+ T cell development. *Immunity.* 3: 359.
24. Pugliese, A., M. Zeller, A. Fernandez, Jr., L.J. Zalcberg, R.J. Bartlett, C. Ricordi, M. Pietropaolo, G.S. Eisenbarth, S.T. Bennett and D.D. Patel. 1997. The insulin gene is transcribed in the human thymus and transcription levels correlated with allelic variation at the INS VNTR-IDDM2 susceptibility locus for type 1 diabetes. *Nat. Genet.* 15: 293.
25. Vafiadis, P., S.T. Bennett, J.A. Todd, J. Nadeau, R. Grabs, C.G. Goodyer, S. Wickramasinghe, E. Colle and C. Polychronakos. 1997. Insulin expression in human thymus is modulated by INS VNTR alleles at the IDDM2 locus. *Nat. Genet.* 15: 289.
26. Talib, S., T.B. Okarma and J.S. Lebkowski. 1993. Differential expression of human nicotinic acetylcholine receptor alpha subunit variants in muscle and non-muscle tissues. *Nucleic. Acids. Res.* 21: 233.
27. Andreetta, F., F. Baggi, C. Antozzi, E. Torchiana, P. Bernasconi, O. Simoncini, F. Cornelio and R. Mantegazza. 1997. Acetylcholine receptor alpha-subunit isoforms are differentially expressed in thymuses from myasthenic patients. *Am. J. Pathol.* 150: 341.
28. Guyon, T., P. Levasseur, F. Truffault, C. Cottin, C. Gaud and S. Berrih Aknin. 1994. Regulation of acetylcholine receptor alpha subunit variants in human myasthenia gravis. Quantification of steady-state levels of messenger RNA in muscle biopsy using the polymerase chain reaction. *J. Clin. Invest.* 94: 16.
29. Sommer, N., N. Willcox, G.C. Harcourt, and J. Newsom Davis. 1990. Myasthenic thymus and thymoma are selectively enriched in acetylcholine receptor-reactive T cells. *Ann. Neurol.* 28: 312.
30. Marx, A., A. Wilisch, A. Schultz, S. Gattenlöhner, R. Nenninger and H.K. Müller-Hermelink. 1997. Pathogenesis of Myasthenia gravis. *Virchows Archive.* 430: 355.

Myasthenia Gravis: Disease mechanisms and immunointervention
P. Christadoss (Ed)

6. Abnormal Thymocyte Development and Neurofilament-Reactive Thymocytes in Thymoma

Viola Hoffacker[1], Anja Schultz[1], Regina Nenninger[1], Socrates Tzartos[2], Hans-Konrad Müller-Hermelink[1] and Alexander Marx[1]

[1]Institute of Pathology, University of Würzburg, Germany

[2]Hellenic Pasteur Institute, Athens, Greece

Introduction

Myasthenia gravis (MG) is an autoimmune disease caused by autoantibodies against the acetylcholine receptor (AChR) at the neuromuscular junction [1, 2]. Mature CD4+ T-cells are involved in the production of these antibodies [3, 4]. The destruction at the neuromuscular endplates leads to the clinical symptom of muscle weakness.

About 90% of MG patients have thymic alterations. The majority (80%) have an inflammatory alteration of the thymus called thymitis [5], and approximately 10% of the patients have a thymoma [6], which is a tumor of epithelial origin [7]. Depending on the alteration of the thymus, the etiology and pathology of the autoimmune disease could be very different. Table 1 describes the most important differences between thymomas and thymitis.

Table 1. Thymic alterations in myasthenia gravis

	Thymitis	Thymoma	References
Pathology	inflammation	epithelial tumor of the thymus	[5, 7]
Epithelial Compartment	normal	abnormal (altered expression of endo genous proteins)	[8–10]
T-cell maturation	normal	abnormal (terminal maturation unknown)	[6, 11, 12]
Autoreactive T-cells	AChR	AChR and ?	[5, 13, 14]
Autoantibodies	AChR	AChR, striational muscle antigens, neuronal structures, interleukins	[15–17]

In summary, certain features concerning thymic microenvironment and T-cell development are changed in thymoma compared to normal thymus or thymitis. For that reason, we suggest that abnormal intratumourous T-cell maturation is related to paraneoplastic MG. To address this hypothesis we ask two questions: Does terminal T-cell maturation take place in thymomas of myasthenia gravis patients? Are intratumourously generated mature T-cells autoreactive against the acetylcholine receptor α subunit or neurofilament?

Materials and Methods

Patients and Cells

The diagnosis of MG was based on clinical features, electromyography and on the detection of anti-AChR autoantibodies as described previously [18, 19]. All tissues were kept on ice immediately after biopsy and cell preparation for FACS analysis or T-cell proliferation assays was done within 15 min to 3 h after surgery. Thymocytes and peripheral blood mononuclear cells (PBMC) were isolated from thymus or thymoma tissue and from blood as described previously [19].

Cell Surface Marker

Staining of surface antigens was performed using the following monoclonal antibodies (mAb) obtained from Becton Dickinson (Heidelberg, Germany): anti CD1a (PE-labelled), anti-CD3 (PerCP-labelled), anti-CD4 (PerCP-labelled) and anti-CD69 (FITC-labelled). Anti-CD3 (FITC-, PE-labelled), anti-CD4 (FITC-labelled) and anti-CD8 (PE-labelled) mAbs were purchased from DAKO (Hamburg, Germany). Anti-CD8 (FITC-labelled), anti-CD27 (unlabelled), anti-CD45RA (FITC-labelled) and donkey-anti-mouse (PE-labelled) mAbs were obtained from Dianova (Hamburg, Germany). Isotype controls as well as anti-CD3 (Quantum-Red-labelled) and anti-CD4 (Quantum Red -labelled) mAbs were purchased from Sigma (Deisenhofen, Germany). Direct or indirect staining was performed as described previously [19].

FACS Analysis

Sampling and analysis were performed using a Becton Dickinson FACS can flow cytometer equipped with a 15-mW, air-cooled, 488-nm argon-ion laser. For each staining, 2×10^5 cells were used. All immunofluorescence profiles were plotted on a 4-decade log scale. Data were analyzed by histograms and dot plots using the Lysis II software (Becton Dickinson).

Cloning and Expression of Recombinant Proteins

Recombinant glutathione-S-transferase (GST)-fusion proteins of the AChR α-subunit (amino acid 1-150, 140-216 and 301-398), of the Glutaminyl-tRNA-Synthetase (Glu-Syn) (amino acid 1-604) and the control protein GST were prepared as described previously [19]. In addition, the mid size-neurofilament cDNA from the pNF-M (36) clone [20] was subcloned into the GST expression system (Pharmacia, Freiburg, Germany). The fusion protein GST-NF-M (459-737) was isolated by the batch method as described by Pharmacia.

Proliferation assay

Thymocytes together with autologous, irradiated PBMC used as antigen presenting cells, were cultured with fusion proteins of NF-M, AChR, Glu-Syn or control protein GST (5 μg/ml) and proliferation was measured [19]. The proliferation rate is shown as stimulation index (SI), i.e. the ratio of counts in the presence of antigen versus counts in the presence of GST [21]. For statistical analyses the Mann-Whitney U test was used [19].

Results

Using FACS analysis we could show that all subsets of thymocyte development, CD4+ and CD8+ single positive (SP) cells and CD4+CD8+ double positive (DP) cells, can be found in both thymitis and thymoma (Fig. 1). In thymoma, it seems that the mature CD4+ SP thymocyte subset is decreased compared to thymitis. Indeed, we found that the percentage of the mature CD4+ T-cell subset is reduced in thymoma (Fig. 2). It was only 55% of these cells in thymoma compared to 82% in thymitis. To further characterize the mature T-cells we looked at the terminal T-cell subset, which acquires CD45RA. In thymoma, this subset is massively reduced compared to normal thymus and residual normal thymus adjacent to thymoma (Fig. 3). These mature CD45RA+ emigrant T-cells might be composed of autoreactive T-cells.

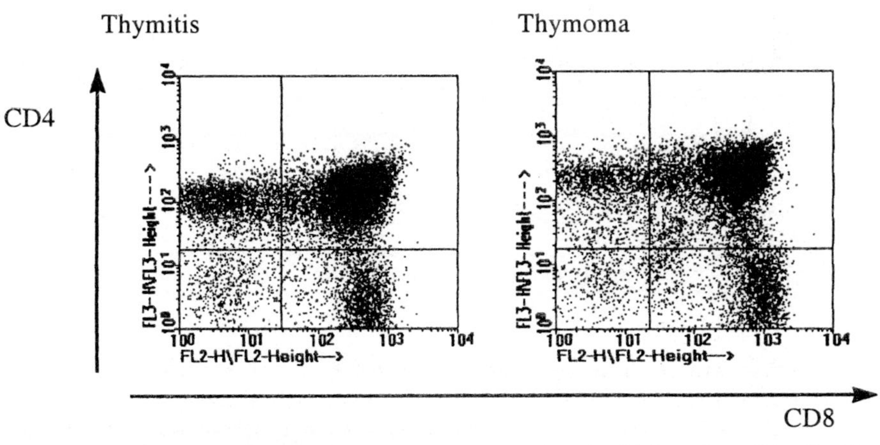

Fig. 1. Flow cytometric analysis of thymocytes gated on the CD3+ subset. Distribution of CD4+ and CD8+ SP, CD4-CD8-cells and CD4+CD8+DP cells in thymitis and thymoma derived thymocytes. All subsets of T-cell maturation can be found both in thymitis and thymoma.

Recently, we also looked for abnormal protein expression in thymoma by immunohistochemistry (data not shown). Interestingly, we found two proteins in these tumors: one which reacts with a mAb directed to the α subunit of the AChR [22] and a second protein, which was stained by a neurofilament-specific antibody mAbNN18 [10]. Since unusual protein expression might result in the generation or activation of autoreactive T-cells against AChR and neurofilament, we performed T-cell proliferation assays using recombinant AChR α subunit

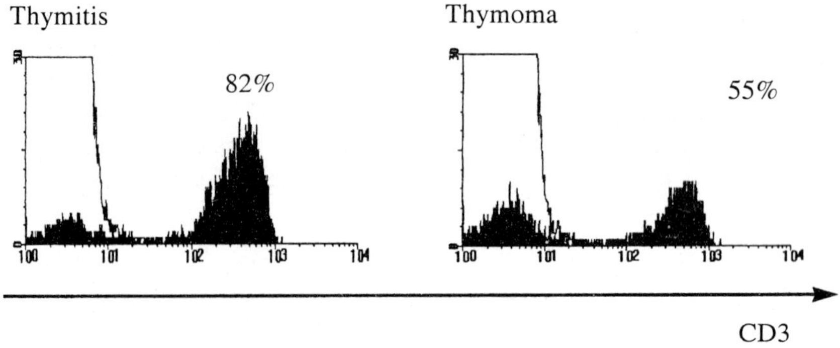

Fig. 2. CD3 profiles of T-cells gated on CD4+/CD8- thymocytes in thymitis and thymoma tissue, analysed by three-color FACS analysis. Mature CD4+ subset is decreased in thymomas.

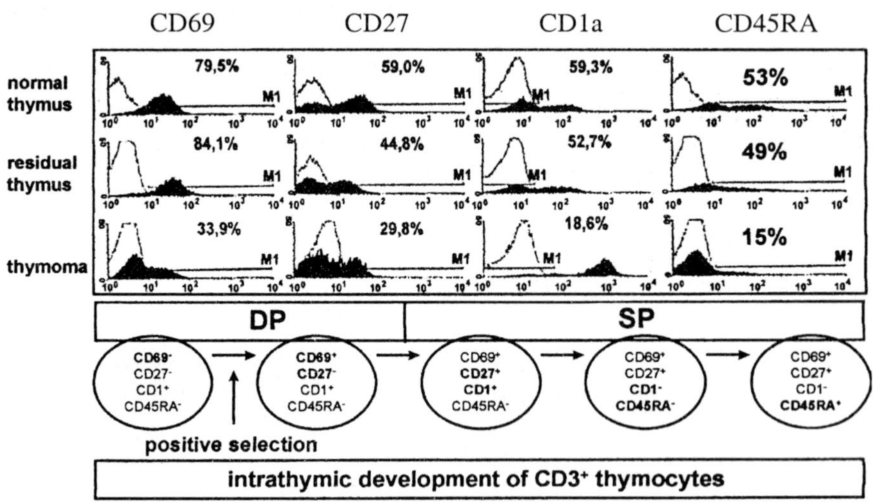

Fig. 3. Flow cytometric analysis of thymocytes gated on the CD3+ subset to characterize the terminal stages of T-cell maturation in thymomas and control tissues [23]. Phenotypically, the CD3+ thymocytes were identical in thymomas compared with controls, but the most terminal T-cell subset was massively reduced in thymomas.

fragments (AChR (1-150), (140-216) and (301-398) and neurofilament (NF-M (459-737) as antigens. While T-cells from normal control thymus showed low reactivities toward different recombinant AChR α-subunit fragments (Fig. 4), T-cells from MG patients with thymoma proliferated in response to these antigens. This is very similar to MG patients with thymitis [21]. As negative control autoantigens we used recombinant glutaminyl-tRNA-synthetase (Glu-Syn) and human myelin basic protein (MBP). Neurofilament-reactive T-cells we found predominently in MG patients with thymoma (Fig. 5).

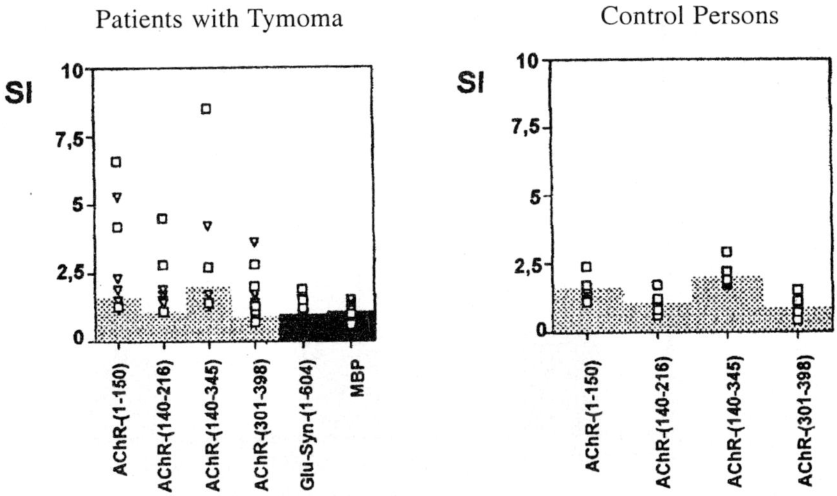

Fig. 4. **Autoantigen-specific proliferation of thymoma-derived thymocytes. Thymocytes were stimulated with various recombinant fragments of the α-subunit of the AChR. Recombinant fragment of glutaminyl-tRNA-synthetase (Glu-Syn) and myelin basic protein (MBP) were used as negative controls. AChR-specific proliferation of thymocytes from thymoma patients were increased compared with cells from control persons. There was only a slightly proliferation after stimulation with the control proteins. Dotted bars indicate the average SI of control patients without MG. Proliferative responses were analysed by proliferation assays and were given as ratio between autoantigen and control antigen (glutathione-S-transferase for fusion proteins, medium for MBP) specific proliferation (SI).**

Conclusions

The present work supports evidence of an abnormal excess of immature over mature CD4+ SP thymocytes in thymoma [12]. However, although T-cell maturation was less efficient in thymomas, the tumors contained the same CD3+ thymocyte subsets as the control tissues, including that with the pre-emigrant phenotype (CD3+, CD69+, CD27+, CD1a-, CD45RA+) [23]. Predominantly, this most mature T-cell subset was massively reduced in thymomas. To elucidate the association with MG in thymoma patients, we looked for autoreactive T-cells against the α subunit of the AChR and neurofilament protein, which shows an abnormal expression in the epithelial cells in thymoma [10]. In agreement with Sommer et al. (1990) we found increased responses of thymoma derived T-cells to recombinant fragments of AChR. In addition, we found the highest specific T-cell responses against neurofilament protein in thymoma patients with MG.

Assuming that autoreactive T-cells can emigrate from thymomas, we conclude, that the abnormal and non-tolerogenic intratumorous T-cell maturation may be related to the pathogenesis of paraneoplastic MG.

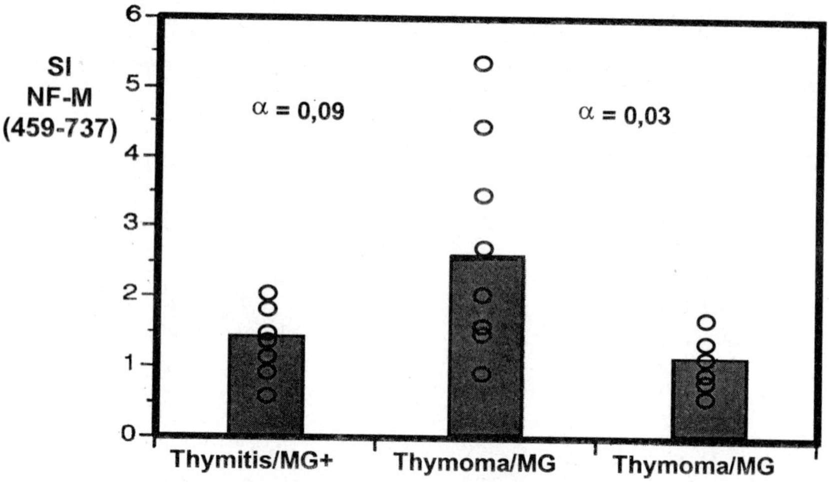

Fig. 5. Increased proliferative responses to the NF-M fragment of thymoma derived T-Cells from MG patients compared to thymoma patients without MG and MG patients with thymitis. The proliferative responses were analysed by proliferation assays and were given as ratio between autoantigen (NF-M) and control antigen (glutathione-S-transferase) specific proliferation (SI). The circles indicate the SI for NF-M responses from individual patients, the bars indicate the average SI for each group of patients.

Acknowledgment

We thank Professor MD B. Schalke, Institute of Neurology, University of Regensburg and Professor MD W. Nix, Institute of Neurology, University of Mainz, for providing us with thymus or thymoma tissues and Mrs. E. Oswald, Mrs. A. Homburger and Mr. E. Schmitt for technical assistance.

This work was supported by grant Ma 1492/2-1 (DFG) and BMBF 2000 (Teilprojekt C-5), Bundesministerium für Bildung und Forschung, Germany.

References

1. Drachman, D.B. 1994. Myasthenia gravis. *N. Engl. J. Med.* 330: 1797.
2. Oosterhuis, H.J. and J.B. Kuks. 1992. Myasthenia gravis and myasthenic syndromes. *Curr. Opin. Neurol. Neurosurg.* 5: 638.
3. Willcox, N. 1993. Myasthenia gravis. *Curr. Opin. Immunol.* 5: 910.
4. Vincent, A. 1994. Aetiological factors in development of myasthenia gravis. *Adv. Neuroimmunol.* 4: 355.
5. Marx, A., A. Wilisch, A. Schultz, S. Gattenlöhner, R. Nenninger and H. K. Müller-Hermelink. 1997. Pathogenesis of Myasthenia gravis. *Virchows Archive* 430: 355.
6. Müller-Hermelink, H.K., A. Wilisch, A. Schultz and A. Marx. 1997. Characterization of the human thymic microenvironment: Lymphoepithelial interaction in normal thymus and thymoma. *Arch. of Hist. and Cyt.* 60: 9.
7. Rosai, J. and G.D. Levine. 1976. *Atlas of tumor pathology: Tumors of the thymus.* Armed Forces Institute of Pathology, Washington,

8. Meinl, E., W.E. Klinkert and H. Wekerle. 1991. The thymus in myasthenia gravis. Changes typical for the human disease are absent in experimental autoimmune myasthenia gravis of the Lewis rat. *Am. J. Pathol.* 139: 995.
9. Marx, A., R. O'Connor, K.I. Geuder, F. Hoppe, B. Schalke, S. Tzartos, I. Kalies, T. Kirchner and H.K. Müller-Hermelink. 1990. Characterization of a protein with an acetylcholine receptor epitope from myasthenia gravis-associated thymomas [see comments]. *Lab. Invest.* 62: 279.
10. Marx, A., A. Wilisch, A. Schultz, A. Greiner, B. Magi, V. Pallini, B. Schalke, K. Toyka, W. Nix, T. Kirchner and H.K. Müller-Hermelink. 1996. Expression of neurofilaments and of a titin epitope in thymic epithelial tumors. Implications for the pathogenesis of myasthenia gravis. *Am. J. Pathol.* 148: 1839.
11. Willcox, N., M. Schluep, M.A. Ritter, H.J. Schuurman, J. Newsom Davis and B. Christensson. 1987. Myasthenic and nonmyasthenic thymoma. An expansion of a minor cortical epithelial cell subset? *Am. J. Pathol.* 127: 447.
12. Takeuchi, Y., Y. Fujii, M. Okumura, K. Inada, K. Nakahara and H. Matsuda. 1993. Characterization of CD4+ single positive cells that lack CD3 in the human thymus. *Cell Immunol.* 151: 481.
13. Hohlfeld, R., K.V. Toyka, K. Heininger, H. Grosse Wilde, and I. Kalies. 1984. Autoimmune human T lymphocytes specific for acetylcholine receptor. *Nature* 310: 244.
14. Sommer, N., G.C. Harcourt, N. Willcox, D. Beeson and J. Newsom Davis. 1991. Acetylcholine receptor-reactive T lymphocytes from healthy subjects and myasthenia gravis patients. *Neurology* 41: 1270.
15. Muller, K.M. 1989. Anti-neuroblastoma antibodies in myasthenia gravis: clinical and immunological correlations. *J. Neurol. Sci.* 93: 263.
16. Marx, A., T. Kirchner, A. Greiner, H.K. Müller-Hermelink, B. Schalke and M. Osborn. 1992. Neurofilament epitopes in thymoma and antiaxonal autoantibodies in myasthenia gravis. *Lancet.* 339: 707.
17. Meager, A., A. Vincent, J. Newsom-Davis, and N. Willcox. 1997. Spontaneous neutralising antibodies to interferon—alpha and interleukin-12 in thymoma-associated autoimmune disease [letter]. *Lancet.* 350: 1596.
18. Müller-Hermelink, H.K., A. Marx and T. Kirchner. 1994. Advances in the diagnosis and classification of thymic epithelial tumors. In *Recent Advances in Histopathology.* P. Anthony and R. MacSween, eds. Edinburgh, Churchill Livingstone, p. 49.
19. Nenninger, R., A. Schultz, V. Hoffacker, M. Helmreich, A. Wilisch, B. Vandekerckhove, T. Hunig, B. Schalke, C. Schneider, S. Tzartos, H. Kalbacher, H.K. Muller-Hermelink and A. Marx. 1998. Abnormal thymocyte development and generation of autoreactive T cells in mixed and cortical thymomas. *Lab. Invest.* 78: 743.
20. Myers, M.W., R.A. Lazzarini, V.M. Lee, W.W. Schlaepfer and D.L. Nelson. 1987. The human mid-size neurofilament subunit: a repeated protein sequence and the relationship of its gene to the intermediate filament gene family. *EMBO J.* 6: 1617.
21. Sommer, N., N. Willcox, G.C. Harcourt and J. Newsom Davis. 1990. Myasthenic thymus and thymoma are selectively enriched in acetylcholine receptor-reactive T cells. *Ann. Neurol.* 28: 312.
22. Tzartos, S.J. and M.S. Remoundos. 1992. Precise epitope mapping of monoclonal antibodies to the cytoplasmic side of the acetylcholine receptor alpha subunit. Dissecting a potentially myasthenogenic epitope. *Eur. J. Biochem.* 207: 915.
23. Vanhecke, D., G. Leclercq, J. Plum and B. Vandekerckhove. 1995. Characterization of distinct stages during the differentiation of human CD69+CD3+ thymocytes and identification of thymic emigrants. *J. Immunol.* 155: 1862.

Myasthenia Gravis: Disease mechanisms and immunointervention
P. Christadoss (Ed)

7. Cellular Mechanisms of Target Antigen Attack in Experimental Autoimmune Myasthenia Gravis

Mathilde Aurélia Poussin and Premkumar Christadoss

Department of Microbiology and Immunology, University of Texas Medical Branch, Galveston, TX 77555-1070, USA

Introduction

Myasthenia gravis (MG) is a T cell-dependent, antibody-mediated autoimmune neuromuscular disease. Autoantibodies directed against the nicotinic acetylcholine receptor (AChR) activate the complement cascade after binding to AChR. This results in a functional decrease in the AChR at the neuromuscular junction, which leads to neuromuscular transmission defects and culminates in weakness and fatigue of skeletal muscles in MG patients.

The ligand of AChR is acetylcholine (ACh), which binds to AChR in the muscle channel that allows release of sodium ions into muscle cells. This process leads to local electrical depolarization of the membrane. The AChR is a complex pentameric structure containing 2 α-subunits, one β and one δ. The last fetal γ-subunit is replaced by an ε before birth. The molecular weights of the subunits range between 45 and 55 kDa (Tzartos, this volume). The α subunit is considered to be the most highly immunogenic region. Both T and B cells in MG patient and rodents with experimental autoimmune myasthenia gravis (EAMG) are predominantly stimulated by or reacting to the α-subunit [1, 2].

The major histocompatibility complex (MHC) is a cluster of genes involved in the rejection of foreign non-self tissues, immune surveillance, and defense against infections. The MHC genes are located on the human 6th chromosome, and they express highly polymorphic cell surface MHC molecules. The MHC class II polymorphism appears to be the strongest risk factor for development of most of the autoimmune diseases, and MG is not an exception [3–5], (Hjelmström et al., this volume). Several other polymorphisms (FcγRIIA, FcγRIIB, CTLA-4, TNF, IL-1β and IL-1 receptor antagonist genes) have also been involved in MG (6-9, Lefvert et al., this volume). However, the precise immunological and cellular mechanisms involved in myasthenia gravis susceptibility and protection are not fully understood. In this review, we will delineate the cellular mechanisms of EAMG pathogenesis.

Experimental Autoimmune Myasthenia Gravis

Much of our present knowledge about the immunopathogenesis of MG has been obtained through studies on animal models of MG. EAMG in mice is a well-documented model of the human disease [10, 11]. In this model, the autoimmune disease is induced in susceptible strains of mice by subcutaneous immunization with AChR purified from *Torpedo californica* (tAChR) emulsified in complete Freund's adjuvant (CFA). The autoimmune destruction of AChR by antibodies and complement in mice produces a defect in the neuromuscular transmission, causing muscle weakness characteristic of that in human MG. Usually, mice develop clinical experimental myasthenia gravis only after the second immunization with AChR in CFA.

Many inbred strains of mice have been studied and their respective susceptibility and resistance to induction of EAMG are well characterized. The mouse MHC is called the H-2 complex and there is evidence for H-2 linkage of the AChR-specific lymphocyte response. MHC class II genes control the lymphocyte proliferative response to AChR [12, 13]. Even in human MG, MHC class II (HLA-DQ, HLA-DR) genes control the *in vitro* lymphoproliferative response [14, 15]. EAMG can be induced in mice carrying the H-2^b haplotype [e.g. C57BL/6 (B6) or C57BL/10 (B10) mice], while mice with H-2^p or H-2^k haplotypes are relatively resistant [16-18]. In mice, several immunodominant T-cell epitopes have been identified. The main pathogenic T-cell epitope is located within amino acids 146-162 of the alpha chain of AChR (α146-162). Either neonatal or adult tolerance to peptide α146-162 prevented AChR-induced EAMG [19, 20].

The Lewis rat is susceptible to the induction of EAMG after immunization with AChR emulsified in CFA, but also by immunization with the sequence 125-147 of the human α chain [21]. EAMG can also be induced in young brown Norway rats by passive transfer of antibodies against the main immunogenic region of the α chain of AChR. In contrast, aged rats are resistant, because they are resistant to antibody-mediated AChR degradation [22, 23]. The Wistar Furth rats are resistant to induction of EAMG, this is related to a decreased T-cell reactivity to peptide 100-116, compared to Lewis rats [24].

EAMG can also be induced in rabbits, and studies using immunogenic peptides synthesized based on the human sequence of the alpha chain of AChR indicate a main pathogenic role for peptides α138-167, α156-187 and α185-199 [25]. *Ex vivo* removal of antibodies specific for AChR from the sera of these animals by immunoadsorption results in clinical improvement [26].

Because of the availability of MHC mutant, transgenic, and gene knockout mice in the B6 and B10 background, EAMG in mice is an attractive model for studying human MG. Further, the mouse model of MG mimics human MG in many clinical and immunopathological manifestations [10, 11]. We, and others, have undertaken further studies to determine precisely the exact cellular mechanisms of target antigen attack in EAMG.

MHC Class II Molecules and CD4 Coreceptor Involvement

The MHC molecules are responsible for the presentation of antigenic peptides processed from endogenous cytosolic proteins (class I) or exogenous antigens (class II). Antigen processing includes degrading the antigen into peptide fragments. This occurs in intracellular organelles. In the Golgi apparatus, MHC class II molecules ($\alpha\beta$) can be found complexed to a polypeptide called the invariant chain (Ii). The $\alpha\beta$-Ii complex is transported through the Golgi complex to an endosomal acidic compartment where Ii is released. This event allows binding on the class II molecule of the peptide, coming from endosomes. MHC class II heterodimers are not expressed on all cells types, but primarily on the specialized antigen-presenting cells (B-lymphocytes, monocytes/macrophages, Langerhans' cells and dendritic cells).

$CD4^+$ T lymphocytes are important immune cells because of their helper function. $CD4^+$ T lymphocytes are involved in myasthenia gravis, as well as in EAMG. *In vitro* administration of anti-CD4 mAb suppressed AChR-specific lymphocyte proliferation. *In vivo* administration of anti-CD4 mAb not only prevented clinical EAMG, but also reversed the established disease [27]. The MHC class II deficiency and therefore $CD4^+$ T cell deficiency in the MHC class II gene disrupted mice completely rendered them resistant to the induction of clinical EAMG. Virtually no anti-AChR antibody or AChR-specific lymphocytes proliferative responses were observed in MHC class II-deficient mice immunized with AChR [28].

CD4 gene knockout mice are also more resistant to EAMG than are wild type mice. The resistance here also is associated with a diminution of antibody production (and the number of anti-AChR IgG-secreting cells) and AChR-reactive, IFN-γ-secreting cells. The lymphoproliferative response is also impaired in $CD4^{-/-}$ mice [29]. Therefore, class II and CD4 deficiency lead to the same result, implying that both class II and $CD4^+$ cells play a crucial role in EAMG development.

Studies on MHC Class II Mutant and Transgenic Mice

The α and β chains of murine MHC class II molecules are encoded by separate genes, located in the I region of the H-2 complex. The Aα and Aβ genes encode, respectively, the α and β chains of the I-A molecule. The Eα and Eβ genes encode the α and β chains of the I-E molecule respectively. The MHC class II molecules present endogenously processed exogenous antigenic peptide to $\alpha\beta$ T cell receptor (TCR) on $CD4^+$ cells. At the same time, the CD4 coreceptor molecule binds to the monomorphic region of MHC class II α and β chains [30]. This interaction is a crucial step for the initiation of MHC class II restricted antigen-specific immune responses.

The I-A subregion genes of the H-2 primarily control the immune responses to AChR *in vitro* and *in vivo* and the I-A gene dose influences the development of clinical EAMG [10, 12, 13, 18]. Treatment of SJL mice ($H\text{-}2^s$) with antibodies to the $I\text{-}A^s$ molecule before immunization with AChR in CFA suppressed the antibody response to tAChR [10].

The first genetic evidence for the importance of the MHC class II molecule in EAMG and induced autoimmune diseases came from the study of B6.C-$H\text{-}2^{bm12}$ (bm12) mice [31, 32]. The bm12 is the first and only I-A subregion mutant. The difference between C57BL/6 and bm12 strains is only 3 amino acids in the β chain of MHC class II I-A molecule ($Ile^{67} \rightarrow Phe$, $Arg^{70} \rightarrow Gln$, $Thr^{71} \rightarrow Lys$).

The Aβ mutation (gene conversion) in bm12 mice suppressed both the cellular and humoral immune response to AChR, and thus prevented the induction of EAMG [13, 32]. It is interesting to notice that in human DQ (equivalent of mouse I-A) polymorphism has been observed in MG (3, Hjelmström et al., this volume). The bm12 mouse T cells give a reduced response to few T cell epitopes: peptide α146-162 [19, 33, 34], α150-169, α181-200, α182-198 and α360-368 [35, 36]. These sequences induce good lymphoproliferation in AChR-immunized C57BL/6 mice. The bm12 mice generate a good lymphoproliferative response after *in vitro* stimulation with the peptide α111-126 [19, 32, 33]. F1 mice (B6 × bm12) develop EAMG with the same frequency as B6 mice. They also recognize the same T-cell epitopes [36]. Bm12 mice MHC class II molecule I-A^{bm12} bind peptide α146-162 with a lower affinity than the MHC class II of C57BL/6 mice does [37]. We hypothesize that resistance of bm12 mice is related to a defect in the processing of AChR and/or recognition of pathogenic epitope α146-162, while their antigen presenting cells (APC) MHC class II molecules can bind α146-162 and the subdominant epitope α111-126 with equivalent affinity. This last epitope would induce a lesser pathogenic response when presented to CD4$^+$ cells than the dominant epitope contained in the region α146-162 (Poussin et al., unpublished).

Mice from the H-2^b haplotype have a constitutive deletion of the Eα gene, and therefore, fail to express the I-E molecule on their cell surface. Two strains of mice can allow us to determine the relative importance of I-A and I-E molecules in the development of EAMG. The Eα^k transgene renders mice (B10. Aα^b: β^b. Eα^k: β^b or B10 A$^+$ E$^+$) more resistant to EAMG than B10. The over incidence of disease in transgenic mice correlates with a lower level of autoantibodies [38]. This could be explained by the fact that the transgene is obtained from a relatively resistant haplotype. Another explanation could be that transgenic mice carry two MHC class II isotypes (I-A and I-E) instead of one (I-A) in B10 mice. Therefore, the I-A^b molecule of B10 A$^+$ E$^+$ mice can present the pathogenic epitopes as in B10 mice, but the hybrid class II I-E (E α^k:β^b) presents some other peptides (Poussin et al., unpublished) leading to two possible effects: (a) presentation of protective epitopes, or (b) polyclonal activation and dilution of the antigenic response against pathogenic epitopes.

Another strain allows us to study the importance of the I-A $\alpha\beta$ genes in EAMG pathogenesis. This strain is transgenic for I-Aα^k in the B10 background. The I-Aα^k transgene product pairs with the endogenous I-Aβ^b chain to lead to the expression of a hybrid MHC class II molecule (I-A α^k: β^b). In B10.TgAα^k transgenic mice, the incidence of disease is reduced and the anti-AChR antibody production is impaired after immunization with AChR [39]. This strain also has two MHC class II isotypes; one hybrid Aα^k: β^b and the other endogenous Aα^b: β^b, but they have no I-E molecule expressed. The explanations for the observed resistance could be the same as for the B10 E$^+$ A$^+$ mice, except the two MHC class II isotypes are encoded by I-A genes. A summary of MHC class II molecules involved in protection is presented in Table 1.

It appears that the expression of susceptible I-A allele (e.g. Aα^b: β^b) is strongly related to susceptibility to the induction of EAMG, as alteration of the

Table 1. Summary of MHC class II molecules involved in EAMG protection [16-18, 28, 31, 38, 39]

Strain	Expression of						EAMG protection
	Gene				Molecule		
	I-Aα	I-Aβ	I-Eα	I-Eβ	I-A	I-E	
C57BL/10	b	b	×	b	$\alpha^b\beta^b$	×	No
B10 · BR	k	k	k	k	$\alpha^k\beta^k$	$\alpha^k\beta^k$	Yes
B10 · Aβ^0	b	×	×	b	×	×	Yes
B10 · TgEα^k	b	b	k	b	$\alpha^b\beta^b$	$\alpha^k\beta^b$	Yes
B10 · TgAα^k	k, b	b	×	b	$\alpha^k\beta^b$, $\alpha^b\beta^b$	×	Yes
Bm12	b	bm12	×	b	$\alpha^b\beta^{bm12}$	×	Yes

×: no gene or molecule

I-A molecule in susceptible strains leads to protection. I-E molecule can have a protective effect if it is expressed at the same time as I-A^b in an H-2^b strain (e.g. B10.Tg E$^k_\alpha$). The protection, in B10.TgEα^k and B10.TgAα^k mice could be explained by the nature and the diversity of epitopes presented during thymic selection, allowing a better deletion/anergy of AChR reactive clones. Protection could also be related to presentation of less pathogenic (maybe protective) epitopes by I-A^{bm12} or I-A α^k β^b molecules, or due to polyclonal activation and dilution of the antigen response against the pathogenic epitopes.

TCR Gene Usage

Several studies have also been performed to determine the TCR genes used in the immune response to AChR. The importance of Vβ6 TCR expression has been demonstrated by the association of reactivity to AChR with expression of *Mls* gene. Mice homozygous for H-2^b (associated to susceptibility), but with a lack of expression of Vβ6 exhibit a low responsiveness to AChR [40]. The α146-162-reactive T cell lines and clones generated from B6 mice expressed predominantly the Vβ6 gene product [41]. Studies comparing B6 and bm12 mice, showed that in bm12 mice Vβ6$^+$ cells do not expand in response to AChR *in vitro,* although non-immune B6 and bm12 mice have similar levels of Vβ6$^+$ cells [40–42]. On the other hand, *in vivo* depletion of Vβ6$^+$ cells neither abrogates *in vitro* responsiveness to AChR, nor prevents clinical EAMG [43]. Moreover, the B10.TCR^c strain (with a genomic deletion of certain TCR Vβ genes, including Vβ6) and the B10.Vβ8.2 strain (transgenic strain with a restricted TCR Vβ8 S2 repertoire) responded to AChR and developed EAMG [43, 44]. The data implicate multiple Vβ genes in the pathogenesis. Vβ8 can also have a pathologic function, since depletion of Vβ8 in B10.Vβ8.2 mice, which show preferential usage of TCRVα1S8 gene, prevented EAMG [44].

MHC Class I Molecules and CD8 Coreceptor Involvement

MHC class I-restricted CD8$^+$ T cells are mostly cytotoxic cells involved in the immune response against intracellular pathogens. In this case processed and T cell recognized antigens have an intracellular origin. But this is not their only function. They are also involved in the immune response by production of cytokines, and some have "helper" function. CD8 gene deficient mice have shown a decreased incidence of EAMG [29]. However, in our hands although we observed suppressed anti-AChR antibody production in CD8 cell deficient mice, there was no significant difference in the clinical incidence of EAMG between wild-type and CD8 cell deficient mice (Goluszko et al., unpublished).The β2 microglobulin-deficient mice ($\beta 2m^{-/-}$) lacking MHC class I molecules and $CD8^+$ T cells have been used to study the potential role of MHC class I-restricted $CD8^+$ T cells in immune response. The MHC class I molecule and CD8 cell deficiency in the $\beta 2m^{-/-}$ mice failed to prevent EAMG and suppress anti-AChR antibody response [45]. On the other hand, the CD8 gene knockout mice ($CD4^+CD8^-$ or $CD4^-CD8^-$) have a reduced anti-AChR antibody response (29). The suppressed anti-AChR antibody response in CD8 cell-deficient mice, but not in MHC class I intact mice could be due to the regulation of anti-AChR antibody production by non-MHC class I-restricted $CD8^+$ T cells.

B-lymphocyte involvement

B-lymphocytes have two important functions in the immune (and autoimmune) response: they differentiate to plasmocytes, the antibody-producing cell, and they are excellent antigen-presenting cells (APC). They have long been suspected to be of major importance in EAMG, as anti-AChR antibodies mediate the disease. Mice deficient for B cells failed to generate anti-AChR antibodies and were completely resistant to induction of EAMG after immunization with AChR [46, 47]. In those mice, clinical EAMG could only be induced by passive transfer with antibodies to the main immunogenic region [46]. Moreover, in those mice the early lymphoproliferative response to AChR and the immunodominant peptide α146-162 was also impaired, but the late lymphoproliferative response (90 days after the first immunization with AChR) of B cell deficient mice and wild-type mice to whole AChR and the dominant peptide α146-162 was equivalent. This indicates that in EAMG B-lymphocytes are essential in the induction of disease because they are antibody-producing cells, and APC. The APC function can be partially compensated for by other APC [46]. Anti-AChR antibody alone is not fully sufficient to cause EAMG. Terminal complement activation is also required for the development of clinical EAMG [47].

Role of Cytokines

Cytokines are small proteins (8 to 80 kDa) involved in the regulation of immune reactions. They are a component involved in the communication in the immune system. They act by binding onto receptors on the cellular membrane. They can have an autocrine as well as a paracrine action. Production of an AChR-induced soluble "helper" factor by cells from AChR-immunized mice was described more than 10 years ago [48]. Since then, many studies have tried to elucidate the roles of known cytokines in the pathogenesis of EAMG.

The production of mRNAs for several cytokines (IFN-γ, IL-4 and TGF-β) has been studied in the rat model of EAMG. Lymphoid organs of rats with EAMG contain AChR-reactive mononuclear cells producing high levels of mRNAs for IFN-γ, IL-4 and TGF-β. Up-regulation of IFN-γ is observed during the early and midterm phase of EAMG, while IL-4 is mainly involved in later stages of the disease. TGF-β is up-regulated in early and late stages of EAMG in rats [49].

One of the easiest and direct ways to study their implication in the development of EAMG is the use of cytokine (or cytokine receptor) gene knockout mice, lacking completely the expression of at least one cytokine (or receptor for cytokines). But this approach does not provide all of the answers. Often the functions can be shared by several cytokines, and compensating mechanisms exist in the immune system. At least, it is possible to determine whether a given cytokine is essential for the development of EAMG. Further, one could specifically neutralize the function of a given cytokine by antibody specific for that cytokine and study its action in pathogenesis.

The influence of IFN-α, which down-regulates MHC class II expression on lymphoid cells, has been studied by treating AChR-immunized mice with IFN-α. IFN-α treatment after immunization with AChR suppressed the development of EAMG in C57BL/6 mice [50]. IFN-α treatment after established disease induced significant remission of disease, with reduction of anti-AChR antibodies belonging to the IgG_1 and IgG_{2b} isotypes [51].

IFN-γ gene knockout mice do not develop muscle weakness after immunization with AChR [52]. The resistance to clinical EAMG is associated with dramatically reduced levels of circulating anti-AChR antibodies, compared to those in wild type mice. Reduction of antibodies affects all the IgG isotypes. AChR-primed IFN-γ knockout mice still develop a good lymphoproliferative response to AChR and dominant peptide α146-162 [52]. IFN-γ receptor gene knockout mice also exhibit a lower incidence of disease than do wild-type littermates. Their production of AChR-specific antibodies is reduced. This is mainly due to a decrease in specific IgG_{2a} antibodies. The lymphoproliferative response to AChR is not affected in IFN-γ receptor gene knockout mice [53].

IL-4 gene knockout mice develop EAMG and have an intact *in vitro* lymphoproliferative response to AChR and peptide α146-162. They also produce *in vitro* more IL-2 and IFN-γ than do wild-type C57BL/6 mice after priming with AChR. Anti-AChR IgG antibody production by IL-4 KO mice *in vivo* is equivalent to that of C57BL/6 mice, but IgG_1 levels are decreased [55]. We did not observe any significant increase in the incidence of clinical EAMG in IL-4 deficient mice. However, Karachunski et al. have observed an increase in the incidence of clinical EAMG in IL-4 deficient mice. This may be due to the different methods used to screen clinical EAMG between the two laboratories ([55], Karachunski et al., this volume).

IL-12 treatment of B6 mice increased lymphoproliferative response and IFN-γ production in cells from AChR-immunized mice stimulated *in vitro* with AChR. AChR-primed IL-12 gene knockout mice have a reduced incidence of EAMG and production of IFN-γ after *in vitro* stimulation with AChR [56].

Data indicate that IL-12 and IFN-γ, but not IL-4 are required for the development of EAMG. However, IL-4 appears to play a role during the mucosal AChR peptide tolerance (Karachunski et al., this volume). All the data obtained with cytokine or their receptor gene knockout mice are summarized in Table 2.

Table 2. Effect of cytokine-or cytokine receptor-gene disruption on EAMG [52, 56]

Knockout	Clinical EAMG (%)	Anti-AChR antibodies	Proliferative response to	
			AChR	α146-162
No	50-80	High IgG_1 and IgG_{2b}	High	High
IFN-γ	0	Low (↓ IgG_1, IgG_{2a} and IgG_{2b})	High	High
IFN-γ R	19-23	Low (↓ IgG_1, IgG_{2a} and IgG_{2b})	High	ND
IL-12	17	Low (↓→ IgG_{2a})	ND	ND
IL-4	60-80	High (↓ IgG_1)	High	High

ND: Not done.

Cellular mechanisms of target antigen attack in EAMG

The afferent limb of an autoimmune response to AChR is schematically shown in Figure 1. First, the autoreactive B cells bind to the AChR (with low affinity?) via B-cell receptor/surface IgG. AChR is processed and presented by B cells and other APC. Dominant (e.g. α146-162) or subdominant (e.g. α111-126 or α182-198) AChR peptides are presented by the I-A^b molecule. Specific $CD4^+$ cells recognize the peptide/MHC class II complex and undergo proliferation. APC secrete IL-1, IL-12 (as IL-1 or IL-12 deficiency have prevented EAMG ([56], Huang and Lefvert, personal communication) and activate the Th cells specific for AChR peptides. Further, not only the above first signal is required, but also the second costimulatory signal via B7/CD28 interaction leads to activation of T cells specific for AChR-dominant peptides (CD28 deficiency partially suppressed EAMG) ([57], Shi et al. this volume).

In second step (Fig. 2), the reaction is amplified by cooperation between T and B cells. This requires production of various cytokines (e.g. IL-2 and IFN-γ but not IL-4, as EAMG is prevented in IFN-γ gene knockout mice but not in IL-4 gene knockout mice) [52-55], and leads to selection of B cells producing antibodies with a higher affinity for AChR. The interactions between B7/CD28 and CD40/CD40L are crucial in the development of primary T and B cell autoimmune response to AChR. The CD40/CD40L interaction is absolutely required in the induction of EAMG, as CD40 gene knockout mice are completely resistant to EAMG ([57], Shi et al., this volume). Anti-AChR antibodies of high pathogenic potential either destroy AChR by antigen modulation and by Ab and complement (C3-C9)-mediated destruction of AChR [47].

Future Prospects to Study EAMG/MG Pathogenesis

Now, we have an increasing knowledge about the cellular mechanisms involved in the target antigen attack in EAMG, and similar mechanisms could operate in myasthenia gravis. The enigma still remains: In humans, what is the initial event which leads to an autoimmune response against AChR? A hypothesis is molecular mimicry by which an immune response to a foreign antigen (e.g. an infectious agent) shares homologies with endogenous AChR.

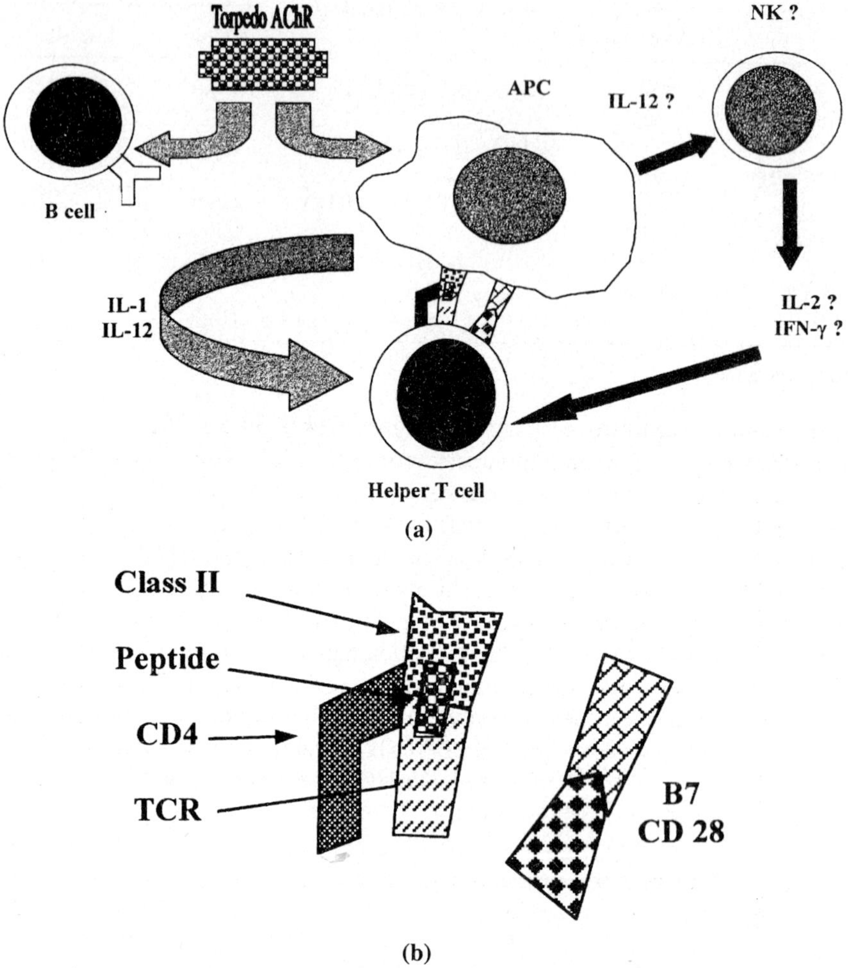

Fig. 1. Hypothetical model of the early events leading to autoimmune response to AChR in EAMG. A: global cellular interaction, B: detail of molecular communication between APC and helper T-cells.

Our future strategy will be to study new generations of HLA class II transgenic mice. At present, two strains have been developed which carry human MHC class II gene (HLA-DQ6 and HLA-DQ8) [58, 59]. EAMG susceptibility and resistance have been associated in the expression of human class II allele. HLA-DQ6 mice are more resistant than HLA-DQ8 mice to the induction of EAMG [60]. Identification of T and B cell AChR epitopes in the HLA transgenic mice will allow us to induce T and B cell tolerance to control EAMG and MG in an antigen-specific manner [1, 61].

The next question is the relevance of the use of AChR from *Torpedo californica* for immunization. The origin of the human disease is not really known and could likely be a cross reactivity between a foreign protein and self-AChR. Considering the main immunogenic role of the α chain of AChR, *Torpedo californica* remains an excellent choice, as there is significant homology between its α chain and human α chain (Fig. 3).

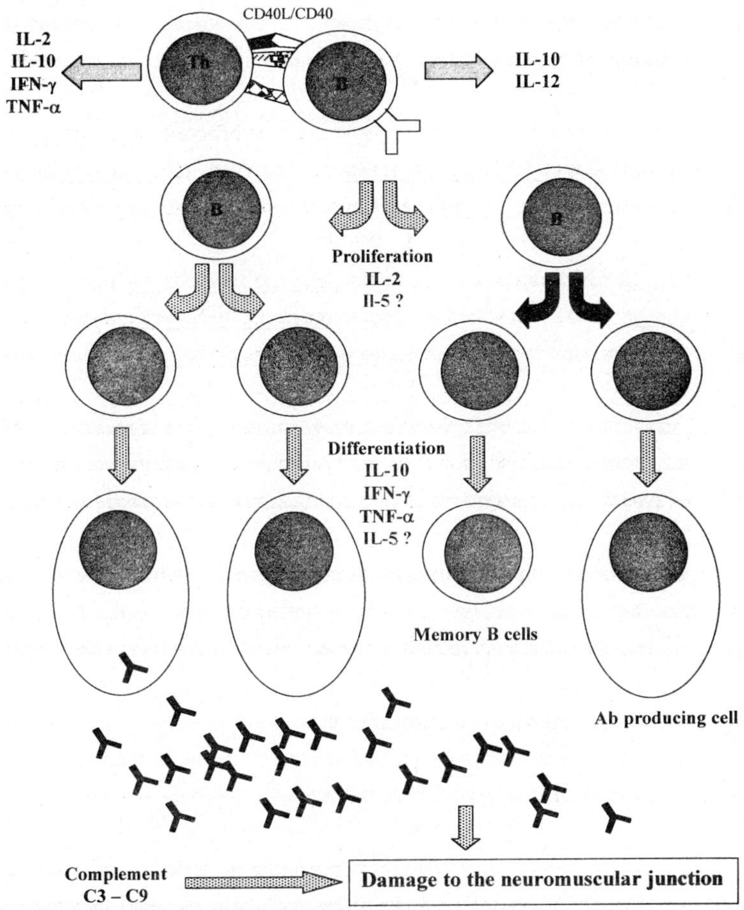

Fig. 2. Hypothetical model of the secondary events leading to the production of pathogenic autoantibodies in EAMG.

In fact, (a) immunization of HLA-transgenic mice with AChR from *Torpedo* and (b) graft of human cells (from peripheral blood lymphocytes or thymus) immune to AChR from *Homo sapiens* to SCID mice (Wang et al., this volume) lead to the same result that there is a reactivity to *Mus* AChR, leading to EAMG. Therefore, there is a high probability that animal models of MG will continue to be used to study pathogenesis of MG as well as to develop specific therapy (mostly antigen-specific tolerance; Baggi et al., Deng et al., Fuchs et al., Karachunski et al. and Pass-Rozner et al., this volume) able to reverse established EAMG/MG.

```
(Human)    MEPWPLLLLFSLCSAGLV----LGSEHETRLVAKLFKDYSSVVRPVEDHRQVVEVTVGLQ   56
(Mouse)    MCGRRGGIWLALAAALLHVS--LQGEFQRRLYKELVKNYNPLERPVANDSQPLTVYFSLS   58
(Torpedo)  MILCSYWHVGLVLLLFSCCGLVLGSEHETRLVANLLENYNKVIRPVEHHTHFVDITVGLQ   60

(Human)    LIQLINVDEVNQIVTTNVRLKQQWVDYNLKWNPDDYGGVKKIHIPSEKIWRPDLVLYNNA  116
(Mouse)    LLQIMDVDEKNQVLTTNIWLQMSWTDHYLQWNMSEYPGVKNVRFPDGQIWKPDILLYNSA  118
(Torpedo)  LIQLISVDEVNQIVETNVRLRQQWIDVRLRWNPADYGGIKKIRLPSDDVWLPDLVLYNNA  120

(Human)    DGDFAIVKFTKVLLQYTGHITWTPPAIFKSYCEIIVTHFPFDEQNCSMKLGTWTYDGSVV  176
(Mouse)    DERFDATFHTNVLVNASGHCQYLPPGIFKSSCYIDVRWFPFDVQQCKLKFGSWSYGGW--  176
(Torpedo)  DGDFAIVHMTKLLLDYTGKIMWTPPAIFKSYCEIIVTHFPFDQQNCTMKLGIWTYDGTKV  180
                          111             126                  146

(Human)    AINPESDQPDLSNFMESGEWVIKESRGWKHSVTYSCCPDTPYLDITYHFVMQRLPLYFIV  236
(Mouse)    SLDLQMQEADISSYIPNGEWDLMGIPGKRNEKFYECCKE-PYPDVTYTVTMRRRTLYYGL  235
(Torpedo)  SISPESDRPDLSTFMESGEWVMKDYRGWKHWVYYTCCPDTPYLDITYHFIMQRIPLYFVV  240
               162                   182                   198

(Human)    NVIIPCLLFSFLTGLVFYLPTDSGEKMTLSISVLLSLTVFLLVIVELIPSTSSAVPLIGK  296
(Mouse)    NLLIPCVLISALALLVFLLPADSGEKISLGITVLLSLTVFMLLVAEIMPATSDSVPLIAQ  295
(Torpedo)  NVIIPCLLFSFLTGLVFYLPTDSGEKMTLSISVLLSLTVFLLVIVELIPSTSSAVPLIGK  300

(Human)    YMLFTMVFVIASIIITVIVINTHHRSPSTHVMPNWVRKVFIDTIPNVMFFSTMKRPSREK  356
(Mouse)    YFASTMIIVGLSVVVTVIVLRYHHHDPDGGKMPKWTRIILLNWCA---WFLRMKRPGEDK  352
(Torpedo)  YMLFTMIFVISSIIITVVVINTHHRSPSTHTMPQWVRKIFIDTIPNVMFFSTMKRASKEK  360

(Human)    QDKKIFTEDIDISDISGKPGPPPMGFHSPLIK----------------------------  388
(Mouse)    VRPACQHKPRRCSLASVELSAGAGPPTSNGNLLYIGFRGLEGMHCAPTPDSGVVCGRLAC  412
(Torpedo)  QENKIFADDIDISDISGKQVTGEVIFQTPLIK----------------------------  392

(Human)    -----------------HFEVKSAIEGIKYIAETMKSDQESNNAAAEWKYVAMVMDHILL  431
(Mouse)    SPTHDEHLMHGTHPSDGDPDLAKILEEVRYIANRFRCQDESEVICSEWKFAACVVDRLCL  472
(Torpedo)  -----------------NPDVKSAIEGVKYIAEHMKSDEESSNAAEEWKYVAMVIDHILL  435

(Human)    GVFMLVCIIGTLAVFAGRLIELNQQG----                                457
(Mouse)    MAFSVFTIICTIGILMSAPNFVEAVSKDFA                                502
(Torpedo)  CVFMLICIIGTVSVFAGRLIELSQEG----                                461
```

Fig. 3. Alignment of the sequences of the *a* chains of AChR from human, mouse and Torpedo. Bold: amino acids common to the three species; bold + italic; amino acids common to human and torpedo sequences, underlined: dominant peptides.

Acknowledgement

Our studies reported in this review were supported by grants from NIH, Muscular Dystrophy Association, Association Française contre les Myopathies (AFM), Myasthenia Gravis Foundation of America, Sealy Foundation and James W. McLaughlin Foundation. M. Poussin is an AFM postdoctoral fellow.

References

1. Tzartos S.J., T. Barkas, M.T. Cung, A. Mamalaki, M. Marraud, P. Orlewski, D. Papanastasiou, C. Sakarellos, M. Sakarellos-Daitsiotis, P. Tsantili, and V. Tsikaris. 1998 . Anatomy of the antigenic structure of a large membrane antigen, the muscle-type nicotinic acetylcholine receptor. *Immunol. Rev.* 163: 89.
2. Vincent A. and N. Willcox. 1994. Characterization of specific T cells in myasthenia gravis. *Immunol. Today* 15: 41.
3. Bell J., L. Rassenti, S. Smoot, K. Smith, C. Newby, R. Hohlfeld, K. Toyka, H. McDevitt and L. Steinman. 1986. HLA-DQ beta-chain polymorphism linked to myasthenia gravis. *Lancet* 8489: 1058.
4. Hjelmström P., R. Giscombe, A.K. Lefvert, R. Pirskanen, I. Kockum, M. Landin-Olsson and C.B. Sanjeevi. 1996. Polymorphic amino acid domains of the HLA-DQ molecule are associated with disease heterogeneity in myasthenia gravis. *J. Neuroimmunol.* 65: 125.
5. Hjelmström P., C. De Weese-Scott, J. E. Penzotti, T. P. Lybrand and C.B. Sanjeevi. 1998. Structural differences between HLA-DQ molecules associated with myasthenia gravis characterized by molecular modeling. *J. Neuroimmunol.* 85: 102.
6. Raknes G., G.O. Skeie, N.E. Gilhus, S. Aadland and C. Vedeler. 1998. Fcgamma RIIA and Fcgamma RIIB polymorphisms in myasthenia gravis. *J. Neuroimmunol.* 8: 173.
7. Huang D., L. Liu, K. Noren, S.O. Xia, J. Trifunovic, R. Pirskanen and A. K. Lefvert. 1998. Genetic association of CTLA-4 to myasthenia. *J. Neuroimmunol.* 88: 192.
8. Hjelmström P., C.S. Peacock, R. Giscombe, R. Pirskanen, A.K. Lefvert, J.M. Blackwell and C.B. Sanjeevi. 1998. Polymorphism in tumor necrosis factor genes associated with myasthenia gravis. *J. Neuroimmunol.* 88: 137.
9. Huang D., R. Pirskanen, P. Hjelmström and A.K. Lefvert. 1998. Polymorphisms in IL-1β and IL receptor antagonist genes are associated with myasthenia gravis. *J. Neuroimmunol.* 81: 76.
10. Kaul R., M. Shenoy and P. Christadoss. 1994. The role of major histocompatibility complex genes in myasthenia gravis and experimental autoimmune myasthenia gravis pathogenesis. *Adv. Neuroimmunol.* 4: 387.
11. Christadoss P., R. Kaul, M. Shenoy and E. Goluszko. 1995. Establishment of a mouse model of myasthenia gravis which mimics human myasthenia gravis pathogenesis for immune intervention. In Immunobiology of proteins and peptides VIII, M.Z. Atassi and G.S. Bixler Eds., Plenum Press, New York.
12. Christadoss P., V.A. Lennon and C.S. David. 1979. Genetic control of experimental autoimmune myasthenia gravis in mice. 1. Lymphocyte proliferative response to acetylcholine receptor is under H-2 linked ir gene control. *J. Immunol.* 123: 2540.
13. Christadoss P., V.A. Lennon and C.S. David. 1981. Genetic control of experimental

autoimmune myasthenia gravis in mice. III. Ia molecules mediate cellular immune responsiveness to acetylcholine receptors. *J. Immunol.* 138: 1141.

14. Hohlfeld R., B. Conti-Tronconi, I. Kalies, J. Bertrams and K.V. Toyka. 1985 Genetic restriction of autoreactive acetylcholine receptor-specific T lymphocytes in myasthenia gravis. *J. Immunol.* 135: 2393.
15. Brocke S., C. Brautbar, L. Steinman, O. Abramsky, J. Rothbard, D. Neumann, S. Fuchs and E. Mozes. 1988. *In vitro* proliferative response and antibody titers specific to human acetylcholine receptor in patients with myasthenia gravis and relation to HLA class II genes. *J. Clin. Invest.* 82: 1894.
16. Christadoss P., V.A. Lennon, E.H. Lambert and C.S. David. 1979. Genetic çontrol of experimental autoimmune myasthenia gravis in mice. In: T and B lymphocytes: recognition and function. Academic press, New York, p. 249.
17. Berman P.W. and J. Patrick. 1980. Linkage between the frequency of muscular weakness and loci that regulate immune responsiveness in murine experimental autoimmune myasthenia gravis. *J. Exp. Med.* 152: 507.
18. Christadoss P., V.A. Lennon, C.J. Krco, E.H. Lambert and C.S. David. 1981. Genetic control of autoimmunity to acetylcholine. Role of Ia molecules. *Ann. NY Acad. Sci.* 377: 258.
19. Shenoy M., M. Oshima, M.Z. Atassi and P. Christadoss. 1993. Suppression of experimental autoimmune myasthenia gravis by epitope-specific neonatal tolerance to synthetic region alpha 146-162 of acetylcholine receptor. *Clin. Immunol. Immunopathol.* 66: 230.
20. Wu B., C. Deng, E. Goluszko and P. Christadoss. 1997. Tolerance to a dominant T cell epitope in the acetylcholine receptor molecule induces epitope spread and suppresses murine myasthenia gravis. *J. Immunol.* 159: 3016.
21. Yoshikawa H., K. Iwasa, K. Satoh and M. Takamori. 1997. FK506 prevents induction of rat experimental autoimmune myasthenia gravis. *J. Autoimmun.* 10: 11.
22. Hoedemackers A., J.L. Bessereau, Y. Graus, T. Guyon, J.-P. Changeux, S. Berrih-Aknin, P. van Breda Vriesman and M. H. De Baets. 1998. Role of the target organ in determining susceptibility to experimental autoimmune myasthenia gravis. *J. Neuroimmunol.* 89: 131.
23. Hoedemackers A., J.L. Bessereau, Y. Graus, T. Guyon, J.-P. Changeux, S. Berrih-Aknin, P. van Breda Vriesman and M.H. De Baets. 1998. Differential susceptibility of young and old rats neuromuscular junctions to antibody mediated AChR degradation in experimental autoimmune myasthenia gravis. *Ann. N. Y. Acad. Sci.* 841: 550.
24. Zoda T.E. and K.A. Krolick. 1993. Antigen presentation and T cell specificity repertoire in determining responsiveness to an epitope important in experimental autoimmune myasthenia gravis. *J Neuroimmunol.* 43: 131.
25. Jacobson L., A. Vincent, P. Shillito and J. Newsom-Davis. 1993. EAMG induced in rabbits by immunization against peptides representing human AChR. In *Myasthenia gravis and related disorders, Ann. N. Y. Acad. Sci.* 681: 295.
26. Hinman C.L. and R. Stevens-Truss. 1998. In-line affinity chromatography of specific antibody from rabbits with experimental myasthenia gravis as a prelude to immunotherapy. *Immunopathol. Immunotoxicol.* 20: 233.
27. Christadoss P. and M.J. Dauphinee. 1986. Immunotherapy for myasthenia gravis. A murine model. *J. Immunol.* 136: 2437.
28. Kaul R., M. Shenoy, E, Goluszko. and P. Christadoss. 1994. Major histocompatibility complex class II gene disruption prevents experimental autoimmune myasthenia gravis. *J. Immunol.* 152: 3152.

29. Zhang G.-X., B.-G. Xiao, M. Bakhiet, P. van Der Meide, H. Wigzell, H. Link and T. Olsson. 1996. Both $CD4^+$ and $CD8^+$ T cells are essential to induce experimental autoimmune myasthenia gravis. *J. Exp. Med.* 184: 349.
30. König R., S. Fleury and R.N. Germain. 1996. The structural basis of CD4-MHC interactions: coreceptor contributions to T cell recognition and oligomerization-dependant signal transduction. *Cur. Topics Microbiol. Immunol.* 205: 19.
31. Christadoss P. 1989. Immunogenetics of experimental autoimmune myasthenia gravis. *Crit. Rev. Immunol.* 9: 247.
32. Christadoss P., J.M. Lindstrom, R.W. Melvold and N. Talal. 1985. Mutation at I-A beta chain prevents experimental autoimmune myasthenia gravis. *Immunogenetics* 21: 33.
33. Infante A.J., P.A. Thompson, K.A. Krolick and K.A. Wall. 1991. Determinant selection in murine experimental autoimmune myasthenia gravis. Effect of the bm12 mutation on T cell recognition of acetylcholine receptor epitopes. *J. Immunol.* 146: 2977.
34. Yang B., K.R. McIntosh and D.B. Drachman. 1998. How subtle differences in MHC class II affect the severity of experimental autoimmune myasthenia gravis. *Clin. Immunol. Immunopathol.* 86: 45.
35. Bellone M., N. Ostlie, S.J. Lei, X.-D. Wu and B. Conti-Tronconi. 1991. The I-A^{bm12} mutation, which confers resistance to experimental myasthenia gravis, drastically affects the epitope repertoire of murine $CD4^+$ cells sensitized to nicotinic acetylcholine receptor. *J. Immunol.* 147: 1484.
36. Karachunski P.I., N. Ostlie, M. Bellone, A.J. Infante and B.M. Conti-Fine. 1995. Mechanisms by which the I-A^{bm12} mutation influences susceptibility to experimental autoimmune myasthenia gravis: a study in homozygous and heterozygous mice. *Scand. J. Immunol.* 42: 215.
37. Oshima M. and M.Z. Atassi. 1995. Effect of amino acid substitutions within the region 62-76 of I-$A\beta^b$ on binding with and antigen presentation of *Torpedo* acetylcholine receptor α-chain peptide 146-162. *J. Immunol.* 154: 5245.
38. Christadoss P., C.S. David, M. Shenoy and S. Keve. 1990. E^k_α transgene in B10 mice suppresses the development of myasthenia gravis. *Immunogenetics* 31: 241.
39. Christadoss P., C.S. David and S. Keve. 1992. I-$A\alpha^k$ transgene pairs with I-$A\beta^b$ gene and protects C57BL10 mice from developing autoimmune myasthenia gravis. *Clin. Immunol. Immunopathol.* 62: 235.
40. Krco C.J., C.S. David and V.A. Lennon. 1992. Mouse T lymphocyte response to acetylcholine receptor determined by T cell receptor for antigen $V\beta$ gene products recognizing Mls-1^α. *J. Immunol.* 147: 3303.
41. Infante A.J., H. Levcovitz, V. Gordon, K.A. Wall, P.A. Thompson and K.A. Krolick. 1992. Preferential use of a T cell receptor $V\beta$ gene by acetylcholine receptor reactive T cells from myasthenia gravis-susceptible mice. *J. Immunol.* 148: 3385.
42. Drachman D.B., K.R. Mc Intosch and B. Yang. 1998. Factors that determine the severity of experimental autoimmune myasthenia gravis. *Ann. N.Y. Acad. Sci.* 841: 262.
43. Wu B., M. Shenoy, E. Goluszko, R. Kaul and P. Christadoss. 1995. TCR gene usage in experimental autoimmune myasthenia gravis pathogenesis. Usage of multiple TCRBV genes in the H-2^b strains. *J. Immunol.* 154: 3603.
44. Kaul R., B. Wu, E. Goluszko, C. Deng, V. Dedhia, G.H. Nabozny, C. S. David, I.J. Rimm, M. Shenoy, T.M. Haqqi and P. Christadoss. 1997. Experimental autoimmune myasthenia gravis in B10.BV8S2 transgenic mice. Preferential usage of TCRAV1 gene by lymphocytes responding to acetylcholine receptor. *J. Immunol.* 158: 6006.

45. Shenoy M., R. Kaul, E. Goluszko, C. David and P. Christadoss. 1994. Effect of MHC class I and CD8 cell deficiency on experimental autoimmune myasthenia gravis pathogenesis. *J. Immunol.* 153: 5330.
46. Dedhia V., E. Goluszko, B. Wu, C. Deng and P. Christadoss. 1998. The effect of B cell deficiency on the immune response to acetylcholine receptor and the development of experimental autoimmune myasthenia gravis. *Clin. Immunol. Immunopathol.* 87: 266.
47. Christadoss P. 1988. C5 gene influences the development of murine myasthenia gravis. *J. Immunol.* 140: 2589.
48. Christadoss P., J.M. Lindstrom, N. Talal, C.R. Duvic, A. Kalantri and M. Shenoy. 1986. Immune response gene control of lymphocyte proliferation induced by acetylcholine receptor-specific helper factor derived from lymphocytes of myasthenic mice. *J. Immunol.* 137: 1845.
49. Zhang G.-X., V. Navikas V. and H. Link. 1997. Cytokines and the pathogenesis of myasthenia gravis. *Muscle & Nerve* 20: 543.
50. Shenoy M., S. Baron, B. Wu, E. Goluszko. and P. Christadoss. 1995. IFN-α treatment suppresses the development of experimental autoimmune myasthenia gravis. *J. Immunol.* 154: 6203.
51. Deng C., E. Goluszko, S. Baron and Christadoss P. 1996. Interferon α therapy is effective in suppressing the clinical experimental myasthenia gravis. *J. Immunol.* 157: 5675.
52. Balasa B., C. Deng, J. Lee, L.M. Bradley, D.K. Dalton, P. Christadoss P. and N. Sarvetnick. 1997. Interferon γ (IFN-γ) is necessary for the genesis of acetylcholine receptor-induced clinical experimental autoimmune myasthenia gravis in mice. *J. Exp. Med.* 186: 385.
53. Zhang G.-X., B.-G. Xia, X.-F. Bai, A. Orn, P.H. van Der Meide and H. Link. 1998. IFN-γ is required to induce experimental autoimmune myasthenia gravis. *Ann. N. Y. Acad. Sci.* 841: 576.
54. Zhang G.-X., B.-G. Xiao, X.-F. Bai, P.H. van Der Meide, A. Orn and H. Link. 1999. Mice with IFN-γ receptor deficiency are less susceptible to experimental autoimmune myasthenia gravis *J. Immunol.* 162: 3775.
55. Balasa B., C. Deng, J. Lee, P. Christadoss and N. Sarvetnick. 1998. The Th2 cytokine IL-4 is not required for the progression of antibody-dependent autoimmune myasthenia gravis. *J. Immunol.* 161: 2856.
56. Moiola L., F. Galbiati F, G. Martino, S. Amadio, E. Brambilla, G. Comi, A. Vincent, L.M. Grimaldi and L. Adorini. 1998. IL-12 is involved in the induction of experimental autoimmune myasthenia gravis, an antibody-mediated disease. *Eur. J. Immunol.* 28: 2487.
57. Shi F.-D., B. He, H. Li, D. Matusevicius, H. Link and H.-G. Ljunggren. 1998. Differential requirements for CD28 and CD40 ligand in the induction of experimental autoimmune myasthenia gravis. *Eur. J. Immunol.* 28: 3587.
58. Neeno T., C.J. Krco, J. Harders, J. Baisch, S. Cheng S and C.S. David. 1996. HLA-DQ8 transgenic mice lacking endogenous class II molecules respond to house dust allergens. *J. Immunol.* 156: 3191.
59. Cheng S., J. Baisch, C. Krco, S. Savarirayan, J. Hanson, K. Hodgson, M. Smart and C. David. 1996. Expression and function of HLA-DQ8 (DQA1*0301/DQB1*0302) genes in transgenic mice. *Eur. J. Immunogenetics* 23: 15.
60. Raju R., W.-Z. Zhan, P. Karachunski, B. Conti-Fine, G.C. Sieck and C. David. 1998. Polymorphism at the HLA-DQ locus determines susceptibility to experimental autoimmune myasthenia gravis. *J. Immunol.* 160: 4169.
61. Godkin A.J., M.P. Davenport, A. Willis, D.P. Jewell and A.V.S. Hill. 1998. Use of complete eluted peptide sequence data from HLA-DR and -DQ molecules to predict T cell epitopes, and the influence of nonbinding terminal regions of ligands in epitopes selection. *J. Immunol.* 161: 850.

Myasthenia Gravis: Disease mechanisms and immunointervention
P. Christadoss (Ed)

8. Anti-Acetylcholine Receptor CD4$^+$ T Cells in Myasthenia Gravis: Epitope repertoire and T cell receptor gene usage

Bianca M. Conti-Fine[1,2,@], Zeng-Yu Wang[1], Raghavanpillai Raju[1,*], James F. Howard Jr.[3] and Duraiswamy Navaneetham[1,2].

[1]Department of Biochemistry, Molecular Biology and Biophysics, University of Minnesota, St. Paul, MN 55108

[2]Department of Pharmacology, School of Medicine, University of Minnesota, Minneapolis, MN 55455

[3]Department of Neurology, University of North Carolina at Chapel Hill, NC 27599

[@]Previously known as Bianca M. Conti-Tronconi

*Present address: Department of Immunology, Mayo Clinic, Rochester, MN 55905

Introduction

Although the symptoms of myasthenia gravis (MG) are due to the binding of auto-antibodies to the nicotinic acetylcholine receptor (AChR) at the neuromuscular junction (reviewed in [1]), the anti-AChR CD4$^+$ T cells have been intensely investigated, because they may be the prime movers in the pathogenesis of MG. Furthermore, specific immunosuppressive treatments targeted on the autoimmune CD4$^+$ cells have proven successful in experimental autoimmune diseases, including the experimental model of MG, mouse experimental autoimmune MG (EAMG) ([2-4] and references therein).

In EAMG, the synthesis of anti-AChR antibodies and development of myasthenic symptoms require CD4$^+$ cells [1]. MG patients have anti-AChR CD4$^+$ cells in the blood and thymus that can be propagated *in vitro* and have T helper functions [1]. Several lines of circumstantial evidence have suggested for a long time that CD4$^+$ T helper cells must have an important role in human MG. First, anti-AChR antibodies in MG patients, including those bound to the neuromuscular junction, are primarily high affinity IgG [1], whose synthesis requires T helper factors. Second, the only obvious and early effect on the anti-AChR immune response of thymectomy—a staple in the treatment of MG—is an immediate, substantial decrease in the anti-AChR reactivity of blood T cells [1]. Third, treatment of MG patients with anti-CD4$^+$ antibodies abolished the T cell response *in vitro* to the AChR and caused clinical and electrophysiological improvement [1].

Recently, experiments in SCID mice engrafted with immune cells from MG patients have proven that also in human MG, anti-AChR CD4$^+$ cells have a crucial role for synthesis of pathogenic anti-AChR antibodies and development of MG symptoms. We engrafted SCID mice with blood mononuclear cell (BMC) from MG patients, or BMC depleted in CD4$^+$ T cells from the same patients, and we investigated the appearance of myasthenic symptoms and of human anti-AChR antibody in the engrafted mice: most mice engrafted with BMC, and none of those engrafted with the CD4$^+$-depleted BMC developed significant muscle weakness, or had significant concentrations of anti-AChR antibodies in the serum and measurable amounts of anti-AChR antibody bound to the muscle AChR [5].

Of the characteristics of the CD4$^+$ cells specific for a given antigen, the epitope repertoire that they recognize on the antigen and the structure of the T cell receptors (TCR) they use are among the most important. Elucidation of these characteristics might provide a foundation for development of specific immunosuppressive approaches, and clues to the events that triggered the autoimmune response. In this chapter we will summarize our work on the sequence regions of the human AChR recognized by the autoimmune CD4$^+$ cells in MG patients, on the TCR Vβ region genes that they use, and on the overall usage of the different TCR Vβ families in the blood and the thymus of MG patients.

T Cell Recognition of the Different Muscle AChR Subunits in Generalized MG Patients

Muscle AChR is formed by four homologous subunits: α, β, γ (or ε) and δ, and it exists in two developmentally regulated isoforms [6]. Embryonic muscle AChR contains α, β, γ and δ subunits [6]. Upon innervation, the γ-subunit is generally replaced by the ε-subunit [6]. Adult extra-ocular muscles still express the γ-subunit, and presumably the embryonic AChR isoform [7-8]. The thymus, which is involved in the pathogenesis of MG, and which might be the place where the anti-AChR sensitization starts [9], expresses an AChR-like protein(s) similar or identical to those in embryonic muscle AChR, containing the γ, not the ε-subunit [10-11]. Thus, if the thymus embryonic-like AChR is the original sensitizing autoantigen in MG, the anti-AChR CD4$^+$ cells of MG patients might not recognize the ε-subunit at all. However, the thymus expresses mRNA for the ε-subunit as well [12], and therefore it might also express an adult-type AChR. The ε-subunit may have gone undetected by the antibodies used to detect the AChR-subunit in the thymus, due to the relatively low sensitivity of that approach.

The α-subunit has an important role in the pathogenesis of MG, because it forms a domain recognized by most anti-AChR antibodies in human MG and rodent EAMG, and several epitopes recognized by CD4$^+$ cells in both MG and EAMG [1].

Little is known about the role of non-α subunits in the anti-AChR response in MG. In rodent EAMG, the anti-AChR response involves subunits other than the α. Rats immunized with individually purified AChR α, β, γ or δ subunits develop EAMG [13], and CD4$^+$ cells of rodents immunized with purified AChR recognize the α-subunit preferentially, but they also recognize other AChR subunits [14-15]. Thus, non-α subunits may also be the target of a pathogenic autoimmune response in human MG.

We have propagated from MG patients CD4$^+$ T cell lines specific for the β, γ and δ-subunit [1]: this suggested a role of those subunits in the anti-AChR CD4$^+$ response but did not prove it, because the high antigen concentration used for propagation of the lines might cause T cell activation *in vitro*, and yield lines that are not representative of the clonal anti-AChR CD4$^+$ population *in vivo* [16].

To determine whether anti-AChR CD4$^+$ cells in MG patients recognize subunits other than the α, we investigated the human muscle AChR subunits recognized by the blood CD4$^+$ cells in 25 patients that had generalized MG (gMG) [17-18]. Three patients had a thymoma. We used CD4$^+$ T cells directly obtained from the blood to avoid misrepresentations of the CD4$^+$ repertoire resulting from biased clonal propagation *in vitro*. As representative antigens of the human AChR subunits, we used pools of overlapping synthetic peptides spanning the sequences of each of the human AChR subunits. We tested the response of CD4$^+$ cells to those AChR subunit peptide pools in proliferation assays *in vitro*.

The synthetic peptides we used were approximately 20 residues long. That length compares with that of naturally processed, class-II restricted epitopes, that are 9-14 residues [19]. Extra residues at either end of the epitope sequence do not affect the attachment of the peptide to the binding cleft of the presenting HLA class II molecules, which is open at both its ends [1]. The peptides overlapped by five-to-ten residues to reduce the risk of missing epitopes "broken" between peptides. Peptides thus designed are a reasonable compromise between the conflicting needs of reducing the risk of missing epitopes and using peptide panels of manageable size.

Most gMG patients without thymomas recognized all AChR-subunits (Fig. 1). The intensity of the T cell response to the AChR peptide pools was comparable to that of the normal response to a strong exogenous antigen, tetanus toxoid. Only six out of 22 gMG patients without thymomas did not recognize all AChR subunits, and they were patients whose disease had started recently: the recent onset of their disease is likely related to the recognition of a limited T epitope repertoire on the AChR (see below). One of the 22 gMG patients without thymoma did not recognize the γ subunit, and one did not recognize the α subunit. In gMG patients without thymoma, the δ subunit was recognized significantly less than the α and γ subunits. The lesser response to the δ subunit of the CD4$^+$ cells might be related to the mechanisms that trigger the anti-AChR response, since the thymus, and especially the thymus of MG patients, might not express the AChR δ subunit [20]. Of the three gMG patients with thymomas, one recognized all AChR subunits strongly, while the other two did not recognize the γ subunit (Fig. 1). Although the number of thymoma patients that we tested is too small to allow firm conclusions, these results suggest that unlike gMG patients without thyomas, those with thymoma might recognize the γ subunit to a lesser extent than the other AChR subunits: this might be related to the unique antigenic properties of the AChR-like protein or proteins expressed in thymoma tissue [9].

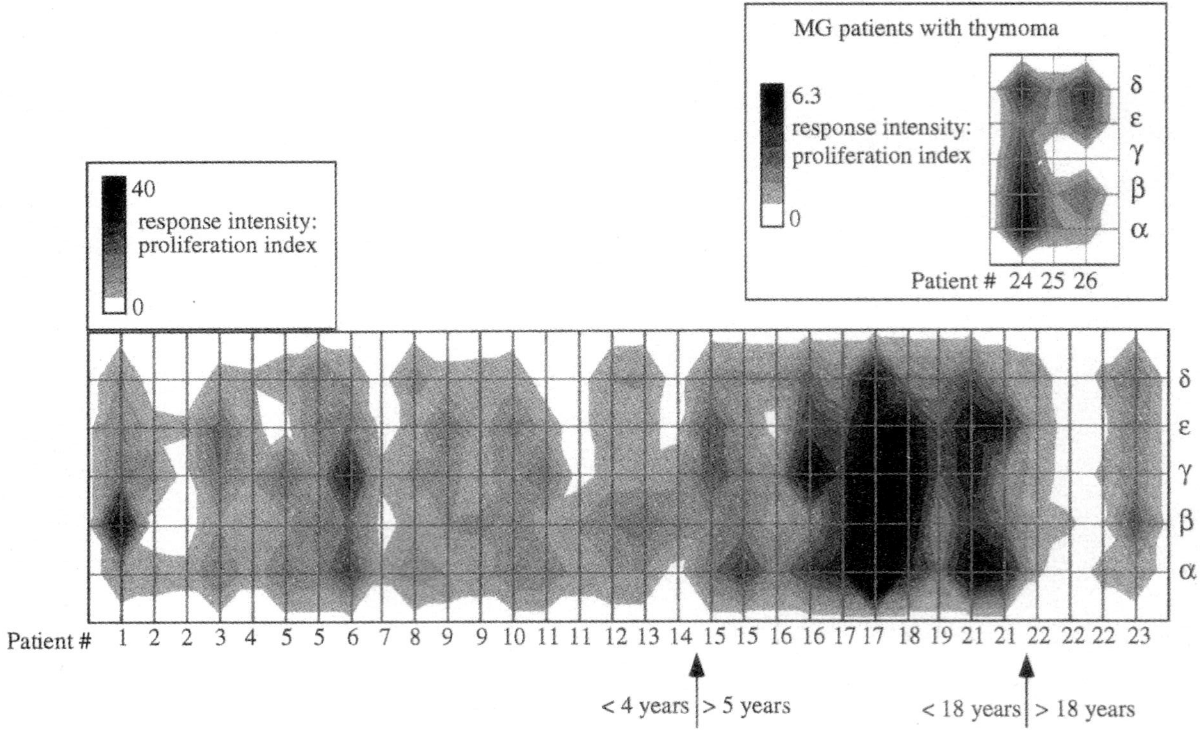

Fig. 1. Spreading of T cell response to all AChR subunits during the course of gMG. Results of proliferation assays using BMC and CD4^{+}-enriched BMC from gMG patients are compared with the years elapsed between the first appearance of symptoms and the time of assay. We report only the proliferative indices that were significant, as compared to the spontaneous cell proliferation: they are represented as a contour map. Each vertical line represents PI obtained with different AChR subunit peptide pools for one subject in one experiment (bottom of plot). Subjects, and the different experiments carried out with same subjects, are arranged in the order determined by the length of time during which they had gMG symptoms, starting at the left with the patients whose symptoms had the most recent onset (bottom of plot). Each horizontal line represents the recognition by the different subjects of one AChR subunit (right of plot). Intensity of the responses to the peptide pools is represented using the color code indicated. Main plot reports the results obtained for gMG patients without thymoma, the insert those for three thymoma patients. Reprinted with permission from B.M.

These results, and those from previous studies that investigated the response to the AChR of either BMC or of anti-AChR T cells lines propagated from MG patients [1, 17], clearly indicate that in gMG the anti-AChR $CD4^+$ response involves all AChR subunits.

Spreading of the Anti-AChR $CD4^+$ Response in MG

How the anti-AChR $CD4^+$ response evolves over time is an important question in the immunobiology of MG. In rat experimental autoimmune encephalomyelitis, the $CD4^+$ response to myelin components may be initiated by sensitization to one epitope, and it spreads later to other epitopes within the same or other myelin antigens [21]. On the other hand, in mouse EAMG hyper immunization with AChR focuses the $CD4^+$ response onto one epitope of the AChR α subunit [22], that is, recognized by highly pathogenic $CD4^+$ cells [23]. Also in Lewis rat EAMG, the pathogenic T cells recognize primarily one epitope on the AChR α subunit [1]. Thus, both paradigms, spreading of the $CD4^+$ response to an increasing number of epitopes, or focusing on a few immunodominant epitopes, might, in principle, apply to the progression of the anti-AChR $CD4^+$ response that occurs in human MG.

We investigated whether or not anti-AChR $CD4^+$ cells in gMG recognize increasingly larger parts of the AChR molecule as the disease progresses. The population of gMG patients without thymoma that we used for the studies described in the previous section comprised patients in which the onset of the symptoms had occurred from one month to 30 years prior to the testing: we compared the ability to recognize the different AChR-subunit peptide pools with the duration of the disease (Fig. 1). Among the patients that had the disease for 5-18 years all but one recognized all AChR subunits, and they had significantly stronger responses to all AChRs subunits than did the patients that had the disease for less than four years. The $CD4^+$ responses to the AChR subunits of the patients that had the disease for 5-18 years compared in their intensity to the responses to a strong exogenous antigen, tetanus toxoid [17, 24]. $CD4^+$ BMC from patients who had developed gMG less than four years prior to the test frequently did not recognize all AChR subunits (Fig. 1): repeated tests over several months revealed recognition of additional subunits.

Thus, the involvement of the entire AChR molecule in the autoimmune $CD4^+$ response of MG patients likely results from spreading of the $CD4^+$ sensitization to increasingly larger parts of the AChR molecule as the disease progresses, and sensitization to an increasing number of AChR-subunits. The higher responses to the AChR subunits of the patients whose disease had lasted for five years or longer as compared to lower responses in those whose disease had lasted for fewer than four years suggest that also the number of T cells that respond to each AChR subunit increases with time. Longitudinal studies of the same patients [25-27] also indicated that the number of AChR epitopes recognized by $CD4^+$ cells and the number of AChR-specific $CD4^+$ cells changes as the disease progresses, consistent with the occurrence of T epitope spreading in MG.

The different characteristics of evolution and epitope repertoire of the anti-AChR $CD4^+$ response in MG, as compared to rodent EAMG, underscores the different immunobiology of spontaneous human autoimmune diseases, as compared to their experimental models induced by immunization with purified autoantigens and adjuvants.

T Cell Recognition of the Muscle AChR Subunits in Ocular MG (oMG) Patients

Frequently, the initial symptoms of MG are diplopia and/or ptosis, caused by weakness of the extraocular muscles (EOM) [1]. In most patients the weakness spreads to the skeletal muscles, but in 16% of all MG patients it remains localized to the EOM [1]. The cause of the lack of spreading of the symptoms in oMG is still unknown.

EOM have intrinsic functional properties that make them especially susceptible to develop MG symptoms when failure of the AChR function occurs: for example, ptosis and limitations of ocular movements are the most common and early manifestations of congenital MG, caused by genetic defects of the AChR expression or structure that affect to a similar extent the AChRs of all muscles [1]. oMG patients have fewer serum anti-AChR antibodies than gMG patients, and ~50% of them do not have measurable serum anti-AChR antibody [1, 28]. In oMG the symptoms might be limited to the EOM simply because the anti-AChR response remains modest in time, with production of anti-AChR antibody in amounts insufficient to compromise the strength of muscles other than the EOM. On the other hand, the preferential involvement of the EOM in MG might be related to some unique antigenic properties of the AChR expressed by the EOM, which appears to include both the embryonic and the adult AChR isotypes [7, 8].

In a first study, we investigated the response to the AChR-subunits of four oMG patients: their $CD4^+$ cells recognized consistently only the embryonic γ subunit, and they never recognized the ε subunit significantly [17]. They occasionally recognized the α, β and δ subunits. These findings suggested that oMG patients might differ in the recognition of the γ and the ε subunits from the gMG patients, for which the T cell sensitization to these two subunits is comparable. Previous findings that some oMG patients have antibodies that uniquely recognize the synapses of the EOM [28], where the *en grappe* synapses of multiterminal toxic fibers and many *en plaque* synapses of singly innervated fibers in the EOM express an embryonic-like AChR in addition to the adult isoform [8], supported the possibility that in oMG the anti-AChR response might focus on the γ subunit.

The findings summarized above raised the possibility that a preferential recognition of the γ subunit was related to the distribution of muscle weakness in gMG and oMG. However, the *levator palpebrae* muscle, which in oMG is affected with a frequency and severity similar to those of the EOM, does not express the γ subunit [29]. Also, other studies found that some oMG patients have $CD4^+$ cells and antibodies specific for the adult AChR isoform [30].

Those discrepancies may be due to a heterogeneity in the characteristics of the $CD4^+$ response in oMG patients, or to the unstable recognition of AChR in oMG, with changes over time of the subunits recognized. An unstable sensitization of $CD4^+$ cells might be insufficient for a vigorous and consistent anti-AChR antibody response, and explain why anti-AChR antibodies are present only in 50% oMG patients, and in low titers [28].

In a second study [18] we tested the CD4⁺ cell recognition of the AChR subunits in a relatively large number of oMG patients, and determined how it evolved over time. We tested CD4⁺-enriched BMC or BMC from 14 oMG patients that had developed oMG from up to 16 years prior to the test. We tested eight patients two or three times, up to 20 months apart. The BMC in most patients recognized one or more AChR-subunits. However, in several patients, including some which had developed the disease four or more years prior to the test, BMC did not recognize some subunits. In most oMG patients the recognition of the AChR subunits was low as compared to that in gMG patients [17, 24]. The recognition of AChR-subunits was not stable over time: in most of the oMG subjects tested more than once, one or more subunits recognized in the first test were not recognized in the later tests.

Consistently, the proliferative responses to the different AChR subunits of the CD4⁺ cells from oMG patients were much lower than those observed for gMG patients [17-18, 24]. A low CD4⁺ T cell response agrees with the low serum concentrations of anti-AChR antibodies observed in oMG patients [1, 28].

We have started investigating how the epitope repertoire of the anti-AChR CD4⁺ cells of oMG patients evolves in time. We examined the γ subunit epitopes recognized by two oMG patients at approximately one-year intervals. We tested one patient three times, and the other twice. The first patient had a vigorous response to the γ subunit in the first experiment, and he recognized, at that time, a number of γ subunit peptides. His response to the γ subunit was substantially less in the other two experiments. In conformity with his lower response to the γ subunit, the CD4⁺ cells at those times recognized a more limited repertoire that included some of the epitopes recognized previously, as well as new epitopes not recognized in the previous experiment(s). We obtained similar results with the CD4⁺ cells of the second patient, who also recognized the γ subunit slightly more strongly in the first experiment. In both experiments, his CD4⁺ cells recognized several γ subunit epitopes. The repertoire identified in the two experiments overlapped to a small extent. Several peptides were recognized in one experiment, but not in the other. These results are consistent with an unstable CD4⁺ recognition that wanders from one AChR epitope to another.

CD4⁺ T Cell Repertoire on the AChR: Immunodominant, Universal Epitope Sequences Recognized by Most or All MG Patients

We have studied the epitope repertoire of AChR-specific CD4⁺ cells in MG patients by testing the response to individual overlapping synthetic AChR peptides spanning the sequence of each AChR subunits of unselected blood CD4⁺ T cells, and of CD4⁺ T cell lines enriched with AChR-specific cells by culture *in vitro* with AChR antigens [1, 24]. The use of those two cell populations has different advantages and limitations. AChR-specific CD4⁺ lines have strong, consistent responses to individual peptides that allow a clear-cut assessment of their epitope repertoire. However, they may have a repertoire different from that of the original CD4⁺ population, due to biased clonal propagation *in vitro*. Also, the denatured antigens, such as synthetic and biosynthetic peptides, that are commonly used for propagation of $CD4^+$ cells specific for rare antigens, may be processed into peptides different from those obtained from processing of the native antigen *in vivo*, and expand $CD4^+$ clones irrelevant for the immune process *in vivo*. The use of unselected T cells or $CD4^+$ T cells from the blood of MG patients avoids the risk of detecting a biased repertoire due to the selective clonal loss or enrichment. However, because of the low frequency of antigen-specific $CD4^+$ cells in the blood, the results obtained from testing non-selected blood $CD4^+$ T cells might be too low to be convincing, especially when assessing the response to individual epitopes.

Due to the "orthogonal" advantages and shortcomings of unselected blood $CD4^+$ cells and of AChR-specific $CD4^+$ lines, it was from the combined results of those two approaches that many AChR sequence regions forming $CD4^+$ epitopes could be identified confidently. We have tested the response to the individual AChR peptides of the anti-AChR cell lines by proliferation assay, and that of unselected blood $CD4^+$ cells by proliferation and enzyme-linked immunospot (ELISPOT) assays. The latter assay detects the antigen-induced secretion of interferon-γ (IFN-γ) by individual $CD4^+$ Th1 cells, demonstrating their role in the anti-AChR $CD4^+$ response. These different approaches have given consistent and complementary results.

We found that a number of sequence regions on each AChR subunit forms $CD4^+$ epitopes (Table 1). Each patient had an individual repertoire, yet a few sequences on each AChR subunit were recognized by all or most patients, irrespective of the MHC haplotype [25-26, 31-35]. The results of studies on the response of the unselected blood $CD4^+$ cells [25-26], or of the blood $CD4^+$ Th1 subset [35], indicated that those "universal" epitope sequences are recognized by high numbers of T cells. Thus, they should be considered both universal and immunodominant epitope sequences (indicated in bold characters in Table 1). Their immunodominance may be related to easy cleavage and processing, and to the ability of human DR molecules to interact with many unrelated peptides, as discussed later.

Thus, while the anti-AChR antibody response in MG is focused on the main immunogenic region (MIR) [1], the anti-AChR $CD4^+$ cells recognize a complex epitope repertoire, that involves a large part of the AChR molecule. This reduces the hope for easy development of specific immunosuppresive procedures targeted on epitopes recognized by autoimmune T cells, because even the immunodominant epitopes recognized by most MG patients are quite a few.

We have studied most extensively the $CD4^+$ epitope repertoire on the α subunit. For this subunit, we have carried out studies using each of the approaches listed above: testing of unselected blood $CD4^+$ cells by proliferation and by IFN-γ immunospot assay, and propagation of α-subunit-specific $CD4^+$ cell lines and determination of their epitope repertoire. We have investigated the $CD4^+$ repertoire on the other AChR-subunits using only one or two of those approaches: although less extensive than those carried out for the α-subunit, those studies yielded repertoires with similar overall characteristics for all of the AChR subunit. Thus, we will describe here in some detail the characteristics of the CD4$^+$ repertoire on the α subunit, which is representative of those we found on the other AChR subunits as well.

Four AChR α subunit sequences, α48-67, α101-137, α304-322 and the carboxyl terminal sequence, α403-437, were recognized by the majority of the MG patients, irrespective of their HLA class II type, and by a high number of cells. We will refer to them as universal epitope sequences. The strong response to those sequences is the "tip" of a response to sequence regions that may include peptide sequences on either side of these universal epitope sequences. The peptide sequences recognized by 50% or more of the MG patients are clustered in five sequence regions. One corresponds to residues α1-14; the second to residues α48-80, comprising peptides α48-67 and α63-80; the third to residues α101-154, consisting of peptides α101-120, α118-137 and α135-154; the fourth to residues α304-337, including peptides α304-322 and α320-337; and the fifth to residues α403-437, comprising peptides α403-421 and α419-437.

Most of the α subunit sequences that form epitopes for the CD4$^+$ cells correlate with sequence regions that form non-transmembrane domains: those regions are believed to be at least partially exposed on the AChR surface [6]. Three universal epitopes sequences should be extracellular, or include extracellular parts. The sequence region α48-80 is neighbors with, and includes, residues α67-76, that are involved in formation of the MIR [1]. The sequence region α101-154 includes a putative extracellular sequence region between two cysteine residues at positions 128 and 142, which must be at least partially exposed on the AChR surface, since it is glycosylated [6]. Sequence regions homologous to the universal epitope sequence α304-322 are exposed on the cytoplasmic surface in other AChRs [36]. The amino terminus of all AChR-subunits is extracellular, although it is not clear whether it is exposed on the AChR surface, because it is accessible to the binding of antibodies only after mild denaturation of the AChR [36]. The universal epitope sequence α403-437 includes the carboxyl terminal region of the α-subunit (residues α428-437), which is hydrophilic and likely exposed on the extracellular surface, and the hydrophobic segment α409-427, which is believed to form a transmembrane α-helix, called M4 [6, 36].

Three other transmembrane segments are believed to exist in the α and in the other AChR subunits, called M1 (residues α211-236), M2 (residues α242-261) and M3 (residues α277-298) (6, 36). These putative transmembrane regions largely correspond to three peptides that were sometimes recognized by the CD4$^+$ cells of MG patients: α214-234, α246-264 and α280-297. Hydrophobic sequences in the core of a protein may form epitopes for human CD4$^+$ T cells, if they are flanked by sequence loops exposed on the surface of the molecule and accessible to the processing enzymes [37].

The universal epitopes sequences identified by the use of CD4$^+$ T cell lines propagated from MG patients by stimulation with the a pool of synthetic peptides spanning the α-subunit sequence [31] and those identified by the use of unselected blood CD4$^+$ cells [25, 35] corresponded very well. This verifies that, as shown in many other human and experimental systems [16], synthetic peptides can be safely used for propagation of antigen-specific CD4$^+$ cell lines. The use of non-

Table 1. Sequence segments of the α, β, γ, δ and ε subunits of human muscle AChR forming epitopes frequently recognized by CD4⁺ cells in MG patients

		α subunit[1]					
Region α1-80	Region α101-168	Region α191-207	Region α293-337	Region α387-437			
α1-14 α19-34 α32-51 α**48-67** α63-80	α**101-120** α**118-137** α135-154 α151-168	α191-207	α293-308 α**304-322** α320-337	α387-405 α**403-421** α**419-437**			
		β subunit[2]					
Region β16-50	Region β181-200	Region β271-290	Region β316-350	Region β361-425			
β16-35 β31-50	β**181-200**	β**271-290**	β**316-335** β**331-350**	β361-380 β376-395 β391-410 β406-425			
				γ subunit[3]			
Region γ30-49	Region γ60-124	Region γ135-154	Region γ248-288	Region γ297-355	Region γ366-400	Region γ411-430	Region γ470-495
γ30-49	γ60-79 γ**75-94** γ90-109 γ105-124	γ135-154	γ248-267 γ263-273 γ269-288	γ297-312 γ306-325 γ**321-340** γ336-355	γ366-385 γ381-400	γ411-430	γ470-489 γ476-495

δ subunit[4]					
Region δ1-20	Region δ61-80	Region δ91-185	Region δ196-290	Region δ346-392	Region δ461-496
δ1-20	δ61-80	δ91-110	δ196-215	δ346-362	δ461-480
		δ106-125	δ213-230	δ363-386	δ476-496
		δ121-140	δ226-245	δ373-392	
		δ136-155	δ241-260		
		δ151-170	δ256-275		
		δ166-185	δ271-290		

ε subunit[5]					
Region ε51-70	Region ε91-110	Region ε121-170	Region ε231-320	Region ε351-370	Region ε431-473
ε51-70	**ε91-110**	ε121-140	ε231-250	ε351-370	ε431-450
		ε141-160	ε241-260		ε451-470
		ε151-170	ε261-280		ε461-473
			ε281-300		
			ε291-310		
			ε301-320		

[1]From [25, 31, 35]; [2]From [32]; [3]From [26, 34]; [4]From [26, 33]; [5]From [27].

Reprinted with permission from B.M. Conti-Fine et al. (1998), Ann. N.Y. Acad. Sci. 841: 283–308. Copyright Annals of the New York Academy of Sciences, 1998.

selected $CD4^+$ blood cells identified a broader repertoire than that detectable with α subunit-specific $CD4^+$ cell lines. This suggests that the use of peptide sequences as stimulators results in preferential propagation of the $CD4^+$ cells specific for the most immunogenic parts of the antigen.

$CD4^+$ Cells that Recognize Universal AChR Epitopes have a Restricted but Individual Usage of TCR Vβ Gene Families

An important question in the biology of T cells is how the structure of the TCR relates to the peptide epitope/MHC molecule complex that is recognized specifically. MG is an ideal system to study the TCR gene usage in human autoimmunity and its relationship with the $CD4^+$ epitope repertoire, because the target autoantigen, the muscle AChR, is known and well characterized.

Anti-AChR $CD4^+$ cells in MG express TCR that are $\alpha\beta$ heterodimers [1]. Each TCR chain includes a variable region, which confers specificity, and a constant region. For the β subunit, the variable region genes result from somatic rearrangement of germline-encoded V (variable), D (diversity) and J (joining) segments. More than 100 different TCR Vβ genes have been reported and are classified into 24 families, based on the extent of sequence similarity.

Studies on the TCR usage of T cells isolated from tissues and blood of autoimmune patients yielded conflicting results [38]. Some studies reported that T cell responses may have a restricted TCR repertoire, but other studies found extreme TCR diversity [38-39]. This was likely due to the use of unselected T cells: even when they had been eluted from the affected tissues, they likely included the "bystander" T cells, in addition to the autoAg-specific T cells. Investigations on these matters should strive to use populations of T cells enriched as much as possible in antigen-specific autoimmune T cells [16, 37].

To determine whether anti-AChR $CD4^+$ cells in MG patients have a restricted usage of the TCR Vβ genes, we used $CD4^+$ T cell lines specific for human AChR epitopes, propagated from gMG patients [31-34, 40]. We determined their Vβ usage using a semiquantitative reverse transcriptase PCR (RT-PCR) assay [41]. We analyzed the TCR Vβ usage of 16 anti-AChR $CD4^+$ polyclonal cell lines [41]. The lines had been propagated from the patients' blood using pools of overlapping peptides corresponding to the sequence of an AChR subunit, or individual synthetic sequences forming immunodominant AChR epitopes: in either case, the lines recognized peptides that formed universal, immunodominant AChR epitopes (see previous sections). The lines had been propagated for short periods of time (twelve lines for less than two months, four lines for less than five months) to reduce the risk of biased clonal propagation. Most lines had limited Vβ usage (Fig. 2): however, in most cases different Vβ regions were used for different epitopes in the same patient, and for the same epitope in different patients. A few patients used the same Vβ regions for recognition of different epitopes. The Vβ4 and Vβ6 regions were used most frequently.

Thus, while the autoimmune $CD4^+$ cells that recognize a given AChR epitope generally have restricted TCR Vβ usage, in any given MG patient the autoimmune anti-AChR T cell population, which recognizes multiple AChR epitopes, generally utilizes a variety of Vβ regions, that differ from patient to patient. These results

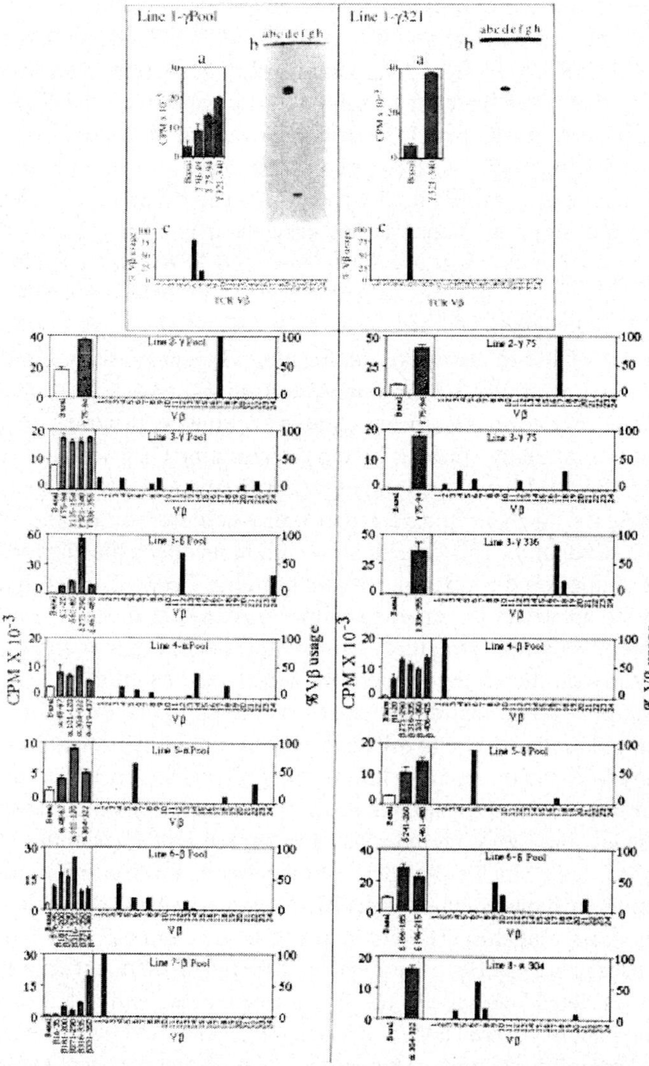

Fig. 2. Epitope specificity and TCR Vβ usage of the AChR-specific CD4⁺ lines. Results of one of at least two consistent RT-PCR assay experiments for each of the CD4⁺ lines, as indicated in each panel. Lines are grouped according to the patient from which they were obtained. For each line we report the result of a proliferation assay, carried out to verify the peptide specificity of the line. This figure reports only the responses of the lines to peptides that were recognized significantly. Basal rate of cell proliferation of each line is also reported.

For the lines of patient #1 (top panels), we report the radiogram (graph b), whose densitometric scan yielded the data used to calculate the percentage of usage of the different Vβ gene families, reported in graph c. Signal-to-noise ratio obtained in this experiment is representative of that obtained in all RT-PCR experiments carried out with the CD4⁺ lines. For all the other lines we report a plot of the relative Vβ usage, determined from densitometric scans of autoradiograms of RT-PCR experiments.

Reprinted with permission from R. Raju et al. (1997) J. Autoimmunity 10: 203–217. Copyright Academic Press, Harcourt Brace & Company Publishers, 1997.

agree well with those of a previous study, which also concluded that there is a restricted but individual heterogeneity among the TCR Vβ and Vα gene transcripts used by anti-AChR T cells from MG patients [42]. Also, they are consistent with another study that investigated the extent of heterogeneity of the TCR Vβ genes in the blood T cells of MG patients: that study found that four of fifteen patients had T cells showing signs of clonal expansion, and in three of them the Vβ12 family might have been preferentially used [43]. The finding that only a few MG patients showed signs of clonal T cell expansion is likely due to the use of unselected blood T cells. Since the antibody-based TCR assay used in that study could detect only five Vβ families, other Vβ regions might have been preferentially used, and be undetected.

The limited Vβ usage that we found for the individual anti-AChR CD4$^+$ lines suggest that the potentially autoimmune T cells that survive clonal deletion have a limited TCR repertoire. Given the complex antigenic structure of the AChR, with recognition of many epitopes by the autoimmune CD4$^+$ cells, the restricted Vβ usage by the CD4$^+$ cells recognizing individual epitopes may be obfuscated by the complexity of their epitope repertoire, when one studies the whole anti-AChR CD4$^+$ population. This consideration might reconcile the disparate findings of previous studies on the Vβ usage of autoimmune T cells in other diseases [38-39]. It may be surmised, by analogy with the AChR, that most or all autoAgs have a complex antigenic structure. This model is supported by the results of an extensive study on the epitope repertoire recognized by human CD4$^+$ cells on myelin basic protein, which identified at least 26 epitopes [44]. If this model is true, then the autoimmune T cells will have a broad variability in clonal composition, because they will include many clones, recognizing the complex repertoire of epitopes present on the autoantigen. Also, when the T cells are eluted from the affected tissues, they may include variable amounts of "bystander" T cells of unrelated specificity, since as few as 2% of the T cells infiltrating tissues affected by autoimmune responses may be specific for the autoAg [38]. The restricted or unrestricted usage found in different studies for autoimmune T cells involved in the same disease may reflect the dishomogeneity of different samples, in the presence of restricted Vβ usage by the T cells recognizing individual autoepitopes.

We found that, in general, different Vβ regions were used for different epitopes in the same patient, and for the same epitope in different patients. These findings do not support an important role for a superantigen in maintenance of the anti-AChR CD4$^+$ response in MG. However, they do not exclude that a superantigen may be involved in the initial triggering of the anti-AChR response, since, in principle, activation of autoimmune CD4$^+$ cells specific for one epitope might start an autoimmune response [45]. The epitope spreading that occurs as autoimmune responses develop [45] may obfuscate the epitope specificity and TCR usage of the CD4$^+$ populations originally expanded by a superantigen.

The TCR usage we found for the anti-AChR CD4$^+$ cells in MG patients agrees well with a model of tolerance which postulates that while most autoreactive T cells are deleted during the ontogenesis of the immune system, some of them survive carrying a limited Vβ repertoire [39].

In both experimental autoimmune encephalomyelitis and EAMG, only CD4$^+$

cells recognizing certain epitopes are effective in causing the disease, while $CD4^+$ cells of other epitope specificities are ineffective [1, 46]. This finding also supports the possibility that in MG, only $CD4^+$ cells recognizing certain AChR epitopes are pathogenic. If so, since they will likely utilize a limited number of Vβ families, TCR-targeted specific immunosuppressive procedures could be developed. The need to block T cells carrying several TCR Vβ families might not impair the immune functions, since elimination of up to 50% of the TCR Vβ families in mice is compatible with normal immune responses [47].

TCR Vβ Usage in the Thymus and Blood of MG Patients

The initial sensitization of anti-AChR $CD4^+$ cells in MG might occur in the thymus [1, 9], which in most MG patients has lymphoid follicular hyperplasia (LFH) or contains a thymoma. Thymectomy is used in the treatment of MG, and it is often followed by long-term improvement of the symptoms [9].

Normal and LFH thymus expresses AChR similar to that of muscle [9-10], that is likely synthesized by the thymus myoid cells (MC) [9]. MC have morphologic and biochemical similarities with striated myotubes [9]. In MG thymuses with LFH, the MC are in contact with HLA-DR-positive reticulum cells, close to or inside germinal centers [9]. This unusual microenvironment is compatible with a role of MC in anti-AChR sensitization [9].

Several lines of evidence support the possibility that an anti-AChR immune response occurs in MG thymuses. Thymuses with LFH have morphological changes that make the thymus structure similar to that of peripheral immune organs [9], including the presence of germinal centers that are identical to the secondary lymph follicles of peripheral lymphoid organs. Thymuses of MG patients have a significant increase in mature T cells, and a significant decrease in immature T cells, as compared to normal thymus tissue [9]. Transplantation of fragments of MG thymus into SCID mice caused the appearance of human anti-AChR antibodies and loss of muscle AChR [48], and thus, MG thymuses contain all the functional components necessary for the anti-AChR antibody response. Anti-AChR T and B cells can be propagated from MG thymuses [1, 9]. Since in EAMG the thymus does not show the pathological changes seen in human MG [49], anti-AChR T cells are present in the thymus of MG patients not just because of homing in the thymus of T cells activated in the periphery.

Microbial superantigens may trigger autoimmune responses [47]. The thymus seems to be an ideal place to search for clues about the intervention of a superantigen in MG. We sought clues about the intervention of a superantigen in MG, by investigating whether unusual expansion or deletion of T cells carrying particular Vβ region families occurs in the thymus and in the blood of MG patients, as compared to the TCR Vβ usage in the thymus and blood of normal subjects.

We have determined the frequency of use of the different TCR Vβ families by the thymus and blood T cells in MG patients and in control subjects [50], using the same multi-primer RT-PCR assay that we had used to determine the TCR Vβ usage by the anti-AChR $CD4^+$ lines propagated from MG patients [41].

We found identical TCR Vβ usage in the thymuses from MG patients without thymoma and from controls, except that Vβ2 was slightly, yet significantly, more used in the thymuses from MG patients (Fig. 3): this might be related to a biased Vβ usage by the AChR-specific CD4$^+$ cells in the MG thymus, but obfuscated by the Vβ usage of the majority, non-AChR specific T cells. Anti-AChR CD4$^+$ cells that preferentially used Vβ2 have been described in both MG patients and healthy subjects [41-42]. Still, the similar Vβ usage in the myasthenic and normal thymuses does not support an important role of the thymus as a place where the anti-AChR sensitization takes place when MG is clinically evident. This agrees with the negative results obtained in another study that attempted identification among the total T cell population of MG thymuses of single, TCR Vβ rearranged bands [51]. Yet another study found an increased usage of Vβ5.1 and Vβ8 in hyperplastic or normal thymuses from MG patients [52]: that study used Abs selective for different Vβ5 subfamilies, and found an increased usage of Vβ5.1. Our assay, that relies on PCR amplification of all the genes of a given Vβ family, might not detect a selective small increase in the use of one subfamily.

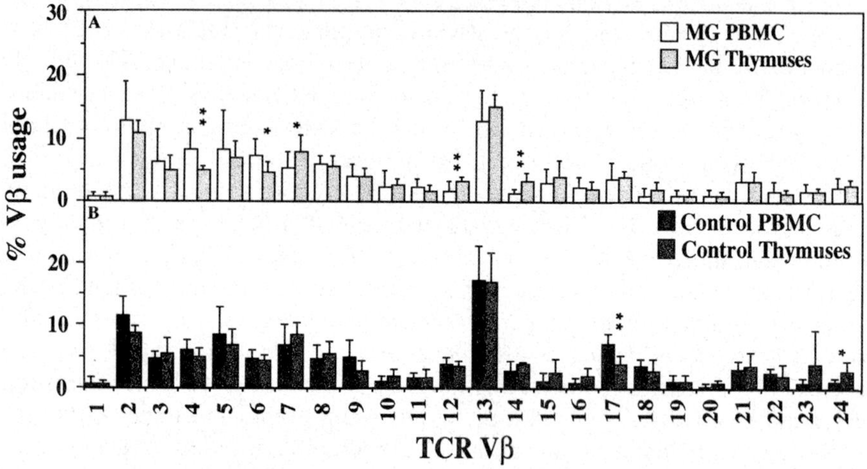

Fig. 3. Comparison of TCR Vβ usage in the thymus and in the blood of MG patients and control subjects. A: average Vβ usage ± S.D. in thymuses (light gray columns; n = 10) and blood T cells (PBMC) (white columns; n = 7) of MG patients. B: average Vβ usage ± S.D. in thymuses (dark gray columns; n = 4) and PBMC (black columns; n = 8) of controls subjects. The stars represent a significant difference in the use of a given Vβ family in PBMC as compared to thymuses (*$p < .05$; **$p < 0.004$). See text for further details. Reprinted with permission from D. Navaneetham et al. (1998), J. Autoimmunity 11: 621–633. Copyright Academic Press, Harcourt Brace & Company Publishers, 1998.

Blood T cells of MG patients without thymoma used Vβ4, Vβ6, Vβ15, Vβ16 and Vβ24 significantly more than the healthy controls, and Vβ12, Vβ14, Vβ17 and Vβ18 significantly less. The increased usage of certain Vβ gene families by the blood T cells of MG patients is consistent with the possibility that a superantigen might be involved in the activation of anti-AChR T cells, and in the pathogenesis of MG. Also, it agrees with our previous finding of a frequent preferential usage of Vβ4 and Vβ6 by anti-AChR T cell lines propagated from MG patients [41]:

the preferential expansion of Vβ4 and Vβ6 in MG patients might reflect the immunodominance of certain AChR epitopes, or the action of a superantigen outside the thymus. The increased usage of Vβ4 and Vβ6 in the thymuses of MG patients suggests a more prevalent usage of these gene families, and of Vβ15, Vβ16 and Vβ24, in the anti-AChR response in MG than suggested by our previous study on the TCR Vβ usage of anti-AChR $CD4^+$ T cell lines [41]. In that study, we found that not all of the epitope-specific anti-AChR $CD4^+$ lines we studied used Vβ4 or Vβ6 preferentially [41]. Furthermore, several MG patients never yielded anti-AChR $CD4^+$ lines that used Vβ4 or Vβ6. Anti-AChR $CD4^+$ cells in MG patients recognize a large epitope repertoire [1, 24]. Our previous study may have underestimated the frequency of usage of Vβ4 and Vβ6, and that of Vβ15, Vβ16 and Vβ24, because it used a small number of MG patients and of anti-AChR $CD4^+$ lines [41]. Another study on the TCR Vβ usage of anti-AChR T cell lines from MG patients and one control found that two of the seven lines studied preferentially used Vβ6 [42]. Other lines used preferentially other Vβ regions [42]. The large repertoire of anti-AChR T cells and the small number of lines investigated in that study [42] may have caused an underestimate of the use of Vβ4 and Vβ6. The finding that the blood T cells of MG patients use some Vβ families (Vβ12, Vβ14, Vβ17 and Vβ18) significantly less than controls is not inconsistent with the action of a superantigen: prolonged activation of T cells by a superantigen may result in their apoptosis. Previous findings that a few anti-AChR T cell lines preferentially used Vβ12, Vβ14, Vβ17 and Vβ18 [41-42] support that possibility.

We observed small differences in the Vβ usage in blood and thymuses of MG patients: MG patients used Vβ4 and Vβ6 significantly more in the blood than in the thymus, while the opposite occurred for Vβ7, Vβ12 and Vβ14 [50]. These small differences are likely due to preferential Vβ usage by the anti-AChR T cells in the blood, discussed above. The healthy subjects used only Vβ17 slightly more in the blood than in the thymus and vice versa for Vβ24: these minimal differences in TCR Vβ usage might be due to expansion in the blood of T cell clones specific for common antigens.

Although these data do not support the hypothesis that a superantigen acting in the thymus has an important role in MG pathogenesis, they cannot exclude that a superantigen in the thymus might have started the anti-AChR response. The AChR-specific $CD4^+$ T cells in the thymus of MG patients are likely a minor population, as compared to the other, non AChR-specific $CD4^+$ and $CD8^+$ T cells. Thus, the finding that the Vβ repertoire was essentially the same in the whole population of T cells in the thymuses of MG patients without thymoma and normal subjects does not exclude that there might be differences in the Vβ repertoire of the selected, AChR-specific $CD4^+$ cells present in the thymus. The slightly yet significantly higher usage of Vβ2 in the thymuses of MG patients without thymoma might be an indicator of a biased Vβ usage by the AChR-specific $CD4^+$ cells.

We studied the Vβ usage from two of the patients that had a thymoma: in one, we studied the TCR Vβ use of the thymus, in the other of the blood. We found a more skewed Vβ use in the thymus with thymoma than in the other MG thymus: it had higher use of Vβ8 and Vβ23, and lower usage of Vβ3, Vβ15 and Vβ24. The other thymoma patient had a higher use of Vβ8 in the blood as compared to the non-thymoma patients, and a lower usage of Vβ7. These findings agree with the described differences in thymus pathology and anti-AChR immune response in MG patients with thymoma, as compared with those that have thymic hyperplasia [9].

In studies on the TCR Vβ usage of AChR-specific CD4$^+$ cell lines from MG patients, which used anti-AChR T cells of limited epitope specificity, CD4$^+$ populations originally expanded by the action of a superantigen [41-42] may have been missed, and the extent of usage of Vβ4 and Vβ6 in MG underestimated. The study of the TCR Vβ usage by the unselected blood CD4$^+$ cells had the shortcoming that the high background due to the many T cells specific for other antigens may have obfuscated the Vβ repertoire of the AChR-specific CD4$^+$ cells. Yet, the lack of bias in T cell selection may have allowed the detection in most or all MG patients of an expansion of Vβ4- and Vβ6-bearing T cells. Such preferential usage might be related to recognition of immunodominant, universal epitopes on the AChR or to the persistent, subtle action of a superantigen, perhaps at a location other than the thymus.

Acknowledgements

This work was partially supported by the NINDS grant NS 23919 and by a research grant from the Muscular Dystrophy Association (to B.M. C.-F.). Dr. Wang was a recipient of a Muscular Disease Research Fellowship from the Muscular Dystrophy Association.

References

1. Conti-Fine, B.M., M. Bellone, J.F. Howard Jr. and M.P. Protti. 1997. Myasthenia Gravis. The Immunobiology of an Autoimmune Disease. Neuroscience Intelligence Unit. R.G. Landes. Austin, TX, USA 1–230.
2. Karachunski, P.I., N. Ostlie. D. Okita, and B.M. Conti-Fine. 1997. Protection from experimental myasthenia gravis in C57Bl/6 mice by sniffing of synthetic CD4$^+$ T cells epitopes. *J. Clin. Invest.* 100: 3027.
3. Wu, B., C. Deng, E. Goluszko and P. Christadoss. 1997. Tolerance to a dominant T cell epitope in the acetylcholine receptor molecule induces epitope spread and suppresses murine myasthenia gravis. *J. Immunol.* 159: 3016.
4. Karachunski, P.I., N.S. Ostlie, D. Okita, R. Garman and B.M. Conti-Fine. 1999. Subcutaneous administration of T epitope sequences of the acetylcholine receptor prevents experimental myasthenia gravis. *J. Neuroimmunol.* 93: 108.
5. Wang, Z.-Y., P.I. Karachunski, J.F. Howard Jr. and B.M. Conti-Fine. 1999. Myasthenia in SCID mice grafted with myasthenic patient lymphocytes. Role of CD4$^+$ and CD8$^+$ cells. *Neurology* 52: 484.
6. Conti-Tronconi, B.M., K.E. McLane, M.A. Raftery, S. Grando and M. P. Protti. 1994. The nicotinic acetylcholine receptor: Structure and autoimmune pathology. *Cri. Rev. Biochem. Mol. Biol.* 29: 69.
7. Horton, R.H., A.A. Manfredi and B.M. Conti-Tronconi. 1993. The "embryonic" γ subunit of the nicotinic acetylcholine receptor is expressed in adult extrinsic ocular muscles. *Neurology* 43: 983.

8. Kaminski, H.J., L.L. Kushner and C.H. Block. 1996. Expression of acetylcholine receptor isoforms at extraocular muscle endplates. *Invest. Opthalmol. Vis. Sci.* 37: 345.
9. Hohlfeld, R. and H. Wekerle. 1994. The thymus in Myasthenia Gravis. *Neurol. Clin. North America* 12: 331.
10. Nelson, S. and B.M. Conti-Tronconi. 1990. Adult thymus expresses an embryonic muscle acetycholine receptor-like protein. *J. Neuroimmunol.* 29: 81.
11. Geuder, K.I., A. Marx, V. Witzemann, B. Schalke, K. Toyka, T. Kirchner, and H.K. Muller-Hermelink. 1992. Pathogenetic significance of fetal-type acetylcholine receptors on thymid myoid cells in myasthenia gravis. *Dev. Immunol.* 2: 69.
12. Kaminski, H.J., R.A. Fenstermaker, F.W. Abdul-Karim, J. Clayman, and R.L. Ruff. 1993. Acetylcholine receptor subunit gene expression in thymic tissue. *Muscle Nerve* 16: 1332.
13. Lindstrom, J., B. Einarson and J. Merlie. 1978. Immunization of rats with polypeptide chains from Torpedo acetylcholine receptor causes an autoimmune response to receptors in rat muscle. *Proc. Natl. Acad. Sci. U.S.A.* 75: 769.
14. Bellone, M., N. Ostlie, P.I. Karachunski and B.M. Conti-Tronconi. 1993. Cryptic epitopes on nicotinic acetylcholine receptor are recognized by autoreactive CD4$^+$cells. *J. Immunol.* 151: 1025.
15. Fujii, Y. and J. Lindstrom. 1988. Specificity of the T cell immune response to acetylcholine receptor in experimental autoimmune myasthenia gravis. Response to subunits and synthetic peptides. *J. Immunol.* 140: 1830.
16. Raju, R., B. Diethelm-Okita, D. Okita and B.M. Conti-Fine. 1996. Epitopes repertoire of human CD4$^+$ T lines propagated with tetanus toxoid or with synthetic tetanus toxoid sequences. *J. Autoimmun.* 9: 79.
17. Wang, Z.-Y., D. Okita, J.F. Howard Jr. and B.M. Conti-Fine. 1998. T cell recognition of the muscle acetylcholine receptor subunits in generalized and ocular myasthenia gravis. *Neurology* 50: 1045.
18. Wang, Z.-Y., B. Diethelm-Okita, D. Okita, J.H. Kaminski, J.F. Howard Jr. and B.M. Conti-Fine. Unstable T cell recognition of the human acetylcholine receptors in ocular myasthenia gravis. In preparation.
19. Stern, L.J., J.H. Brown, T.S. Jardetzky, J.C. Gorga, R.G. Urban, J.L. Strominger and D.C. Wiley. 1994. Crystal structure of the human class II MHC protein HLA-DR1 complexed with an influenza virus peptide. *Nature* 368: 215.
20. Marx, A., A. Willisch, V. Hoffacker, A. Schultz, S. Tzaetos and H.K. Muller-Hermelink 1999. Lack of acetylcholine receptor delta subunit message and protein in human thymuses suggests the occurence of 'triplet receptors' in the thymic myoid cells. This book.
21. Miller, S.D., B.L. McRae, C.L. Vanderlugt, K.M. Nikcevich, J.G. Pope, L. Pope and W.J. Karpus. 1995. Evolution of the T-cell repertoire during the course of experimental immune-mediated demyelinating diseases. *Immunol. Rev.* 144: 225.
22. Bellone, M., N. Ostlie, P.I. Karachunski and B.M. Conti-Tronconi. 1993. Cryptic epitopes on nicotinic acetylcholine receptor are recognized by autoreactive CD4$^+$cells. *J. Immunol.* 151: 1025.
23. Shenoy, M., E. Goluszko and P. Christadoss. 1994. The pathogenic role of acetylcholine receptor α chain epitope within α146-162 in the development of experimental autoimmune myasthenia gravis in C57BL6 mice. *Clin. Immunol. Immunopathol.* 73: 338.
24. Conti-Fine B.M., D. Navaneetham, P.I. Karachunski, R. Raju, B. Diethelm-okita, D.K. Okita, J.F. Howard Jr. and Z.-Y. Wang. 1998. T-cell recognition of the acetylcholine receptor in myasthenia gravis. *Ann. N.Y. Acad. Sci.* 841: 283.

25. Manfredi, A.A., M.P. Protti, X.D. Wu, J.F. Howard Jr. and B.M. Conti-Tronconi. 1992. CD4$^+$ T-epitope repertoire on the human acetylcholine receptor α subunit in severe myasthenia gravis. A study with synthetic peptides. *Neurology* 42: 1092.
26. Manfredi, A.A., M.P. Protti, M.W.M. Dalton, J.F. Howard Jr. and B.M. Conti-Tronconi. 1993. T helper cell recognition of muscle acetylcholine receptor in myasthenia gravis: epitopes on the γ and δ subunits. *J. Clin. Invest.* 92: 1055.
27. Wang, Z.-Y., D. Okita, J.F. Howard Jr. and B.M. Conti-Fine. 1998. CD4$^+$ T cell recognition of the ε subunit of human muscle acetylcholine receptor in myasthenia gravis. *J. Neuroimmunol.* 91: 33.
28. Oda, K. and Y. Ito. 1981. Myasthenia gravis: antibodies to acetylcholine receptor in ocular myasthenia gravis. *J. Neurol.* 225: 251.
29. Kaminski, H.J., L.L. Kusner, K.V. Nash, and R.L. Ruff. 1995. The γ-subunit of the acetylcholine receptor is not expressed in the levator palpebrae superioris. *Neurology* 45: 516.
30. MacLennon, C., D. Beeson, A.-M. Buijs, A. Vincent and J. Newsom-Davis. 1997. Acetylcholine receptor expression in the human extraocular muscles and their susceptability to myasthenia gravis. *Annal. Neurol.* 41: 423.
31. Protti, M.P., A.A. Manfredi, C. Straub, J.F. Howard Jr. and B.M. Conti-Tronconi. 1990. Immunodominant regions for T helper sensitization on the human nicotinic receptor subunit in myasthenia gravis. *Proc. Natl. Acad. Sci. U.S.A.* 87: 7792.
32. Moiola, L., P. Karachunski, M.P. Protti, J.F. Howard Jr. and B.M. Conti-Tronconi. 1994. Epitopes on the subunit of human muscle acetylcholine receptor recognized by CD4+ cells of myasthenia gravis patients and healthy subjects. *J. Clin. Invest.* 93: 1020.
33. Protti, M.P., A.A. Manfredi, X.D. Wu, L. Moiola, J.F. Howard Jr. and B.M. Conti-Tronconi. 1991. Myasthenia Gravis: T epitopes of the δ subunit of human muscle acetylcholine receptor. *J. Immunol.* 146: 2253.
34. Protti, M.P., A.A. Manfredi, X.D. Wu, L Moiola, M.W.M. Dalton, J.F. Howard Jr., and B.M. Conti-Tronconi. 1992. Myasthenia Gravis. CD4$^+$ T epitopes on the embryonic γ subunit of human muscle acetylcholine receptor. *J. Clin. Invest.* 90: 1558.
35. Wang, Z.-Y., D.K. Okita, J.F. Howard Jr, and B.M. Conti-Fine. 1997. Th1 epitope repertoire on the α subunit of human muscle acetylcholine receptor in myasthenia gravis. *Neurology* 48: 1643.
36. Conti-Fine, B.M., K.E. McLane and S. Lei. 1996. Antibodies as tools to study the structure of membrane proteins. the case of the nicotinic acetylcholine receptor. *Ann. Rev. Biophys. Biomol. Struc.* 25: 197.
37. Raju, R., D. Navaneetham, D.K. Okita, B. Diethelm-Okita, D. McCormick, and B.M. Conti-Fine. 1995. Epitopes for human CD4$^+$ T cells on diphtheria toxin: structural features of sequence segments forming epitopes recognized by most subjects. *Eur. J. Immunol.* 25: 3207.
38. Navarrete, C. and G.F. Bottazzo 1993. In search of TCR restriction in autoreactive T cell in human autoimmunity: why is it so elusive? *Clin. Exp. Immunol.* 91: 189.
39. Casanova, J. and J.L. Maryanski. 1993. Antigen-selected T-cell receptor diversity and self-nonself homology. *Immunol. Today* 14: 391.
40. Moiola, L., M.P. Protti, J.F. Howard and B.M. Conti-Tronconi. 1994. Myasthenia Gravis: Residues of the α and γ subunits of muscle acetylcholine receptor involved in formation of immunodominant CD4$^+$ epitopes. *J. Immunol.* 152: 4686.
41. Raju, R., D. Navaneetham, M.P. Protti, R.M. Horton, B.L. Hoppe, J. F. Howard Jr. and B.M. Conti-Fine. 1997. Preferential TCR Vβ usage by acetylcholine receptor specific CD4$^+$ T cells in myasthenia gravis. *J. Autoimmun.* 10: 203.

42. Melms, A., J.R. Oksenberg, G. Malcherek, R. Schoepfer, C.A. Müller, J. Lindstrom and L. Steinman. 1993. T cell receptor gene usage of acetylcholine receptor-specific T-helper cells. *Ann. N.Y. Acad. Sci.* 681: 313.
43. Grunewald, J., R. Ahlberg, A.-K. Lefvert, H. Dersimonian, H. Wigzell and C. H. Janson. 1991. Abnormal T-cell expansion and V-gene usage in myasthenia gravis patients. *Scand. J. Immunol.* 34: 161.
44. Meinl, E., F. Weber, K. Drexler, G. Morelle, M. Ott, G. Saruhan-Direskeneli, N. Goebels, B. Ertl, G. Jechart, G. Giegerich, S. Schonbeck, N. Bannwarth, H. Wekerle and R. Hohlfeld. 1993. Myelin basic protein-specific T lymphocyte repertoire in multiple sclerosis. Complexity of the response and dominance of nested epitopes due to recruitment of multiple T cell clones. *J. Clin. Invest.* 92: 2633.
45. Vanderlugt, C.J. and S.D. Miller. 1996. Epitope spreading. *Current Opin. Immunol.* 8: 831.
46. Lider, O., A. Miller, S. Miron, R. Hershkoviz, H.L. Weiner, X. Zhang and E. Heber-Katz. 1991. Nonencephalitogenic $CD4^-CD8^-$ $V\alpha2$ $V\beta8.2^+$ anti-myelin basic protein rat T lymphocytes inhibit disease induction. *J. Immunol.* 147: 1208.
47. Woodland, D.L. and M.A. Blackman. 1992. Retroviral Super-Antigens and T cells. *Intl. Rev. Immunol.* 8: 311.
48. Schoenbeck S., F. Padberg, R. Hohlfeld and H. Wekerle. 1992. Transplantation of thymic autoimmune microenvironment to severe combined immunodeficiency mice. A new model of myasthenia gravis. *J. Clin. Invest.* 90: 245.
49. Meinl, E., W.E.F. Klinkert and H. Wekerle. 1991. The thymus in myasthenia gravis: Changes typical for the human disease are absent in experimental autoimmune myasthenia gravis of the Lewis rat. *Am. J. Pathol.* 139: 995.
50. Navaneetham, D., A.S. Penn, J.F. Howard Jr. and B.M. Conti-Fine. 1998. TCR-$V\beta$ usage in the thymus and blood of myasthenia gravis patients. *J. Autoimmun.* 11: 621.
51. Tesch, H., R. Hohlfeld and K.V. Toyka. 1989. Analysis of immunoglobulin and T cell receptor gene rearrangements in the thymus of myasthenia gravis patients. *J. Neuroimmunol.* 21: 169.
52. Truffault, F., S. Cohen-Kaminsky, I. Khalil, P. Levasseur and S. Berrih-Aknin. 1997. Altered intrathymic T-cell repertoire in human myathenia gravis. *Ann. Neurol.* 41: 731.

Myasthenia Gravis: Disease mechanisms and immunointervention
P. Christadoss (Ed)

9. Molecular Mechanisms of MHC Associations with Myasthenia Gravis

Peter Hjelmström[1,2] and Carani B. Sanjeevi[3]

[1]Department of Epidemiology and Public Health, Yale University School of Medicine, New Haven, CT 06520, USA.

[2]Department of Neurology, Yale University School of Medicine; Neuroscience Research Center, Veterans Administration Medical Center, West Haven, CT 06516, USA

[3]Department of Molecular Medicine, Center for Molecular Medicine, CMM, L8:03, Karolinska Hospital, S-171 76 Stockholm, Sweden

Introduction

Myasthenia Gravis is a Complex Genetic Disease Trait

Myasthenia gravis (MG) is a disease characterized by muscle weakness due to autoimmunity against the nicotinic acetylcholine receptor (nAChR) at the neuromuscular junction. The disease is relatively rare with a prevalence rate of approximately 80 persons per million and an incidence rate of approximately 5 persons per million in Caucasian populations [1]. MG has a complex pattern of inheritance, and several genetic and environmental factors are important in conferring susceptibility to the disease. Genes play an important role in MG; the autoimmune disease is familial in 4–7% of the cases [2] and the concordance rate among monozygotic twins is approximately 40% [3]. No concordance has been observed in dizygotic twins, and the large discrepancy in concordance between monozygotic and dizygotic twins suggests that there are multiple genes that confer susceptibility to MG. Several genes have indeed been found to confer susceptibility to MG, which therefore could be defined as a polygenic disease. This review will focus on reports published in the last years that have contributed to our understanding of the associations between MG and genes in the human leukocyte antigen (HLA) complex.

An Introduction to the HLA Complex

The HLA complex (also called the major histocompatibility complex; MHC) is located on the short arm of chromosome 6 in humans. It spans a region of about four million base pairs, and it contains over 100 genes. The HLA complex can be divided into class I, II and III regions (Fig. 1). The class I genes are located telomeric in the complex and encode, for instance, the α-chain of the classical antigen-presenting HLA-A, -B, and -C molecules. The centromeric class II genes encode classical antigen-presenting HLA-DP, -DQ, and -DR molecules, but also other genes such as proteasomes (LMP) and peptide-transporters (TAP). The HLA class III region genes encode proteins with many functions, many of them important in the immune system, such as complement system proteins and tumor necrosis factor (TNF) family proteins.

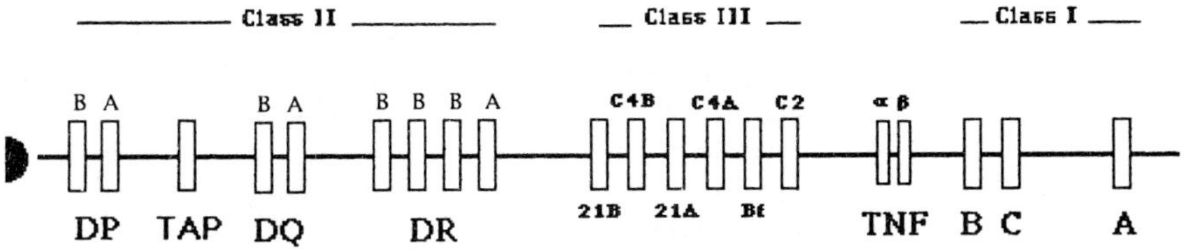

Fig. 1

Many of the genes in the HLA complex are polymorphic and exist in several allelic forms in the population. One of the most conspicuous properties of the HLA complex is that some alleles occur more frequently together than expected by chance. The non-random pairing of alleles in the HLA complex is called linkage disequilibrium (LD), and it is influenced by the low recombination rate in the region. The LD could extend over the whole HLA complex and, for instance, the alleles A1, B8, TNFa1, DR3, DQ2, TAP*0101 and DPB1*0101 are known to be inherited together as the "8.1 ancestral" or "extended DR3" haplotype.

HLA Polymorphisms in MG

Generalized MG in Caucasians is Associated with the Extended DR3 Haplotype

The association between HLA genes and MG was discovered over 25 years ago, and since then numerous studies have been published examining HLA associations with MG. In Caucasians, almost all studies have found MG to be associated with alleles on the extended DR3 haplotype. However, many studies have been done with too few patients or controls, and in other studies, the controls have not been properly matched ethnically with the patients. Furthermore, most studies have been performed with serological typing techniques, which do not allow precise characterization of the genetic polymorphisms. Recent studies using DNA-based techniques have allowed a more precise definition of the HLA associations with MG (Table 1). Even though DQA1*0101-DQB1*0201/0301 heterodimers [8], DQA1*0101 [12], DQB1*0604 [6, 9] and DR2 [5] also have been found to be increased in MG patients in some studies, alleles on the extended DR3 haplotype still show the strongest positive association with generalized MG in Caucasians. It is interesting to note that two independent studies indicate a role for DQA1*0101 in myasthenia gravis in the French population [8, 12]. Not many studies have reported negative HLA associations with MG, but in most of the DNA-based typing studies the DQA1*0103 allele has been found to be decreased in MG patients compared to healthy controls.

Table 1. DNA-based HLA typing studies of Caucasian myasthenia gravis patients

Study (reference)	Population	Association (positive)
[4]	Caucasian (U.K.)	DQb RFLP fragment
[5]	Caucasian (Sweden)	DR3; DQ2
[6]	Caucasian (Norway)	DR3; DQ2
[7]	Caucasian (Australia)	TNFB*1
[8]	Caucasian (France)	DQA1*01-DQB1*0201/0301
[9]	Caucasian (France)	B8; DR3; DQB1*0604
[10]	Caucasian (U.K.)	B8; DR3
[11]	Caucasian (Sweden)	DQ2
[12]	Caucasian (France)	DR3; DQ2; DQA1*0101
[13]	Caucasian (Italy)	DQB1*0502
[14]	CAucasian (Sweden)	TNFB*01; TNFa2
[15]	Caucasian (Germany)	DR3, TNFB*01, B8

The HLA associations with MG are different in different ethnic populations

The HLA associations with MG are different in different ethnic groups (Table 2). There have not been many DNA-based typing studies performed in non-Caucasian populations, and the HLA associations are not as clear as in Caucasians, but the HLA-B8 allele on the extended DR3 haplotype shows a trend to be positively associated with MG in several populations. It is important to note, however, that the clinical features of MG are different in different populations. In Asian populations, the average age of onset of MG is lesser than in Caucasians, and ocular MG is more prevalent (see references in Table 2).

Table 2. HLA associations with MG in different populations

Population	HLA association	Study (reference)
American Black	B8, DR5	[16]
Brazilian	A1, B8	[17]
Caucasian	B8, TNFa2, DR3, DQ2	[9, 11, 14]
Chinese	B46, DR9	[18]
Jamaican	B8, B13, DQ4	[19]
Japanese	DR9, DQB1*03	[20, 21]
North Indian	A9, B21, B35	[22]

The HLA Associations with MG are Different in Different Disease Subgroups

MG is a heterogeneous disease, and it is possible to divide the patients into different subgroups depending on age at onset, clinical features, and thymic pathology. In a landmark paper from 1980, Compston and colleagues showed that it also is possible to subgroup MG patients depending on their HLA associations [23]. Several DNA-based studies in Caucasian populations have now confirmed that alleles on the extended DR3-haplotype are increased almost exclusively in generalized MG patients with thymic hyperplasia, but not in the other patient subgroups [5–7, 9, 10, 24]. The patients with thymic hyperplasia are often females with an early disease onset (below 35 years), and they tend to have an increased frequency of other organ-specific autoimmune diseases also associated with alleles on the extended DR3-haplotype. No consistent HLA associations have been reported in patients with thymoma or normal thymic atrophy, even though some studies have found HLA-B7, DR2 and DQB1*0604 to be increased in these subgroups in Caucasians.

Where is the Susceptibility Gene on the Extended DR3 Haplotype Located?

The alleles on the extended DR3 haplotype are in strong LD, and it has therefore been difficult to determine where on the extended DR3 haplotype the strongest association with MG with thymic hyperplasia is located. The centromeric DP polymorphisms are not associated with MG [9, 10], and stratification analysis of the associations between more telomeric TAP alleles and MG have shown that these are due to LD [25]. Traditionally, the HLA class I allele B8 has been more strongly associated with MG than the HLA class II allele DR3, and it was therefore surprising that the centromeric DQ2 was more strongly associated with MG than DR3 [11]. Degli-Esposti and colleagues proposed after mapping of ancestral haplotypes that there might be two markers on the extended DR3 haplotype that confer susceptibility to MG: one of them located between HLA-B and TNF and the other in the HLA class II region [7]. In a recent study of TNF polymorphisms in thirty-two Swedish MG patients with thymic hyperplasia, we also found evidence that there might be two alleles on the extended DR3 haplotype that are associated with MG [14]. The strongest association was indeed found for the TNFa2 microsatellite marker, located 3.5 kb upstream of the lymphotoxin alpha (LT-α; also called TNF-β) gene, which was present in 23/32 (72%) patients and 33/90 (37%) controls (Odds ratio = 4.41; Pc < 0.01). The findings by Degli-Esposti et al. and Hjelmstrom et al. are in marked contrast to those by Manz et al., where there seems to be no primary TNF associations with MG [15]. However, only bi-allelic RFLP polymorphisms were included in that study, and no stratification analysis was done, which makes it difficult to reach any conclusions. Further genetic studies with more markers in the HLA class III region [26], and a larger number of patients, are clearly needed, in addition to functional studies of expression and regulation of some of the genes in the region, to determine the role of the TNF associations with MG.

Are the TNF Associations with MG Due to Lymphoid Neogenesis?

It is not known what is causing the TNF associations with MG, but it is tempting to speculate that the associations might be due to an increased secretion of the proinflammatory and immunomodulatory cytokines LT-α, LT-β and TNF-α. These cytokines have important functions in the development of secondary lymphoid organs (reviewed in [27]), and it is possible that they also might be involved in the formation of the lymphoid follicular infiltrates in chronic inflammatory autoimmune diseases in a process termed "lymphoid neogenesis" [28]. Several histologic features of the hyperplastic thymus in MG, such as germinal center formation, T and B cell compartmentalization, presence of high endothelial venules, and expression of the extracellular matrix component tenascin, indicate that a new tertiary lymphoid organ indeed has been formed. This new lymphoid organ in the hyperplastic thymus might contribute to exacerbation and perturbation of the myasthenia, a notion that is supported by several findings. Tissue from hyperplastic thymus transplanted into mice with severe combined immunodeficiency syndrome (SCID) gives rise to production of nAChR Abs and myasthenia [29]. Thymectomy of patients with thymic hyperplasia often leads to amelioration, and even remission, of the myasthenia [30]. Interestingly, a recent retrospective study of the impact of HLA on long-term outcome after thymectomy show that alleles on the extended DR3-haplotype indeed are associated with improvement after thymectomy [31].

Role of HLA Molecules in Presenting nAChR Peptides for TCRs in MG

Genes in the HLA-DQ Region are of Particular Importance in MG and EAMG

Results from our group indicate that genes in the HLA-DQ region are important in conferring susceptibility to and protection from MG [11]. These results are in good agreement with findings in the mouse model experimental autoimmune myasthenia gravis (EAMG), where the homologue to DQ, H-2A, seems to be particularly important in determining susceptibility to the disease ([32], Poussin et al., this volume). Recently, a new experimental system to evaluate the role of DQ molecules in MG and EAMG was created by Raju and colleagues [33]. In this model, transgenic mice express either the human DQ8 (DQA1*0301-DQB1*0302) or the human DQ6 (DQA1*0103-DQB1*0601) molecule, but not any endogenous mouse class II molecules. HLA-DQ8 transgenic mice are susceptible, but HLA-DQ6 mice are resistant, to EAMG induced by *Torpedo* acetylcholine receptor immunization. This is additional strong evidence for an important role of HLA-DQ in the development of EAMG and MG.

Molecular Modeling of the DQ Molecules Associated with MG

No crystal structure has yet been reported of a human HLA-DQ molecule, but as HLA-DQ molecules share approximately 60% sequence identity to several available human DR crystal structures, these could be used as templates for homology (comparative) computer-based model building of DQ proteins. We recently analyzed the structural differences between a modeled HLA-DQ2 (DQB1*02) molecule, positively associated with MG, and a DQ6 (DQB1*0603) molecule, negatively associated with MG [34]. The differences in the peptide-binding properties between these molecules were primarily localized to peptide-anchor pocket P7, which has a positively charged lysine at residue 71 in DQ2, and pocket P9, which is much smaller and more polar in DQ6. Our modeling results are in good agreement with previously experimentally determined peptide binding motifs for DQ2 and DQ6.

Docking of the VICE-Peptide from nAChR *a*-subunit 373–380 into DQ Molecules

Based on our molecular modeling of DQ2 and DQ6 molecules and the peptide binding motifs for these molecules, we screened the autoantigen nAChR for peptides that might bind DQ2, but not DQ6 molecules. An interesting candidate peptide that we found was the so-called "very immunogenic cytoplasmic epitope"; "VICE," from nAChR α-subunit 373–380 [35]. The VICE-peptide is cross reactive with a 153-kDa protein found primarily in the thymus and muscles. For our modeling and other experiments we extended the VICE-peptide with two residues at the N-terminus and three residues at the C-terminus, resulting in the final sequence EVKSAIEGIKYIA. The peptide was docked manually *in silico* into the DQ binding groove with the anchor residues placed in the same polyproline II conformation as observed in other peptides bound to MHC class II molecules. Backbone torsion angles of the peptide were slightly adjusted, and anchor residue side chains were rotated for better accommodation. Limited energy minimization and low-temperature molecular dynamics of first only the peptide, and subsequently both the peptide and the binding groove region of the DQ molecules were performed to relieve any residual unfavorable contacts. The membrane proximal domains of the DQ molecules were fixed during the minimization and molecular dynamics process. The resulting models show that the VICE-peptide fits well into both the MG positively associated DQ2 (DQA1*0501-DQB1*0201 and DQA1*0201-DQB1*0201) molecules (Fig. 2), but not into the negatively associated DQ6 (DQA1*0103-DQB1*0603) molecule. This is primarily due to the smaller fifth pocket (position 9) in the groove of the DQ6 molecule. The DQ6 molecule has a preference for smaller aliphatic and hydroxyl amino acids at this position and the large aromatic tyrosine in the VICE peptide is therefore not suitable for the DQ6 pocket.

Further Studies of the VICE-Peptide

In preliminary studies done in collaboration with Dr. Lefvert and colleagues of *in vitro* T-cell responses against the VICE-peptide in peripheral blood from MG patients, we find that patients homozygous for DQ2, but not patients homozygous for DQ6, have a proliferative response against the peptide. The VICE-peptide was recently shown to be of minor importance in MG patients with thymoma [36], in agreement with our findings, as these patients in general do not express DQ2; however, it might thus be of importance in other patient subgroups. Further studies in patients expressing DQ2 are needed to determine if indeed the DQ2 molecule binds different autoantigenic peptides than the negatively associated molecules, or else binds them in an altered binding motif such that different residues would be presented to the T cell receptor (TCR).

Role of Trimolecular Complex of HLA, Peptide and T Cell Receptor in MG

MG has in several studies been associated with abnormal TCR variable (V) gene usage, even though no convincing V gene usage restriction has been observed. However, these studies have been done in peripheral blood, with a small number

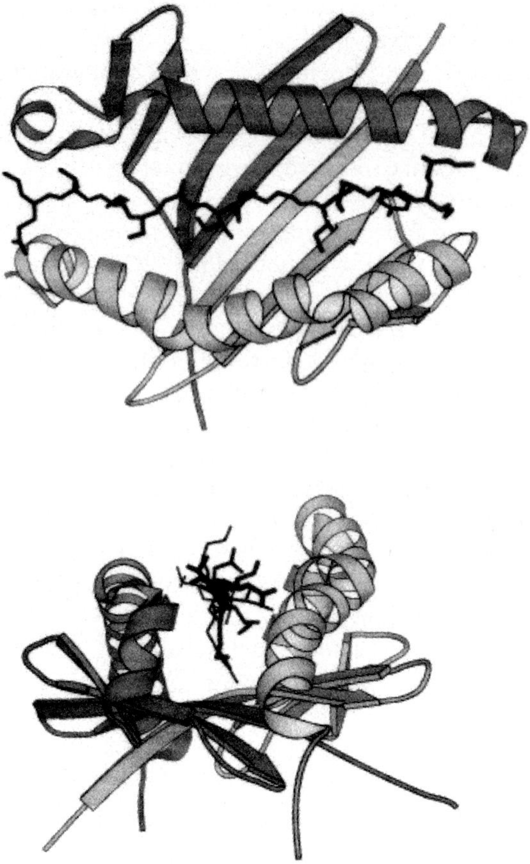

Fig. 2

of patients and a small number of monoclonal antibodies against TCRs. Nevertheless, in a recent large study of twenty-nine Swedish patients with MG, we confirm that there is no restricted V gene usage in peripheral blood of MG patients, even though fourteen of the patients (48%) had T cells showing signs of abnormal TCR V-gene expansions [37]. We did not find any correlation between the HLA genotype and TCR V elements. Peripheral blood may poorly represent events involved in the pathogenesis of MG; a recent study by Truffault and colleagues of the intrathymic T cell repertoire in MG patients shows very interesting results [38]. They found an increased intrathymic expression of Vβ5.1 and Vβ8 subfamilies in MG patients, compared to control subjects, primarily in patients with thymic hyperplasia, and, most importantly, a link between Vβ5.1 expression and alleles on the extended HLA-DR3 haplotype. It is unlikely that this skewing is due to peripheral events, and it further implicates the MG thymus as a site of inflammation and activation of autoreactive T cells. These findings may be an important step in understanding the role of the whole trimolecular complex of HLA molecule, peptide and TCR in the pathogenesis of MG.

Conclusions

MG is a polygenic disease, and it is clear from over twenty-five years of HLA studies that HLA alone cannot account for all the genetic contribution to MG susceptibility. Other genes have indeed been found to confer susceptibility to MG; in particular those in patients that do not have the extended DR3 haplotype. However, it is often difficult to reach a sufficiently high number of patients and controls for simultaneous analysis of several genetic markers, as it is necessary to statistically correct for multiple comparisons, so many of the proposed non-HLA genetic associations with MG need further investigation. Furthermore, there is an apparent lack of genome-wide studies in MG and EAMG. The most convincing genetic association with MG remains the strong association with alleles on the extended DR3 haplotype in MG patients with thymic hyperplasia, who are often females with an early disease onset. This association is actually so strong in certain populations that in the future it might be worthwhile to HLA-type MG patients for one allele on the extended DR3 haplotype to help diagnose the subtype of MG, determine appropriate therapeutic strategy, and predict the outcome of thymectomy and other treatments.

Due to the strong LD in the HLA complex, we still do not know where on the extended DR3 haplotype the susceptibility gene for myasthenia gravis with thymic hyperplasia is located. It is possible that there are two susceptibility genes on the extended DR3 haplotype, one located in the HLA class II region and the other in the HLA class III region, between TNF and HLA-B [7, 14, 24]. Further genetic studies of the HLA class III region around the TNF genes in MG patients with thymic hyperplasia are clearly needed, in addition to functional studies testing if the lymphoid follicular hyperplasia in MG is due to lymphoid neogenesis through localized overproduction of TNF family proteins such as LT-α. The role of TNF family proteins could also be tested in the animal model of myasthenia gravis using mice deficient in selected TNF proteins and receptors through genetic manipulation. We have in this review proposed the new hypothesis that the TNF associations with MG with thymic hyperplasia might be due to an increased intrathymic production of TNF proteins, and that this abnormal production gives rise to the formation of a new tertiary lymphoid organ in the thymus. If this hypothesis is correct it might be possible to design new therapies for MG. For example, specific antagonists to the TNF protein LT-α could be used as an addition or alternative to thymectomy in MG patients with thymic hyperplasia at an early stage of the disease, in particular in patients with the extended DR3 haplotype.

MG is one of the few human autoimmune diseases where the major autoantigen, the nAChR, is known and well characterized. As the candidate antigen-presenting HLA class II molecules (HLA-DQ2, and perhaps DR3), and TCRs (Vβ5.1 and Vβ8) are known, it is now possible to design experiments testing the role of the whole tertiary complex in the pathogenesis of MG. These experiments might ultimately lead to the development of antigen-specific therapies that can be used to vaccinate or treat some MG patients.

Acknowledgment

We thank Drs. Terry P. Lybrand and Julie E. Penzotti for helpful guidance and discussions regarding molecular modeling. This work was supported by grants from Erik and Edith Fernström's Foundation to PH and from the Swedish Medical Research Council to CBS. PH was supported by a fellowship from the Swedish Foundation for International Cooperation in Research and Higher Education.

References

1. Phillips, L.H. and J.C. Torner. 1996. Epidemiologic evidence for a changing natural history of myasthenia gravis. *Neurology* 47: 1233.
2. Pirskanen, R. 1976. Genetic associations between myasthenia gravis and the HL-A system. *J. Neurol. Neurosurg. Psychiat.* 39: 23.
3. Murphy, J. and S.F. Murphy. 1986. Myasthenia gravis in identical twins. *Neurology* 36: 78.
4. Bell, J., L. Rassenti, S. Smoot, K. Smith, C. Newby, R. Hohlfeld, K. Toyka, H. McDevitt and L. Steinman. 1986. HLA-DQ beta-chain polymorphism linked to myasthenia gravis. *Lancet* 1: 1058.
5. Carlsson, B., J. Wallin, R. Pirskanen, G. Matell and C. I. Smith. 1990. Different HLA DR-DQ associations in subgroups of idiopathic myasthenia gravis. *Immunogenetics* 31: 285.
6. Spurkland, A., Gilhus, N.E., Rønningen, K.S., Aarli, J.A. and Vartdal, F. 1991. Myasthenia gravis patients with thymus hyperplasia and myasthenia gravis patients with thymoma display different HLA associations. *Tissue Antigens* 37: 90.
7. Degli-Esposti, M.A., A. Andreas, F.T. Christiansen, B. Schalke, E. Albert and R.L. Dawkins. 1992. An approach to the localization of the susceptibility genes for generalized myasthenia gravis by mapping recombinant ancestral haplotypes. *Immunogenetics* 35: 355.
8. Khalil, I., S. Berrih-Aknin, V. Lepage, M.-N. Loste, P. Gajdos, J. Hors, D. Charron and L. Degos. 1993. *Trans*-encoded DQab heterodimers confer susceptibility to myasthenia gravis disease. *C.R. Acad. Sci. Paris* 316: 652.
9. Vieira, M.L., S. Caillat-Zucman, P. Gajdos, S. Cohen-Kaminsky, A. Casteur and J.F. Bach. 1993. Identification by genomic typing of non-DR3 HLA class II genes associated with myasthenia gravis. *J. Neuroimmunol.* 47: 115.
10. Ratanachaiyavong, S., D. Fleming, M. Janer, A.G. Demaine, N. Willcox, J. Newsom-Davis and A.M. McGregor. 1994. HLA-DPB1 polymorphisms in patients with hyperthyroid Graves' disease and early onset myasthenia gravis. *Autoimmunity* 17: 99.
11. Hjelmström, P., R. Giscombe, A.K. Lefvert, R. Pirskanen, I. Kockum, M. Landin-Olsson and C.B. Sanjeevi. 1995. Different HLA-DQ are positively and negatively associated in Swedish patients with myasthenia gravis. *Autoimmunity* 22: 59.
12. Djabiri, F., S. Caillat-Zucman, P. Gajdos, J.P. Jais, L. Gomez, I. Khalil, D. Charron, J.F. Bach and H.J. Garchon. 1997. Association of the AChRalpha-subunit gene (CHRNA), DQA1*0101, and the DR3 haplotype in myasthenia gravis. Evidence for a three-gene disease model in a subgroup of patients. *J. Autoimmun.* 10: 407.
13. Baggi, F., C. Antozzi, F. Andreetta, P. Confalonieri, E. Ciusani, A. B. Begovich, H.A. Erlich, F. Cornelio and R. Mantegazza. 1998. Identification of a novel HLA class II association with DQB1*0502 in an Italian myasthenic population. *Ann. N.Y. Acad. Sci.* 841: 355.

14. Hjelmström, P., C.S. Peacock, R. Giscombe, R. Pirskanen, A.K. Lefvert, J.M. Blackwell and C.B. Sanjeevi. 1998. Polymorphism in tumor necrosis factor genes associated with myasthenia gravis. *J. Neuroimmunol.* 88: 137.
15. Manz, M.G., A. Melms, N. Sommer, and C.A. Muller. 1998. Myasthenia gravis and tumor necrosis factor b polymorphisms: linkage disequlibrium but no association beyond HLA-B8. *J. Neuroimmunol.* 90: 187.
16. Christiansen, F.T., M.S. Pollack, M.J. Garlepp and R.L. Dawkins. 1984. Myasthenia gravis and HLA antigens in American blacks and other races. *J. Neuroimmunol.* 7: 121.
17. Dias-Tosta, E., R.N. Morato-Fernandez and J.A. Villaca. 1990. Correlation of HLA and myasthenia gravis in a Brazilian population. *Arq. Neuro-Psiq.* 48: 49.
18. Chan, S.H., C.B. Tan, Y.N. Lin, G.B. Wee, M.A. Degli-Esposti and R. L. Dawkins. 1993. HLA and Singaporean Chinese myasthenia gravis. *Int. Arch. All. Immunol.* 101: 119.
19. Barton, E.N., M. Smikle and O.S. Morgan. 1992. Myasthenia gravis and HLA phenotypes in Jamaicans. *South. Med. J.* 85: 904.
20. Horiki, T., H. Inoko, J. Moriuchi, Y. Ichikawa and S. Arimori. 1994. Combinations of HLA-DPB1 and HLA-DQB1 alleles determine susceptibility to early-onset myasthenia gravis in Japan. *Autoimmunity* 19: 49.
21. Matsuki, K., T. Juji, K. Tokunaga, M. Takamizawa, H. Maeda, M. Soda, Y. Nomura and M. Segawa. 1990. HLA antigens in Japanese patients with myasthenia gravis. *J. Clin. Invest.* 86: 392.
22. Mehra, N.K., G.K. Ahuja, V. Taneja and M. C. Vaidya. 1983. HLA antigens and myasthenia gravis in north India. *J. Neurol. Neurosurg. Psychiat.* 46: 361.
23. Compston, D.A., A. Vincent, J. Newsom-Davis and J.R. Batchelor. 1980. Clinical, pathological, HLA antigen and immunological evidence for disease heterogeneity in myasthenia gravis. *Brain* 103: 579.
24. Hjelmström, P., C.S. Peacock, R. Giscombe, R. Pirskanen, A.K. Lefvert, J.M. Blackwell and C.B. Sanjeevi. 1998. Myasthenia gravis with thymic hyperplasia is associated with polymorphisms in the tumor necrosis factor region. *Ann. N.Y. Acad. Sci.* 841: 368.
25. Hjelmström, P., R. Giscombe, A.K. Lefvert, R. Pirskanen, I. Kockum, M. Landin-Olsson and C.B. Sanjeevi. 1997. TAP polymorphisms in Swedish myasthenia gravis patients. *Tissue Antigens* 49: 176.
26. Hsieh, S.L., R.E. March, A. Khanna, S.J. Cross and R.D. Campbell. 1997. Mapping of 10 novel microsatellites in the MHC class III region: application to the study of autoimmune disease. *J. Rheumatol.* 24: 220.
27. Chaplin, D.D. and Y. Fu. 1998. Cytokine regulation of secondary lymphoid organ development. *Curr. Opin. Immunol.* 10: 289.
28. Kratz, A., A. Campos-Neto, M.S. Hanson and N.H. Ruddle. 1996. Chronic inflammation caused by lymphotoxin is lymphoid neogenesis. *J. Exp. Med.* 183: 1461.
29. Schonbeck, S., F. Padberg, R. Hohlfeld and H. Wekerle. 1992. Transplantation of thymic microenvironment to SCID mice: A new model of myasthenia gravis. *J. Clin. Invest.* 90: 245.
30. Lindberg, C., O. Andersen, S. Larsson and A. Oden, 1992. Remission rate after thymectomy in myasthenia gravis when the bias of immunosuppressive therapy is eliminated. *Acta. Neuro. Scand. 86:323.*
31. Machens, A., C. Loliger, U. Pichlmeier, T. Emskotter, C. Busch and J.R. Izbicki. 1998. The impact of HLA on long-term outcome after thymectomy for myasthenia gravis. *J. Neuroimmunol.* 88: 177.

32. Christadoss, P. 1989. Immunogenetics of experimental autoimmune myasthenia gravis. *Crit. Rev. Immunol.* 9: 247.
33. Raju, R., W.Z. Zhan, P. Karachunski, B. Conti-Fine, G.C. Sieck and C. David. 1998. Polymorphism at the HLA-DQ locus determines susceptibility to experimental autoimmune myasthenia gravis. *J. Immunol.* 160: 4169.
34. Hjelmström, P., C. DeWeese-Scott, J.E. Penzotti, T.P. Lybrand and C.B. Sanjeevi. 1998. Structural differences between HLA-DQ molecules associated with myasthenia gravis characterized by molecular modeling. *J. Neuroimmunol.* 85: 102.
35. Tzartos, S.J. and M.S. Remoundos. 1992. Precise epitope mapping of monoclonal antibodies to the cytoplasmic side of the acetylcholine receptor a subunit. *Eur. J. Biochem.* 207: 915.
36. Nagvekar, N., L.W. Jacobson, N. Willcox and A. Vincent. 1998. Epitopes expressed in myasthenia gravis (MG) thymomas are not recognized by patients' T cells or autoantibodies. *Clin. Exp. Immunol.* 112: 17.
37. Hjelmström, P., R. Giscombe, A.K. Lefvert, J. Grünewald, R. Pirskanen, I. Kockum, M. Landin-Olsson and C.B. Sanjeevi. 1997. HLA-DQ associations in relation to T-cell receptor V-gene usage in peripheral blood from Swedish myasthenia gravis patients. *Eur. J. Immunogenet.* 24: 179.
38. Truffault, F., S. Cohen-Kaminsky, I. Khalil, P. Levasseur and S. Berrih-Aknin. 1997. Altered intrathymic T cell repertoire in human myasthenia gravis. *Ann. Neurol.* 41: 731.

Myasthenia Gravis: Disease mechanisms and immunointervention
P. Christadoss (Ed)

10. Non-MHC Genetic Polymorphisms in Human Autoimmune Myasthenia Gravis

Ann Kari Lefvert, DeRen Huang and Biying Xu

Immunological Research Unit, Center of Molecular Medicine,
Department of Medicine, Karolinska Institutet, Sweden

Introduction

The concordance rate for myasthenia gravis (MG) in identical twins is around 30% and this suggests that part of the pathogenesis of MG is determined by genetic factors. However, the reported positive associations with HLA Class I and II are weak, with average odds ratios (OR) of about 3. This suggests the contribution of other genetic factors and to elucidate this, several candidate genes have been examined. The congenital myasthenic syndromes are clearly associated to mutations/variations in the genes for the acetylcholine receptor subunits on chromosome 2, and variations in the α-subunit gene are associated also with acquired autoimmune MG [1, 2].

IgCH Gm allotypes genes located in the variable region of the Ig heavy chain loci have been suggested to confer susceptibility for MG, and there are two studies showing certain allotypes to be associated with MG, especially with high autoantibody concentrations [3, 4]. There are a few studies of the genes of the T cell receptor chains, showing overexpression of selected TCR Vβ gene families [5, 6] and association to T-cell receptor V alpha and C alpha alleles [7, 8]. The Fc gamma receptors, FcgammaRIIA and FcgammaRIIIB contain polymorphisms with differing capacities for IgG binding and phagocytosis, and certain genotypes were increased in MG patients with thymoma [9]. The functional implications of these polymorphisms and their importance for the disease manifestations in MG are not clear.

Our own present studies concern especially the polymorphisms of the genes for the pro- and anti-inflammatory cytokines, genes of the T cell cofactors, and the β2 adrenergic receptor gene. The reason behind this selection of candidate genes is our intention to explore mechanisms beside the autoantibodies against the acetylcholine receptor that contributes to the disease manifestation. The autoantibodies against the acetylcholine receptor are present in 90% of patients with generalized MG and in 70% of patients with ocular disease, and are undoubtedly important for the symptoms [10]. However, the poor correlation between antibody concentration and disease severity challenges the concept of a simple cause and effect relationship between antibodies and disease. Acetylcholine receptor antibodies are found in several non-myasthenic conditions, including thymomas [11], healthy first-degree relatives [12], the healthy twin in a monozygotic pair of twins discordant for MG [13], and primary biliary cirrhosis [14]. Treatment with anti-CD4 antibody abolishes the T cell reactivity by the autoantigen and leads to a long-lasting remission without affecting the level of the autoantibodies [15]. This suggests that mechanisms involving T cells, macrophages and/or their products could contribute to the disease mechanisms. Patients with MG have autoantibodies against both the $\beta 1$ and b2-adrenergic receptors, as well as T cells that are stimulated by these receptors [16, 17]. The density of $\beta 2$-receptors on peripheral blood mononuclear cells is decreased, probably by the direct action of the autoantibodies [18]. Since the $\beta 2$-receptors are present on the cells of the immune system, as well as on skeletal muscle cells, and regulate many functions of these cells, there is a possibility that these immune reactions might act to modulate the disease.

Results and Discussion

TNF-α

The genes for TNF (including TNF-α, lymphotoxin α and β) are tandemly arranged in the central region of the MHC, HLA class III region. This location and the potent proinflammatory and immunomodulatory function of TNF have prompted speculations about the TNF in the etiology of MHC-associated diseases.

In the TNF-α gene there is a bi-allelic polymorphism for which the presence of an A (allele 2, A2), instead of a G (allele 1, A1), allele is associated with higher inducible levels of TNF-α. Our study of a Swedish Caucasian population showed that the frequency of TNF-α-308 A2/A2 genotype was increased (OR = 5.65, $p < 0.05$), while the frequency of genotype A1/A1 was decreased (OR = 0.31, $p < 0.0005$) in patients compared to that in healthy individuals [19]. This association was determined by female patients having an early onset of disease and hyperplasia of the thymus and was confirmed in another study [20].

TNF-α-308 A2 is strongly linked with HLA-A1, B8, DR3, 8.1 ancestral haplotype. The similarity of the association of TNF- α-308 A2 with MG to that of HLA-B8 was investigated and was possibly stronger than that of HLA-DR3 [19].

In reporter gene assays, the TNF-α-308 A2 has higher constitutive and inducible levels of transcription of the gene when compared to the more common allele A1 [21]. Functional studies also suggest that this polymorphism affects TNF-α production, which we also showed in our own study [19].TNF-α is a true pleiotropic cytokine [21]. Transgenic mice carrying a reporter construct, in which TNF coding sequence and introns were replaced by the chloramphenicol acetyltransferase (CAT) coding sequence, constitutively expressed CAT activity in the thymus indicating the biosynthesis of TNF in the thymus of normal animals, and suggesting a role for this protein in the development or regulation of the immune response [22]. The impact of TNF-α-308 A2 may result in malregulation of immune system in the patients with thymic hyperplasia and early onset of the disease.

Non-MHC Genes

The IL-1 Family

IL-1 is an important proinflammatory cytokine. The two IL-1 agonists, IL-1α and IL-1β, function through one of the two members of IL-1 receptor family: IL-1 receptor I. The IL-1 receptor antagonist (IL-1Ra) is a high-affinity antagonist that blocks the binding of IL-1α and IL-1β. IL-1 and IL-1Ra genes are located on the long arm of chromosome 2. The balance between IL-1 and IL-1Ra has been shown to be of importance in both normal and disease states.

A penta-allelic polymorphism in human IL-1Ra gene intron 2 is caused by variable numbers of an 86-bp tandem repeat (VNTR). Individuals with different copy numbers of this repeat sequence have correspondingly different numbers of protein binding sites. Allele 2 is associated with autoimmune diseases, including multiple sclerosis, inflammatory bowel disease and systemic lupus, and is related to an enhanced production of IL-1Ra. The results from different investigations are, however, not consistent.

A bi-allelic polymorphism within the IL-1β gene, a TaqI restriction fragment length polymorphism (RFLP) in exon 5, influences the production of IL-1β protein, with the 13.4 kb allele, allele 2, being a 'high-secretor' phenotype.

In our study of a Swedish Caucasian MG population, the frequencies of the genotype A2/A2 (OR = 4.63, $p < 0.01$) and the allele 2 were increased and that of A1 decreased [23].

Interesting results emerged when carriage of IL-1β TaqI RFLP was studied in relation to carriage of HLA-B8 [23]. The percentage of IL-1β TaqI RFLP allele 2 carriage in patients negative for HLA-B8 was significantly higher than that in healthy individuals (OR = 2.504, $p < 0.01$). The frequency of genotype A2/A2 was even higher in HLA-B8 negative MG group (OR = 5.47, $p < 0.01$), while that of A1/A1 was decreased (OR = 0.40, $p < 0.01$). Thus, IL-1β TaqI RFLP allele 2 plays a more important role in patients negative for HLA-B8. However, IL-1β TaqI RFLP also contributes to development of MG in HLA-B8 positive individuals when allele 2 homozygous individuals were considered. MG patients might thus be genetically divided into several subgroups, among which one is mainly associated with MHC genes, another with IL-1β TaqI RFLP. These two subgroups do not seem to be completely independent.

The IL-1β TaqI RFLP allele 2 carriage was then studied in relation to carriage of IL-1Ra allele 2 [23]. MG patients who were non-carriers of IL-1Ra allele 2 had a higher percentage of IL-1β allele 2 carriers than healthy individuals (OR = 3.09, $p < 0.01$). The frequencies of IL-1β TaqI RFLP allele 2 carriage in the group of IL-1Ra allele 2 carriers were almost the same for MG and healthy individuals. Thus, individuals who do not carry IL-1Ra allele 2 and may have low capacity of IL-1Ra production, IL-1β 'high-secretor' (allele 2) gives even more risk for developing MG. The position of the IL-1β gene in proximity to the IL-1Ra gene and the important immunoregulatory action of both cytokines in the host defense suggest that the IL-1β /IL-1Ra ratio may partially define a biological basis for predisposition to MG. These results also suggest an intrinsic dysregulation of IL-1 molecules in MG.

IL-1β TaqI RFLP allele 2 represents an IL-1β 'high-secretor' phenotype. The expression of IL-1β was increased in hyperplastic thymuses from MG patients [24]; however, our study did not show a higher percentage of allele 2 carriage in MG patients with thymic hyperplasia. As the highest MHC gene-association was observed in patients with early onset disease and thymic hyperplasia, IL-1β TaqI RFLP allele 2 may be less important in this subgroup.

Recently, IL-1α and IL-1β were found to be colocalized with postsynaptic components in innervated mature muscle fibers [25]. Cytokines such as IFN and IL-2 have been shown to directly influence the neuromuscular transmission and patients with MG have mononuclear cell infiltration of skeletal muscle and at the neuromuscular junction [26]. Myasthenia gravis-like syndrome occurs in transgenic mice expressing IFN-γ in the neuromuscular junction [27]. Taking these findings together, we speculate that subtype(s) of MG associated with gene(s) located in the IL-1 gene family might have a pathological mechanism that is completely different from that in subtype(s) associated with MHC genes. In an IL-1 gene associated subtype(s) of MG, IL-1 might affect the neuromuscular junction directly. Alternatively, IL-1 has multiple biologic effects and can influence both cellular and humoral immunological responses [28, 29].

IL-4

Interleukin-4 (IL-4) is important for the maturation of B cells. IL-4 induces human B cell clones to proliferate and switch to IgE and IgG4 synthesis. The human IL-4 gene consists of 4 exons and 3 introns and is found on chromosome 5, within the region coding also for IL-13, IL-5, IL-3 and GM-CSF. There is a dinucleotide repeat microsatellite (4R1) located in the second intron, and this is strongly associated with atopic diseases and serum IgE concentration. A variable number of tandem repeat (VNTR) polymorphisms located in the third intron of IL-4 gene are associated with late onset of multiple sclerosis. In our study of a Swedish MG population there was no difference in these polymorphic sites between patients and healthy individuals [30].

In view of the anti-inflammatory function of IL-4, the patients were subgrouped according to the presence of allele 2 in TNF-α NcoI and IL-1β TaqI RFLP, both representing "high secretor" phenotypes of the TNF-α and IL-1β, respectively. There was no difference in genotypic and allelic distribution between either TNF-α NcoI RFLP allele 2-positive and -negative subgroups or IL-1β TaqI RFLP allele 2 positive and negative subgroups [30].

IL-10

Interleukin-10 (IL-10) displays a broad spectrum of biological activities including immunosuppressive, anti-inflammatory and B-cell-stimulating properties [31]. IL-10 decreases the expression of MHC class II molecules on the surface of antigen-presenting cells and down-regulates co-stimulatory factors such as intercellular adhesion molecules and CD80 and CD86. IL-10 exerts its anti-inflammatory function by inhibiting the synthesis of proinflammatory cytokines (e.g. TNF-α, IL-1α, IL-1β) from T cells and monocytes/macrophages.

The IL-10 gene is situated on chromosome 1 and contains several polymorphisms. At position –1082 (relative to the transcriptional start site), a bi-allelic polymorphism is associated with different levels of IL-10 production. Presence of the A allele correlates with lower IL-10 secretions, while homozygosity for the G allele is related to higher secretions [32]. There are 2 CA repeats located in the promoter region of IL-10, an area in which many potential cytokine response elements cluster. An allelic imbalance between SLE patients and healthy individuals at one of the two CA repeats, IL10.G, was observed, although the functional properties of this polymorphism are not clear. This bi-allelic polymorphism and 2 CA repeat microsatellites located in the promoter region of IL-10 gene were analyzed in our Swedish Caucasian MG patients and ethnically matched, healthy individuals [33]. The prevalence of a "high secretor" phenotype of IL-10 (IL-10 1 G/G) was higher in IL-1β TaqI polymorphism allele 2 positive-healthy individuals "high secretor" phenotype for IL-1β) than in healthy individuals negative for this genotype. This normally occurring balance between proinflammatory (IL-1β) and anti-inflammatory cytokine (IL-10) genes did not survive in MG patients.

In one of the microsatellites, IL10.R, allele 112 was associated with patients having a normal thymic histology. In another microsatellite, IL10.G, allele 134 was associated with patients having higher serum levels of autoantibodies. The percentage of patients heterozygous for allele 134 and 136 was significantly higher in patients with the highest level of antibodies against the acetylcholine receptor (35.6%, 16/45) than that in HC (8.3%, 9/109) ($p < 0.0001$). Thus, these results demonstrate novel genetic markers within the IL-10 gene, indicating different mechanisms for IL-10 involved in the disease.

The fact that the prevalence of the "high secretor" phenotype of IL-10 was higher in healthy individuals positive for the "high secretor" phenotype for IL-1β, while this balance between proinflammatory and anti-inflammatory cytokine was lost in MG patients emphasizes the notion that the balances between IL-1 and IL-1 receptor antagonist and IL-1 and IL-10 are important, and genetic variations which influence any of these counterparts may result in the bias of the balances. The outcome can include deregulation of inflammatory reactions, thus providing an event at the neuromuscular junction that might trigger an autoimmune response.

Our data show a novel genetic association of MG to the IL-10 gene on 1q31-32. The association is rather sophisticated, as it is seen in patients with high autoantibody levels to IL10.G allele 134 and patients with normal thymic histology to IL10.R allele 112. This indicates that IL-10 plays different role in subgroups of patients and that MG is a heterogenetic disease.

CTLA-4

The "Cytotoxic T Lymphocyte Associated Antigen-4" (CTLA-4) has a pivotal role in the regulation of the immune response. CTLA-4 signaling mediates a negative regulation of both the cellular and the humoral response [34]. Blockade of B7-CTLA-4 interaction with anti-CTLA-4 antibodies increases T cell proliferation and anti-CTLA-4-monoclonal antibodies, that can crosslink CTLA-4, inhibit T cell responses induced by anti-CD3 in the presence of CD28 costimulation. Animals deficient for CTLA-4 show a massive T cell lymphoproliferative disorder with increased numbers of activated T cells and elevated basal levels of serum Ig, resulting in autoimmune-like tissue destruction [35]. The gene for CTLA-4 (*Ctla-4*) is located on the human chromosome 2q33 and is closely linked to the CD28 gene, located at a distance of 25-150 kilobases. The *Ctla-4* includes an (AT)n microsatellite within the 3´- untranslated region of exon 3. Allele 106 in the polymorphic (AT)n region in the *Ctla-4* has been reported to confer susceptibility to Graves′ disease, and insulin-dependent (type I) diabetes mellitus.

We have studied *Ctla-4* polymorphisms in healthy individuals and MG patients [36]. Totally 16 alleles were observed, with sizes ranging from 86 to 128 bp. The allele with the highest frequency in both healthy individuals and MG patients had a length of 86 bp in PCR products, followed by an allele of 104 bp. There was no significant difference in the allelic distribution between healthy controls and patients as a whole. The frequency of the shortest allele, 86, in MG patients with thymoma was decreased compared to patients with hyperplasia and normal thymic histology.

To uncover the possible contribution of *Ctla-4* in different subgroups of MG patients, the patients were divided into subgroups according to the "high secretors" of TNF-α -308 NcoI RFLP A2 and IL-1β TaqI A2. The percentage of allele 104 was significantly increased in patients with the IL-1β A2+ phenotype compared to the patients negative for this allele.

Patients with thymomas constitute a distinct clinical entity in whom the usually severe disease starts in middle age and is as common in men as in women. These patients frequently have autoantibodies against muscle proteins, especially against titin, and frequently have mononuclear cell infiltrations in the skeletal muscles [38]. In this regard, it is of special interest to note that mice deficient for the *Ctla-4* show a massive lymphocyte infiltration in skeletal muscles. The association between Ctla-4 and MG patients with thymoma and no association between *Ctla-4* and MG patients with hyperplasia and normal thymic histology found in the present study further confirms the hypothesis that the pathogenesis of myasthenia in patients with thymoma appears to be different from that in other subgroups of the disease.

AT-rich regions in the 3′untranslated regions have an influence on mRNA stability, especially in cytokine genes [39]. The lethal phenotype of animal homozygous for null mutation in *Ctla-4* strongly supports a critical role for CTLA-4 in down-regulating T cell activation and maintaining immunological homeostasis. Although it is difficult to make a statistical conclusion about those rare alleles other than 86 and 104, it is reasonable to speculate that mRNA from the shorter alleles of *Ctla-4* might be more stable and that from longer alleles less stable. Thus, the distribution of *Ctla-4* alleles in patients with thymomas might lead to an instability of *Ctla-4* mRNA, a defect of *Ctla-4* expression and thus an imbalance between the positive (CD28) and the negative (CTLA-4) co-stimulation. The insufficiently opposed CD28 signal pathway triggers T and B cell activation and autoantibody secretion in vivo, resulting in propagation of the disease.

This association of *Ctla-4* and myasthenia gravis patients with thymomas further supports the notion that MG is a heterogenous disease, with partially different disease mechanisms operating in subgroups of patients.

The β2-Adrenergic Receptor

The β2-adrenergic receptor (β2-AR) is a G protein-coupled receptor which has a typical structure of an extracellular amino terminal, seven transmembrane domains and an intracellular carboxyl-terminal. The gene encoding for β2-AR is an intronless gene that is present at q31-32 of chromosome 5. Three loci at amino acid positions 16, 27 and 164 have been found to significantly alter receptor function [40]. Since patients with MG have antibodies and T cells reacting with both the β1-and β2 receptors and a decreased density of receptors on peripheral blood mononuclear cells [16, 17, 18], it was of interest to determine the polymorphisms at amino acid positions 16, 27 and 164 [41]. In our Swedish Caucasian population, we found an increased prevalence of homozygosity for Arg16 in patients with generalized MG (OR = 3.60, $p < 0.01$). The frequencies of gene polymorphisms at amino acid positions 27 and 164 were the same in patients and healthy individuals. The association between MG and homozygosity for Arg16 was present in patients with early disease onset and males with late disease onset and in those with generalized disease but not in patients with only ocular symptoms. It is of special interest that the two groups of patients with early and late onset had similar associations, since the MHC-associations are clearly different for these disease subgroups [42]. This emphasizes that polymorphisms at amino acid position 16 constitute an additional genetic factor contributing to the susceptibility for MG.

Associations to the polymorphisms at amino acid position 27 emerged when patients were stratified according to immunosuppressive treatment and the presence of β2-adrenergic receptor antibodies and acetylcholine receptor antibodies. No patient with β2-AR antibodies in serum was homozygous for Glu27. An explanation for this might be that individuals homozygous for Glu27 do not express the receptor in the fully mature form, in contrast to those homozygous for Gln27. The receptor homozygous for Glu27 might thus be less immunogenic and less capable of inducing antibody formation in vivo. In asthma, there was a strong association between the polymorphisms at amino acid position 27 with IgE levels. MG patients homozygous for Glu27 had a lower prevalence of β2-AR antibodies and were less often treated with immunosuppressive drugs than other patients. Our previous study showed that patients with β2-AR antibodies generally had a more severe disease and were thus more often treated with immunosuppressive drugs [17]. This finding is thus now supported at the gene level. One may hypothesize that the β2-AR antibodies may activate the immune system via the receptor on lymphocytes, and that patients with β2-AR antibodies may thus have a more active immune system than patients without antibodies. Taken together, the results indicate that homozygosity for Glu27 might lead to a less severe disease and to lack of autoantibodies against the β2-AR. Patients with AChR antibodies were more often homozygous for Gln27. Thus, these gene polymorphisms seem to affect the immune response in the disease, possibly via the receptor on the immune cells.

Conclusions

We have addressed the genetic associations of human myasthenia gravis to the genes for the pro-and anti-inflammatory cytokines, to the T cell cofactor CTLA-4, and to the gene of the β2-adrenergic receptor. From these studies, some very interesting associations emerged. The association of the gene for TNF-α-308 allele A2 and disease in young female patients with thymic hyperplasia seems to be stronger than that of DR3 and similar to that of B8. Patients with this allele also had both spontaneous and induced higher secretions of the TNF-α. This cytokine can have multiple effects on the immune system, although its role in MG still has to be clarified.

The genes for the IL-1 family are located on chromosome 2 and the IL-1β TaqI RFLP allele 2, a variant with high secretion of the cytokine, was associated with MG. Most interestingly, this allelic association was more pronounced in patients without HLA-B8, and thus also lower in young female patients with thymic hyperplasia. There was no difference in the IL-1Ra VNTR allelic distribution in MG patients compared with that in healthy individuals. However, MG patients who did not have the high secretor variant IL-Ra allele 2 had a significantly higher percentage of IL-1β TaqI RFLP allele 2 carriage. This suggests the possibilities of an intrinsic disregulation, and an insufficiently opposed action of IL-1β in these individuals. Thus, the genetic association of the IL-1 family to MG is most pronounced in individuals with the lowest MHC association and constitutes a new genetic marker.

The association of the polymorphisms of the IL-10 gene were complex, and since the functional correlation of these polymorphisms are incompletely known, the findings are not easy to interpret. The most important result is probably the fact that MG patients lack the naturally occurring balance between the "high secretor" phenotypes for IL-10 and IL-1β. That this balance has been lost in MG patients emphasizes the notion that the balances between proinflammatory and anti-inflammatory cytokines are important, and genetic variations which influence any of these counterparts may result in the bias of the balances. The association of certain genotypes to high concentrations of antibodies against the acetylcholine receptor shows that also the specific immune response is affected by the IL-10 gene.

The association of (AT)n in the CTLA-4 gene with thymona was a most interesting finding. Alleles, longer than the most common that has 86 bp, can be expected to lead to decreased expression of CTLA-4 protein, and thus to an insufficiently opposed T cell activation via the CD28 pathway. Patients with thymoma constitute a separate disease entity, with usually severe disease, autoantibodies against muscle proteins and infiltrations of mononuclear cells in the striated muscle. Thus, there are some similarities between patients with thymomas and the CTLA-4 knock-out mouse. In a separate study (Huang D. et al, submitted), we have been able to show this increased activation of T cells as correlated to the length of the (AT)n repeats.

The relation of MG to certain polymorphisms in the β2-AR is quite unclear from the functional point of view. Of importance is, however, that the relation to Arg16 is present in all patients with generalized disease, despite their MHC-relation or not.

To summarize, our findings support the notion that MG is a true polygenic disease, with subgroups of patients having quite different genetic backgrounds. Furthermore, this might lead to better treatment design, in order to influence the activity/expression of certain cytokines, T cell cofactors and the β2-AR system.

References

1. Djabiri, F., S. Caillat-Zucman, P. Gajdos, J.P.Jais, L. Gomez, I. Khalil, D. Charron, J.F. Bach and H.J. Garchon. 1997. Association of the AChR-alpha-subunit gene (CHRNA), DQA1*0101, and the DR3 haplotype in myasthenia gravis. Evidence for a three-gene disease model in a subgroup of patients. *J. Autoimm.* 10(4): 407.
2. Heckmann, J.M., K.E. Morrison, B. Emeryk-Szajewska, H. Strugalska, J. Bergoffen, N. Willcox and J. Newsom-Davis. 1996. Human muscle acetylcholine receptor alpha-subunit gene (CHRNA1) association with autoimmune myasthenia gravis in black, mixed-ancestry and Caucasian subjects. *J. Autoimm.* 9(2): 175.
3. Smith, C. I.E., R. Grubb, L. Hammarstrom and R. Pirskanen. 1984. Gm allotypes in Finnish myasthenia gravis patients. *Neurology* 34(12): 1604.
4. Chiu, H.C.G., G. de Lange, N. Willcox, A.Vincent, J. Newsom-Davis, K.H. Hsieh and T.P. Hung. 1988. Immunoglobulin allotypes in caucasian and Chinese myasthenia gravis: differences from Japanese patients. *J. Neurol. Neurosurg. & Psychiat.* 51(2): 214.
5. Gigliotti, D., A.K. Lefvert, M. Jeddi-Tehrani, S. Esin, V. Hodara, R. Pirskanen,. H. Wigzell and R. Andersson. 1996. Overexpression of seleced TCR Vβ gene families within CD4+ and CD8+ T cell subsets of myasthenia gravis patients: A role for superantigens? *Mol. Med.* 2: 452.
6. Mantegazza, R., J.R. Oksenberg, F. Baggi, C. Antozzi, M.T. Illeni, G. Pellegris, F. Cornelio and L. Steinman. 1990. Increased incidence of certain TCR and HLA genes associated with myasthenia gravis in Italians. *J. Autoimm.* 3(4): 431.
7. Oksenberg, J.R., M. Sherritt, A.B. Begovich, H.A. Erlich, C.C. Bernard, L.L Cavalli-Sforza and L. Steinman. 1989. T-cell receptor V alpha and C alpha alleles associated with multiple and myasthenia gravis. *Proc. Natl. Acad. Sci. USA* 86(3): 988.
8. Oksenberg, J.R., C.N. Gaiser, L.L Cavalli-Sforza and L. Steinman. 1988. Polymorphic markers of human T-cell receptor alpha and beta genes. Family studies and comparison of frequencies in healthy individuals and patients with multiple sclerosis and myasthenia gravis. *Hum. Immunol.* 22(2): 111.
9. Raknes, G., G.O. Skeie, N.E. Gilhus, S. Aadland and C. Vedeler. 1998. FcgammaRIIA and FcgammaRIIIB polymorphisms in myasthenia gravis. *J. Neuroimm.* 81(1-2): 173.
10. Lefvert, A.K., K. Bergström, G. Matell, P.O. Osterman and R. Pirskanen. 1978. Determination of acetylcholine receptor antibodies in myasthenia gravis: Clinical usefulness and pathogenetic implications. *J. Neurol.Neurosurg. Psychiat.* 41: 394.
11. Aarli J. A., A.K. Lefvert and O. Tonder. 1981 Thymoma-specific antibodies in sera from patients with myasthenia gravis demonstrated with indirect hemagglutination. *J. Neuroimmunol.* 1: 421.
12. Lefvert, A.K., R. Pirskanen and E. Svanborg. 1985 Anti-idiotypic antibodies, acetylcholine receptor antibodies and disturbed neuromuscular function in healthy relatives to patients with myasthenia gravis. *J. Neuroimmunol.* 9: 41.

13. Lefvert, A.K., R. Pirskanen, H. Eng, A.C. Sundewall and E. Svanborg. 1989 B cell and autoantibody repertoire in a pair of monozygotic twins discordant for myasthenia gravis. *Clin. Immunol. Immunopathol.* 53: 161.
14. Sundewall, A.C., A.K. Lefvert and R. Olsson R. 1985. Anti-acetylcholine receptor antibodies in primary biliary cirrhosis. *Acta Med. Scand.* 217, 519.
15. Åhlberg, R., Q. Yi, R. Pirskanen, G. Matell, C. Swerup, P. Rieber, G. Riethmuller, G. Holm and A.K.Lefvert. 1994. Treatment of myasthenia gravis with anti-CD4 antibody: Improvement correlates to changes in T cell reactivity. *Neurology* 44: 1732.
16. Yi, Q., W. He, G. Matell, R. Pirskanen, Y. Magnusson and A.K. Lefvert. 1996. T and B lymphocytes reacting with the extracellular loop of the β2-adrenergic receptor are present in the peripheral blood of patients with myasthenia gravis. *Clin. Exp. Immunol.* 103: 133.
17. Xu, B., R. Pirskanen and A.K. Lefvert. Antibodies against β1 and β2 adrenergic receptors in myasthenia gravis. 1998 *J. Neuroimmunol.*91(1-2): 82.
18. Xu, B., Q. Yi, R. Pirskanen, G. Matell H. Eng and A.K. Lefvert. 1997. Decreased β2 adrenergic receptor density on peripheral blood mononuclear cells in myasthenia gravis. *J. Autoimmun.* 10(4): 401.
19. Huang, D., R. Pirskanen, G. Matell and A.K. Lefvert. 1999. Tumour necrosis factor-α polymorphism and secretion in myasthenia gravis *J. Neuroimmunol.*94: 165.
20. Hjelmström, P., C.S. Peacock, R. Giscombe, A.K. Lefvert, R. Pirskanen, J.M. Blackwell and C.B. Sanjeevi. 1998. Polymorphism in tumor necrosis factor genes associated with myasthenia gravis. *J. Neuroimmunol.* 88(1-2): 137.
21. Wilson, A.G., J.A. Symons, T.L. Mcdowell, F.S. di Giovine and G.W. Duff. 1994. Effects of a tumour necrosis factor (TNFα) promoter base transition on transcriptional activity. *Br. J. Rheumatol.* 33: 89.
22. Giroir, B.P., T. Brown and B. Beutler. 1992. Constitutive synthesis of tumour necrosis factor in the thymus. *Proc. Natl. Acad. Sci.* USA 89: 4864.
23. Huang, D., R. Pirskanen, P. Hjelmström and A.K. Lefvert. 1998. Polymorphisms in IL-1b and IL-1 receptor antagonist genes are associated with myasthenia gravis. *J. Neuroimmunol.* 81: 76.
24. Emilie, D., M.C. Crevon, S. Cohen-Kaminsky, M. Peuchnaur, O. Devergne, S. Berrih-Aknin and P. Galanaud. 1991 In situ production of interleukins in hyperplastic thymus from myasthenia gravis patients. *Hum. Pathol.* 22, 461.
25. Askanas, V., W.K. Engel and R.B. Alvarez. 1998. Fourteen newly recognized proteins at the human neuromuscular junction and their non-junctional accumulation in inclusion-body myositis. *Ann. NY Acad. Sci. vol.* 841: 28.
26. Maselli, R.A., D.P. Richman and R.L. Wollmann. 1991. Inflammation at the neuromuscular junction in myasthenia gravis. *Neurology 41:1497.*
27. Gu, D., L. Wogensen, N.A. Calcutt, C. Xia, S. Zhu, J.P. Merlie, H.S. Fox, J. Lindstrom, H.C. Powell and N. Sarvetnick. 1995. Myasthenia gravis-like syndrome induced by expression of interferon g in the neuromuscular junction. *J. Exp. Med.* 181: 547.
28. McLellan, A.D., R.V. Sorg, L.A. Williams and D.N. Hart. 1996. Human dendritic cells activate T lymphocytes via a CD40: CD40 ligand- dependent pathway. *Eur. J. Immunol.* 26: 1204.
29. Dinarello, C.A. 1996. Biologic basis for interleukin-1 in disease. *Blood. 87:2095*
30. Huang, D., S. Xia, Y. Zhou, R. Pirskanen, L. Liu and A.K. Lefvert. 1999. No evidence for Interleukin-4 gene conferring susceptibility to myasthenia gravis. *J. Neuroimm.* 92: 208.

31. Lalani, I., K. Bhol and A.R. Ahmed. 1997. Interleukin-10: biology, role in inflammation and autoimmunity. *Ann. Allergy Asthma Immunol.* 79: 469.
32. Turner, D.M., D.M. William, D, Sankaran, M. Lazarus, P.J. Sinnott and I.V. Hutchinson. 1997. An investigation of polymorphism in the interleukin-10 gene promoter. *Eur. J. Immunogenetics.* 24: 1.
33. Huang, D., S. Xia, Y. Zhou, R. Pirskanen, L. Liu and A.K. Lefvert. 1999. Markers in the promotor region of Interleukin-10 (IL-10) gene in myasthenia gravis: Implications on diverse effects of IL-10 in the pathogenesis of the disease. *J. Neuroimmunol.* 94: 82.
34. Rulifson, I.C., A.I Sperling, P.E. Fields, F.W. Fitch and J.A. Bluestone. 1997. CD28 co-stimulation promotes the production of Th2 cytokines. *J. Immunol.* 158: 658.
35. Tivol, E.A., F. Borriello, A.N. Schweitzer, W.P. Lynch, J.A. Bluestone and A.H. Sharpe. 1995. Loss of CTLA-4 leads to massive lymphoproliferation and fatal multiorgan tissue destruction, revealing a critical negative regulatory role of CTLA-4. *Immunity* 3: 541.
36. Huang D., L. Liu, K. Norén, S. Xia, J. Trifunovic, R. Pirskanen and A.K. Lefvert. 1998. Genetic association of *Ctla-4* to myasthenia gravis with thymoma. *J. Neuroimmunol* 88(1-2): 192.
38. Aarli, J.A., K. Stefansson, L.S.G. Marton and R.L. Wollmann. 1990. Patients with myasthenia gravis and thymoma have in their sera IgG autoantibodies against titin. *Clin. Exp. Immunol.* 82: 284.
39. Shaw, G. and R. Kamen. 1986. A conserved AU sequence from the 3′untranslated region of GM-CSF mRNA mediates selective mRNA degradation. *Cell* 46: 659.
40. Green, S., J. Turki, M. Innis and S.B. Liggett. 1994. Amino-terminal polymorphisms of the human β2-adrenergic receptor impart distinct agonist-promoted regulatory properties. *Biochemistry* 33: 9414.
41. Xu B.Y., D. Huang, R. Pirskanen and A.K. Lefvert. β2-adrenergic receptor gene polymorphisms in myasthenia gravis. Submitted.
42. Vieira, M.L., S. Caillat-Zucman, P. Gajdos, S. Cohen-Kaminsky, A. Castiu and J.F. Bach. 1993. Identification by genomic typing of non-DR3 HLA class II genes associated with myasthenia gravis. *J. Neuroimmunol.* 47: 115.

Myasthenia Gravis: Disease mechanisms and immunointervention
P. Christadoss (Ed)

11. Experimental Myasthenia Gravis in Mice: The role of costimulatory molecules

Fu-Dong Shi[1,2], Bing He[1], Hulun Li[1], Darius Matusevicius[1], Hans Link[1] and Hans-Gustaf Ljunggren[2]

[1]Division of Neurology, Karolinska Institute, Huddinge University Hospital, Stockholm, Sweden

[2]Microbiology and Tumor Biology Center (MTC), Karolinska Institute, Stockholm, Sweden

Introduction

Activation of T-cells requires two signals. One signal is provided by the cognate TCR/MHC-peptide interaction. The second costimulatory signal is mediated through ligation of CD28 by B7 [1]. The CD28 molecule is a 44-kD glycoprotein, which is expressed on all murine and human T cells, while its counter receptor pair B7-1 (CD80) and B7-2 (CD86) are expressed mainly on antigen presenting cells (APCs) [1]. In addition to the conventional signals 1 and 2, a direct signal delivered to T-cells via triggering or cross-linking of the CD40 ligand (CD40L) is also required for full activation of T cells to perform effector functions and to produce cytokines [2]. T-helper cells activate resting B-cells through TCR recognition of MHC class II-peptide complexes and costimulation through CD40L/CD40 interactions [2]. CD40L is a 33-kDa membrane protein that is preferentially expressed on activated CD4+ T cells [2], while the counter-receptor for CD40L is CD40, expressed on APCs [2]. The mechanisms for CD28 and CD40L in the regulation of the immune system at the cellular and molecular levels are just beginning to be elucidated. Interactions of CD28-B7 and CD40-CD40L have been implicated in T cell-mediated autoimmune diseases such as experimental allergic encephalomyelitis (EAE) and insulin-dependent diabetes mellitus [3-6].

Myasthenia gravis (MG) and experimental autoimmune myasthenia gravis (EAMG) are caused by autoantibodies against the nicotinic acetylcholine receptor (AChR) in the neuromuscular junctions [7]. The production of autoantibodies to AChR is dependent on the help of T cells [7]. However, the costimulation requirements in the activation of AChR-specific T cells and initiation of pathogenic antibody production remain unexplored. We therefore utilized two genetically altered mouse strains, CD28- and CD40L-deficient mice (CD28-/-, CD40L-/-), to examine and compare the contributions of CD28 and CD40L in the development and progression of EAMG.

Results and Discussion

The present study has addressed the roles of the costimulatory molecules CD28 and CD40L in the genesis of AChR-induced, antibody mediated EAMG. Compared to wild type mice, CD28-/- mice are less susceptible, and CD40L-/- mice are completely resistant to EAMG induction. This indicates that CD28 and CD40L are differentially required for EAMG induction. Functions of T helper cells, as reflected by cytokine responses and anti-AChR IgG antibody production, were regulated differentially by CD28 and CD40L, underlining the differences in the susceptibility to EAMG in these two mutant strains.

Influence of CD28 and CD40L Gene Disruption on AChR Induced Clinical EAMG

To determine and compare the effects of CD28-B7 and CD40-CD40L interactions on the development of AChR-induced EAMG, we immunized C57BL/6 (B6), CD28-/-, CD40L-/-, and littermate control mice with 20 μg of AChR in CFA on day 0 and again on days 30 (first boost) and 60 (second boost). The mouse EAMG model is characterized by a relatively low incidence of disease even after multiple immunizations [8]. Therefore, we collected large numbers of mice in each group. Sixteen out of 22 B6 mice developed muscle weakness before (3 mice) or after (13 mice) the first boosting (73%). Ten mice deteriorated progressively, and one died. Wild type littermate control mice exhibited a similar incidence and severity of myasthenia as did B6 mice (data not shown), and hence B6 mice were used as controls in subsequent studies. In contrast, only 7 out of 22 CD28-/- mice developed muscle weakness before (1 mouse) or after (6 mice) the first boosting (32%, $p < 0.01$). Two mice progressively deteriorated, and one died. There was no difference regarding the time of onset of clinical disease between CD28-/- and B6 mice. The mean severity of disease was mild in CD28-/-, compared to B6 mice (0.46 vs 1.69, $p < 0.01$). CD40L-/- mice remained completely resistant to EAMG induction (0%, $p < 0.001$). These results indicate that both CD28 and CD40L signaling influence the genesis of EAMG, and that CD40L has more pronounced effects.

CD28 and CD40L Gene Disruption Impaired AChR- and Peptide-Induced Lymphocyte Proliferation and Altered Th1/Th2 Cytokine Response

To learn whether the decreased susceptibility to EAMG in CD28-/- and CD40L-/- mice results from inability to evoke T cell responses to AChR and its dominant α146-162 peptide [9], mice were immunized with 20 μg of AChR in CFA. Seven days later, draining lymph node T cell responses were analyzed in vitro for the ability to proliferate and secrete IFN-γ in response to AChR and the α146-162 peptide. As shown in Fig. 1A, the AChR and α146-162 peptide-induced proliferative responses were impaired in the CD28-/- and CD40L-/- mice. MNC from B6 and CD40L-/- mice showed vigorous proliferation upon stimulation with Con A (SI: 35.6 ± 6 and 27.4 ± 6.5, respectively). Thus, the intrinsic potential of T cells to respond to antigen is largely preserved in CD40L-/- mice [10, 11]. In contrast, CD28-/- mice displayed a strong reduction in proliferative response to Con A (SI 16.2 ± 5.1 $p < 0.01$), which is in accordance with previous findings [12].

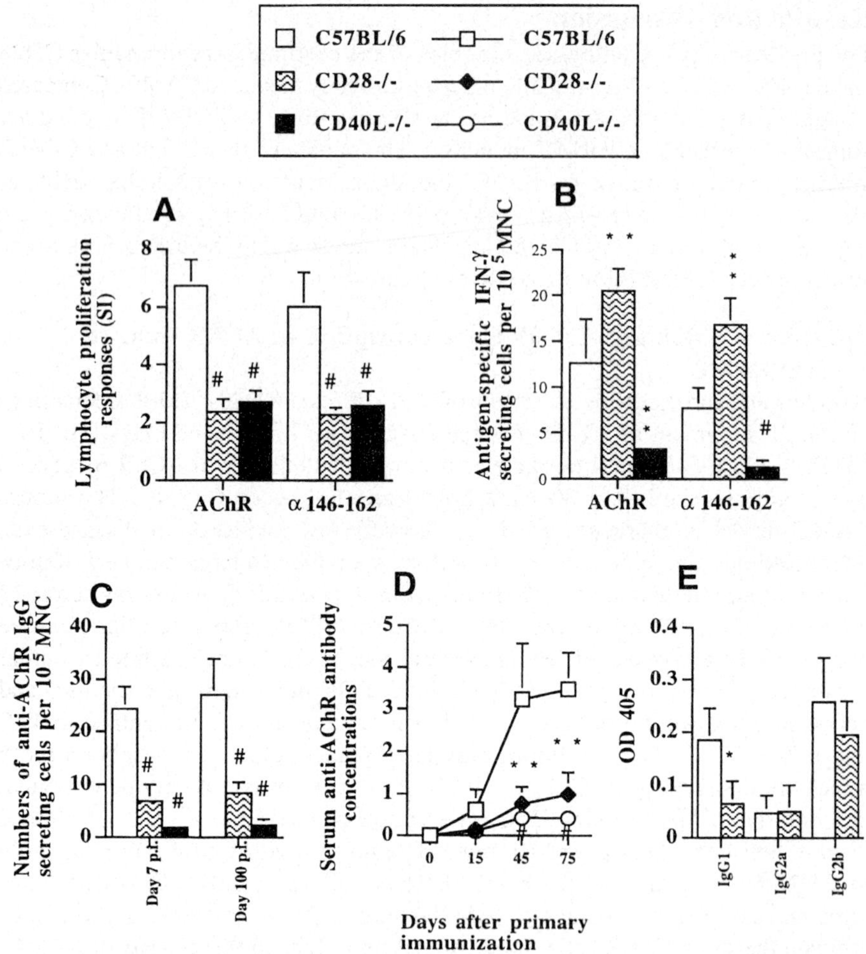

Fig. 1. Influence of CD28 and CD40L gene disruption on autoreactive T and B cell responses. Mice were immunized with 20 mg AChR in CFA into footpads and thigh regions. After 7 days p.i., mice were sacrificed and mononuclear cells were isolated from popliteal and inguinal lymph nodes (PILN). A: Results of proliferative responses are expressed as SI. B: IFN-γELISPOT are expressed as numbers of IFN-γ-secreting cells per 10^5 MNC. Results presented are averages of 4 mice per group and are representative of three independent experiments. C: A significant decrease in the numbers of anti-AChR IgG antibody-secreting cells per 10^5 MNC in CD28-/- and CD40L-/- mice. MNC were isolated from PILN from mice sacrificed on day 7 (4 mice per group, results drawn from the average of three independent experiments) and day 100 p.i. D: Serum anti-mouse AChR antibody levels are greatly decreased in CD28-/- and CD40L-/- mice. Antibody concentrations were measured by RIA and expressed as moles of α-bungarotoxin binding sites bound per liter of serum. Results are averages of 10 mice per group. E: Anti-AChR IgG antibody isotypes. Results are averages of 10 mice per group. For figures A-E, symbols refer to mean values, and bars to S.D. $*p < 0.05$, $**p < 0.01$, $\#p < 0.001$.

Compared to B6 mice, AChR-induced IFN-γ production, reflected by numbers of IFN-γ-secreting cells (Fig. 1B) and protein levels (Table 1) in the culture supernatant, were higher in CD28-/- mice. In contrast, levels of IFN-γ production were lower in CD40L-/- mice. Levels of IL-4 and IL-10 production were lower in both CD28-/- and CD40L-/- mice, compared to B6 mice (Table 1). These data clearly suggest that CD28-/- mice are selectively deficient in their ability to develop or amplify Th2-type responses, and may deviate toward a Th1 phenotype. CD40L-/- mice demonstrated low cytokine production for both Th1 and Th2 type; thus there was no switch toward any Th subset.

Table 1. Cytokine production in the supernatant cultured with and without AChR[a]

	IFN-γ (ng/ml)		IL-4 (pg/ml)		IL-10 (pg/ml)	
Mice	–[b]	AChR	–	AChR	–	AChR
B6	7.2 ± 3.3	33.2 ± 7.4	11.4 ± 5.6	33.6 ± 12.1	86.4 ± 22.2	732 ± 76.2
CD28-/-	37.8 ± 11.3[d]	57.5 ± 8.9[d]	0.00 ± 0.00	7.34 ± 2.21[c]	24.7 ± 8.8[c]	325 ± 93.5[c]
CD40L-/-	0.00 ± 0.00[d]	12.6 ± 4.7[c]	0.00 ± 0.00	9.85 ± 3.21[c]	21.7 ± 4.4[c]	221 ± 47.7[d]

[a]Mice were immunized with 20 μg AChR in CFA into footpads and thigh regions. After 7 days p.i., the mice were sacrificed and mononuclear cells were isolated from popliteal and inguinal lymph nodes (PILN). The supernatants were collected after 48 h of culture. Cytokine productions were determined by ELISA.
[b]no antigen stimulation; [c]$p < 0.05$, [d]$p < 0.01$.
The comparisons were made between the mutant mice and B6 mice.

Role of Th1 Versus Th2 Cytokines in EAMG

In CD28-/- mice, CTLA-4/B7 interactions might function to costimulate T cells in response to AChR and α146-162. Other costimulatory molecules, such as CD43 or signals provided by a set of cytokines or adhesion molecules [13–15], may also act as a substitute for CD28 in these animals. However, these substitutions may not be sufficient to "rescue" AChR-specific T cell activity. In the present model, Th1 cytokine IFN-γ production was enhanced in CD28-/- mice but diminished in CD40L-/- mice, while Th2 responses were diminished in both mutant strains, indicating that the cytokine balance, which is crucial for development of autoimmune diseases [16], can be differentially regulated by CD28 and CD40L. These results agree with previous studies demonstrating that the differentiation of Th precursors into the Th2 subset, but not Th1 subset, is dependent upon CD28 signaling [3, 17]. Of note is that CD28 gene disruption promoted the progression of autoimmune diabetes in NOD diabetic mice strains, associated with enhanced IFN-γ and diminished IL-4 production [3]. Unlike diabetes in CD28-/- NOD mice, EAMG was actually partially prevented in CD28-/- mice, despite the fact that this strain also showed a similar cytokine pattern.

Upon activation by cognate ligand, naïve Th cells differentiate into distinct functional subgroups which are characterized by their pattern of cytokine secretion

[16]. AChR-specific mouse T cells secrete Th1 and Th2 cytokines [18, 19]. Besides the role of Th2 cytokines in EAMG [18], mice with IFN-γ deficiency failed to mount significant AChR-specific Ab responses and became resistant to EAMG induction, indicating that the Th1 cytokine IFN-γ is also required for the generation of a pathogenic anti-AChR humoral immune response [20]. Therefore, it appears that both Th1 and Th2 cytokines provide help for B cells to produce anti-AChR Abs. In contrast to diabetes in CD28-/- NOD mice, immune deviation from Th2 to Th1 cytokine contributes to the reduced incidence and severity of EAMG in CD28-/- mice. Thus, enhanced IFN-γ production could not enhance AChR-specific Abs responses and aggravate disease when the Th2 cytokines IL-4 and IL-10 were diminished.

CD28 and CD40L Gene Disruption Regulated AChR-Specific IgG Antibody and its Isotypes Response

The basic pathology of EAMG is end-plate AChR reduction, caused entirely by anti-AChR Abs [7]. Therefore, the reduced susceptibility to EAMG in the CD28-/- and CD40L-/- mice should be associated with low anti-AChR antibody levels. Thus, we examined the MNC from PILN-secreting IgG on day 7 p.i. as well as on day 100 p.i., i.e., after the second boost. High levels of anti-AChR IgG antibody-secreting cells were detected in B6 mice, which also had a high incidence of muscle weakness upon immunization with AChR + CFA (Fig. 1C). Numbers of anti-AChR IgG antibody-secreting cells were lower in the CD28-/- mice ($p < 0.001$), and reduced to an even greater extent in the CD40L-/- mice ($p < 0.001$) (Fig. 1C). Consistent with the numbers of anti-AChR IgG-secreting cells, levels of serum anti-mouse AChR antibodies were markedly reduced in the CD28-/- and CD40L-/- mice as measured on day 45 and 75 p.i. (Fig. 1D).

Serum from CD28-/- mice contained lower levels of the Th2-dependent IgG1 isotype than did serum from B6 mice. In contrast, CD28-/- mice and B6 mice both had low levels of serum IgG2a (Fig. 1F). The major component of antibodies in CD28-/- mice appeared to be the Th1-dependent IgG2b isotype. These results may reflect an enhanced Th1 but reduced Th2 responses to AChR in the CD28-/- mice. All three isotypes were undetectable in serum from CD40L-/- mice examined at the same dilution as CD28-/- and B6 mice (data not shown).

Both CD28-/- and CD40L-/- mice exhibit defects in isotype switching of thymus dependent Ags [10, 12]. The basis for these defects is that both CD28 and CD40L are crucial for germinal center formation [21, 22]. Then, what accounts for the difference in the susceptibility to EAMG in these two strains? The impairments of isotype switching are not complete in CD28-/- and CD40L-/- mice, because all IgG isotypes in response to thymus-dependent antigen can still be detected in both strains [21, 23]. Our data show that CD28-/- mice still had substantial amounts of IgG2b, which could not be detected in the CD40L-/- mice. Anti-AChR antibodies of IgG2b isotype are suggested to be pathogenic in rat and mouse EAMG [19, 24]. Thus, the difference in IgG2b production may, in part, account for the difference in EAMG susceptibility in these types of mutant mice. In addition, the CD40L-/- mice showed reduction of both Th1 and Th2 cytokines, instead of switching from a Th2 to a Th1 cytokine response, as observed in the CD28-/- mice. The CD40L provides a mitogenic signal to B cells, the potency of which is enhanced by cytokines, notably IL-4 and IL-5 in the mouse [25], and IL-4 and IL-10 in the human [26]. These cytokines and CD40L also provide costimulatory signals that induce secretion of polyclonal Ig of multiple isotypes [25-27]. Thus, the help provided by IFN-γ, as well as by IL-4 and IL-10, was not sufficient for AChR-reactive B cells to produce sufficient amounts of pathogenic antibodies. The lack of CD40L, together with the lack of cytokines, conferred resistance to EAMG in the CD40L-/- mice.

CD28 and CD40L Gene Disruption Regulated B7 Expression Differentially

The difference in the susceptibility to EAMG induction, cytokine patterns and anti-AChR antibody responses seen in CD28-/- and CD40L-/- mice could indicate that other costimulatory activities are differentially regulated by CD28 and CD40L, which in turn affect autoreactive T cell priming, as were the expression of B7-1 and B7-2 on lymph node MNC. Elevated levels of B7-1 and B7-2 expression were observed in CD28-/- mice, suggesting that CTLA4/B7 interactions may be upregulated in the absence of CD28 (Fig. 2). CD40L-/- mice had, in contrast to

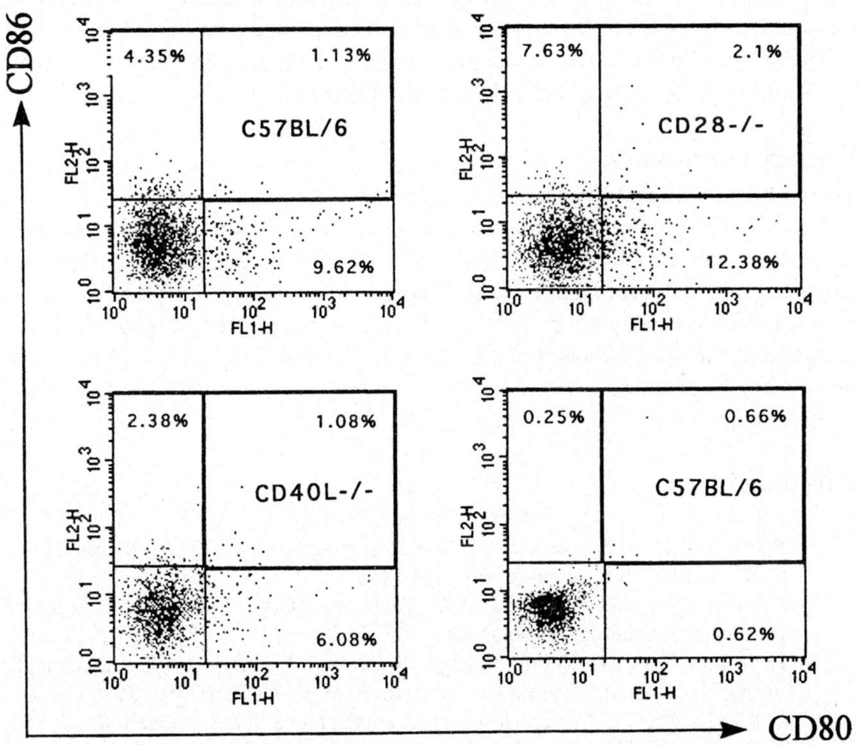

Fig. 2. **Two-color flow cytometry shows expression of CD80 (B7-1) and CD86 (B7-2) and double-stained cells on lymph node MNC from mice immunized with AChR and CFA (day 7 p.i.). Isotype control antibody staining was shown in low left panel.**

CD28-/- mice, a reduced expression of B7-1 and B7-2 (Fig. 2). It is likely that in this setting, the impairments of AChR-reactive T cell priming were due to the lack of CD40-CD40L interactions for the induction of costimulatory activity B7-1 and B7-2, as supported by the observation that B7 costimulation appears to be augmented by CD40 signaling in part by increasing B7 expression on APCs [28].

Conclusion

We demonstrate that compared to wild type mice, the CD28-/- mice became less susceptible, and CD40L-/- mice were completely resistant to EAMG induction. Analysis of T helper functions, reflected by cytokine responses, revealed a switch to a Th1 profile in CD28-/- mice. Consistently, levels of serum AChR-specific antibodies of the IgG1 isotype were decreased in CD28-/- mice. In the CD40L-/- mice, both Th1 and Th2 cytokine responses were diminished, and T cell-dependent, AchR-reactive B cell responses were severely impaired. Thus, CD28 and CD40L are differentially required for induction of EAMG. These results also imply that disruption of CD28-B7 interaction may result in different outcomes in EAMG versus T cell-mediated autoimmune diseases, while interfering with CD40-CD40L signaling may have a similar influence in these two conditions, because neither EAE nor diabetes could be elicited in mice with CD40L deficiency [8, 10]. Since CD40L is expressed preferentially on activated T cells, targeting this T cell population may have therapeutic potentials in MG.

Acknowledgments

We thank Drs P. Christadoss and B.J. Chambers for reading the manuscript, and Professor B. Wahren and Dr. M. Levi, Swedish Institute for Infectious Disease Control, Stockholm, Sweden, for providing α146-162 peptide. This study was supported by grants from the Swedish Medical Research Council, the Petrus and Augusta Hedlund Foundation, the Lars Hierta Foundation, the Magnus Bergwall Foundation, the Åke Wiberg Foundation, the Swedish MS Society (NHR), and the Karolinska Institute.

References

1. Sperline, A.I. and J.A. Bluestone,. 1996. The complexities of T-cell co-stimulation: CD28 and beyond. *Immunol. Rev.* 153: 155.
2. Grewal, I.S. and R.A. Flavell. 1996. The role of CD40 ligand in costimulation and T-cell activation. *Immunol. Rev.* 153: 85.
3. Lenschow, D.J. K.C. Herold, L. Rhee, B. Patel, A. Koons, H.Y. Qin, E. Fuchs, B. Singh, C.B. Thompson and J.A. Bluestone, 1996. CD28/B7 regulation of Th1 and Th2 subsets in the development of autoimmune diabetes. *Immunity* 5: 285.
4. Kuchroo, V.K., M.P. Das, J.A. Brown, A.M. Ranger, S.S. Zamvil, R.A. Sobel, H.L. Weiner, N. Nabavi and L.H. Glimcher, 1995. B7-1 and B7-2 costimulatory molecules activate differentially the Th1-Th2 development pathways: application to autoimmune disease therapy. *Cell* 80: 707.
5. Grewal, I.S., H.G. Foellmer, K.D. Grewal, J. Xu, F. Hardardottir, J.L. Baron, Jr.

C.A. Janeway, and R.A. Flavell, 1996. Requirement for CD40 ligand in costimulation induction, T cell activation, and experimental allergic encephalomyelitis. *Science* 273: 1864.

6. Balasa, B., T. Krahl, G. Palstone, J. Lee, R. Tisch, H.O. McDevitt and N. Sarvetnick, 1997. CD40 ligand-CD40 interactions are necessary for the initiation of insulitis and diabetes in nonobese diabetic mice. *J. Immunol.* 159: 4620.
7. Drachman, D., 1994. Myasthenia gravis. *N. Engl. J. Med.* 330: 1797.
8. Berman, P.W. and J. Patrick, 1980. Experimental myasthenia gravis murine system. *J. Exp. Med.* 151: 204.
9. Shenoy, M., M. Oshima, M.Z. Atassi and P. Christadoss, 1993. Suppression of experimental autoimmune myasthenia gravis by epitope-specific neonatal tolerance to synthetic region of α146–162 of acetylcholine receptor. *Clin. Immunol. Immunopathol.* 66: 230.
10. Renshaw, B.R., W.C. Fansbow III, R.J. Armitage, K.A. Camphell, D. Liggitt, B. Wright, B.L. Davison and C.R. Maliszewski, 1994. Humoral immune responses in CD40 lignad deficient mice. *J. Exp. Med.* 180: 1889.
11. Grewal, I.S., J. Xu, and R.A. Flavell, 1995. Impairment of antigen-specific T-cell priming in mice lacking CD40 ligand. *Nature* 378: 617.
12. Shahinian, A., K. Pfeffer, K.P. Lee, T.M. Kundig, K. Kishihara, A. Wakeham, K. Kawai, P.S. Ohashi and T.W. Mak, 1993. Differential T cell costimulatory requirements in CD28-deficient mice. *Science* 261: 609.
13. Liu, Y. and P.S. Linsley. 1992. Costimuation of T lymphocyte growth. *Curr. Opin. Immunol.* 4: 256.
14. Sperling, A.I., J.M. Green, R.L. Mosley, P.L. Smith, J.A. Bluestone and C.B. Thompson, 1995. CD43 is a murine T cell costimulatory receptor that functions independently of CD28. *J. Exp. Med.* 182: 139.
15. Schwartz, R.H., 1992. Costimulation of T lymphocytes: role of CD28, CTLA-4 and B7 in interleukin-2 production and immunotherapy. *Cell* 71: 1065.
16. Mosmann, T.R. and S. Sad, 1996. The expanding universe of T cell subsets: Th1, Th2 and more. *Immunol. Today* 17: 138.
17. Seder, R.A., R.N. Germain, P.S. Linsley and W.E. Paul. 1994. CD28-mediated costimulation of interleukin 2 (IL-2) production plays a critical role in T cell priming for IL-4 and interferon gamma production. *J. Exp. Med.* 179: 299.
18. Zhang, G.X., B.G. Xiao, M. Bakhiet, P.H. van der Meide, H. Wigzell, H. Link and T. Olsson. 1996. Both CD4+ and CD8+ T cells are essential to induce experimental autoimmune myasthenia gravis. *J. Exp. Med.* 184: 349.
19. Wu, B., C. Deng, E. Goluszko and P. Christadoss, 1997. Tolerance to a dominant epitope in the acetylcholine receptor molecule induces epitope spread and suppresses murine myasthenia gravis. *J. Immunol.* 159: 3016.
20. Balasa, B., C. Deng, J. Lee, L.M. Bradley, D.K. Dalton, P. Christadoss, and N. Sarvetnick, 1997. Interferon *g* (IFN-*g*) is necessary for the genesis of acetylcholine receptor-induced clinical experimental autoimmune myasthenia gravis in mice. *J. Exp. Med.* 186: 385.
21. Teresa, M.F., J.D. Laman, J.A. Ledbetter, A. Aruffo, E. Claassen and R.J. Noelle, 1994. Gp39-CD40 interactions are essential for germinal center formation and development of B cell memory. *J. Exp. Med.* 180: 157.
22. Ferguson, S.E., S. Han, G. Kelsoe and C.B. Thompson, 1996. CD28 is required for germinal center formation. *J. Immunol.* 156: 4576.
23. Ma, J., J. Xu, M.P. Madaio, Q. Peng, J. Zhang, I.S. Grewal, R.A. Flavell and J. Craft, 1996. Autoimmune *lpr/lpr* mice deficient in CD40 ligand: spontaneous Ig class switching with dichotomy of autoantibody responses. *J. Immunol.* 157: 417.

24. Shi, F.D., X. Bai, H. Li, Y. Huang, P.H. van der Meide and H. Link, 1998. Nasal tolerance in experimental autoimmune myasthenia gravis (EAMG): induction of protective tolerance in primed animals. *Clin. Exp. Immunol.* 111: 506.
25. Maliszewski, C.R., K. Grabstein, W.C. Fanslow, R. Armitage, M.K. Spriggs and T.A. Sato, 1993. Recombinant CD40 ligand stimulation of murine B cell growth and differentiation: cooperative effects of cytokines. *Eur. J. Immunol.* 23: 1044.
26. Aritage, R.J., B.M. Macduff, M.K. Spriggs, and W.C. Fanslow, 1993. Human B cell proliferation and Ig secretion induced by recombinant CD40 ligand are modulated by soluble cytokines. *J. Immunol.* 150: 3671.
27. Xu, J., T.M. Foy, J.D. Laman, E.A. Elliott, J. Dunn, T.J. Waldschmidt, J. Elsemore, R.J. Noelle and R.A. Flavell. 1994. Mice deficient for CD40 ligand. *Immunity* 1: 423.
28. Yang, Y. and J.M. Wilson. 1996. CD40 ligand-dependent T cell activation: Requirements of B7-CD28 signaling through CD40. *Science.* 273: 1862.

Myasthenia Gravis: Disease mechanisms and immunointervention
P. Christadoss (Ed)

12. Passive Myasthenia Gravis Induced in SCID Mice by Transfer of Blood Cells from Myasthenic Patients

Zeng-Yu Wang[1], Peter I. Karachunski, James F. Howard Jr.[2] and Bianca M. Conti-Fine[1*]

[1]Department of Biochemistry, Molecular Biology and Biophysics, University of Minnesota, St. Paul, MN 55108; Department of Pharmacology, School of Medicine, University of Minnesota, Minneapolis, MN 55455,

[2]Department of Neurology, University of North Carolina at Chapel Hill, NC

*Previously known as Bianca M. Conti-Tronconi

Introduction

More than 25 years ago, experiments that involved daily injections into mice of immunoglobulins purified from serum of myasthenia gravis (MG) patients demonstrated that this procedure reproduced in the mice the characteristic clinical and electrophysiologic features of MG [1]. During the same years other seminal experiments demonstrated that administration to mice of purified monoclonal antibodies against the acetylcholine receptor (AChR) also reproduced the clinical and electrophysiologic symptoms of MG (rev. in [2]). Those findings proved that autoantibodies against the AChR at the neuromuscular junction cause the symptoms of MG.

The pathogenic anti-AChR autoantibodies in MG patients are high affinity IgG, whose synthesis requires the intervention of $CD4^+$ T helper cells. In rodent experimental MG (EMG), induced by immunization with purified AChR, synthesis of pathogenic anti-AChR antibodies and development of the myasthenia-like symptoms does not occur in the absence of $CD4^+$ T helper cells ([rev. in [2]).

AChR-specific $CD4^+$ cells are present in MG patients, and can be isolated and propagated *in vitro* from the blood and the thymus tissue of MG patients (rev. in [2]). AChR-specific $CD4^+$ lines propagated from the blood of MG patients could stimulate the secretion of polyclonal anti-AChR antibodies *in vitro* [3–4]. However, an AChR-specific helper T cell function *in vivo* and a pathogenic role of $CD4^+$ cells in human MG, postulated for a long time by analogy with EMG, were not proven until recently [5].

MG patients do not have anti-AChR cytotoxic phenomena (rev. in [2]). Consequently, it has been assumed that $CD8^+$ cells do not have a pathogenic role in MG (rev. in [2]), or that they have a protective, regulatory role [6]. However,

$CD8^+$ cells may be involved in the pathogenesis of rodent EMG, and they might have a helping role in the synthesis of anti-AChR antibodies [7-8]. Depletion of $CD8^+$ cells suppressed EMG development and reduced the synthesis of anti-AChR antibodies in Lewis rats [7]. Mutant C57Bl/6 mice that lacked $CD8^+$ cells did not develop EMG and had reduced anti-AChR antibody responses [8]. In contrast with those findings, another study showed that mice deficient in MHC class I molecules, and in $CD8^+$ cells, were highly susceptible to EMG, and concluded that $CD8^+$ cells do not have a pathogenic role in EMG [9]. In summary, the results obtained with rodent EMG suggest that the role of $CD8^+$ cells in the anti-AChR response might be complex, and raise the possibility that also in MG $CD8^+$ cells might be necessary for effective production of pathogenic anti-AChR antibodies.

The study of the role of different components of the immune system in human autoimmune diseases poses difficult challenges. This crucial question cannot be directly addressed *in vivo* for obvious ethical reasons. *In vitro* systems are suitable for the study of certain aspects of the immune response, but they cannot substitute for studies in the whole organism, which is the only system in which the complex interactions between the effectors of the immune response and the target organs can occur, and their ability to cause a pathologic phenotype can be assessed. The passive transfer model, so suitable to investigate the effects of human autoantibodies if they cross react between species, is difficult to extend to investigations of the effect of transfer of immune cells, because communication between immune cells is species-specific, and even specific to immune cells carrying the same MHC molecules. We have used transgenic mice whose immune system is partially "humanized" to investigate certain aspects of the $CD4^+$ T cell function in the development of an anti-AChR response that leads to myasthenic symptoms [10-11]. Those partially "humanized" mice express a certain human class II HLA molecule, whereas they do not express the mouse class II molecules, whose genes had been "knocked out". Still, the "humanized" mice are still far too different from humans to be used as recipients of human immune cells, where such cells could carry out their full function.

To directly investigate the roles in human MG of $CD4^+$ and $CD8^+$ T cells, and of $CD4^+$ cells specific for the AChR, we have taken advantage of a different animal system—mice with severe, combined immunodeficiency [5]. The severe combined immunodeficiency (*scid*) mutation causes aberrant rearrangements of the genes encoding the immunoglobulin and the T cell receptor, and deletion of the entire J region: homozygous *scid/scid* (SCID) mice do not have mature B and T cells, and cannot develop antigen-specific immune responses [12]. They tolerate xenografts, and can be transplanted with human tissues or lymphocytes [13-14]. Because the transplanted immune cells can survive and interact with each other, the SCID mice are a useful system to investigate the mechanisms of autoimmune diseases. Human blood mononuclear cells (BMC), which include macrophages, B cells and T cells, survive in the peritoneal cavity of SCID mice for three or more months, and retain their phenotype and function, including production of human antibodies [13-14]. SCID mice, and other mouse mutants with severe combined immunodeficiency, proved to be suitable for passive transfer of several human and experimental autoimmune diseases, including rheumatoid arthritis [15], autoimmune hair loss [16], experimental autoimmune encephalomyelitis [17] and diabetes (in NOD. *SCID* mice) [18].

Previous studies suggested that SCID mice might be a suitable system to study and dissect the anti-AChR immune response that causes human MG: SCID mice engrafted with thymus [19] or BMC from MG patients [20] developed human anti-AChR antibodies in the blood, had human antibodies bound to the mouse muscle and had ultrastructural damage at the end plate. However, those early studies could not demonstrate the appearance of clinical signs of MG in the engrafted SCID mice.

Passive Transfer of Myasthenic Symptoms in a Chimeric Human-Mouse Model of MG in SCID Mice Engrafted with BMC from MG Patients

As a first step towards investigating the role of $CD4^+$ and $CD8^+$ T cells in the human anti-AChR autoantibody response, we determined the conditions necessary to achieve transfer of the myasthenic phenotype in the SCID, not just of the anti-AChR antibody synthesis, after engraftment of immune cells from MG patients. As a cell population that includes all the component necessary for an antigen-specific antibody response, we used BMC, which includes antigen-presenting cells (the macrophages and any activated B cells), $CD8^+$ and $CD4^+$ T cells, and B cells. These studies are reported in detail in [5].

We used BMC from 19 patients with generalized MG and five healthy subjects. One MG patient did not have detectable serum anti-AChR antibody. We tested the BMC of some patients two or more times: at the time of the different experiments some of these patients had symptoms of similar severity, in others the severity of the symptoms had changed.

Only 6% of the SCID mice engrafted with BMC from MG patients developed obvious myasthenic symptoms (hunched posture, respiratory distress, death), which appeared when most AChR at the mouse muscle synapses was destroyed (rev. in [2]). Thus, a more sensitive, yet non-invasive test, was necessary to reveal myasthenic weakness, and follow its intensity over time.

A suitable test for that purpose is the pancuronium-sensitized hanging grid test, which we describe in detail in [21]. This is a forced exercise test sensitized by administration of a minute amount of pancuronium bromide (0.03 mg/kg intraperitoneum) just before the test. The small amount of pancuronium inactivates a fraction of the mouse muscle AChR; this does not affect the muscle strength of normal mice, but it reveals subclinical myasthenic weakness and allows its measurement. The mice hang from a grid suspended above a soft padding, and we measured the time it took the mouse to fall three times (holding time). The test is parametric, and gives a quantitative assessment of the mouse weakness. We verified the myasthenic nature of the weakness by injecting intraperitoneum edrophonium chloride, a cholinesterase inhibitor that immediately improved the strength of myasthenic mice

We tested the mice weekly using the pancuronium-sensitized hanging grid test. Fig. 1A summarizes the results we obtained testing 62 mice engrafted with BMC from 17 MG patients and 25 mice engrafted with BMC from five healthy

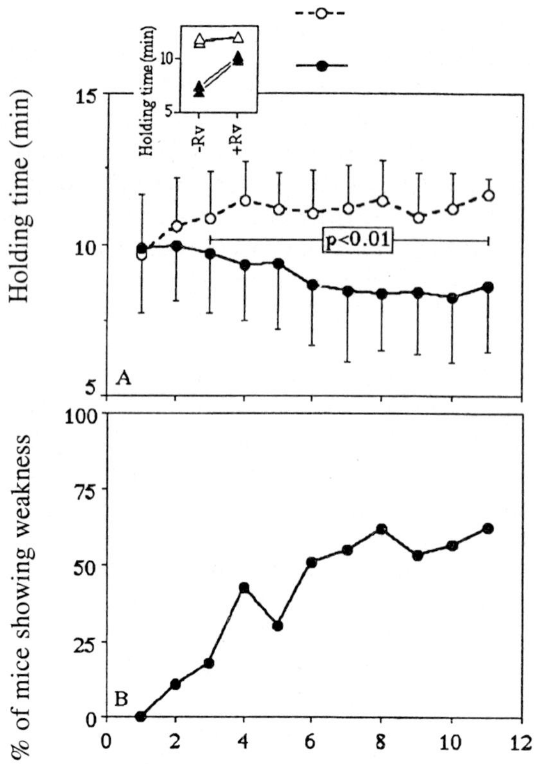

Fig. 1. **A: Results of weekly tests of subclinical muscle weakness, using pancuronium sensitized hanging grid test, from one to 11 weeks after engraftment of BMC from MG patients (black symbols) and healthy subjects (white symbols). Data are the averages ±standard deviation of the holding time of 62 mice engrafted with BMC from 17 MG patients and 25 mice engrafted with BMC from five healthy subjects. Mice engrafted with BMC from healthy subjects did not develop any strength deficit as compared to normal, untreated mice. Average holding time of mice engrafted with BMC from MG patients decreased moderately but steadily during the observation period. From week three onwards the average holding times of the mice engrafted with BMC from MG patients were significantly lower ($p < 0.01$) than those of mice engrafted with BMC from normal subjects. Inset: Improvement of the muscle strength of affected mice after administration of Reversol (black symbols). Reversol did not increase the muscle strength of mice that had normal holding time (white symbols). –Rv, before administration of Reversol; +Rv, after administration of Reversol. B: Frequency of significant muscle weakness in mice engrafted with BMC from MG patients, revealed by the hanging grid test. We considered significantly affected mice with holding times shorter by two standard deviations than the average holding time of all the SCID mice injected with BMC of normal subjects, tested the same time after engraftment. Frequency of the mice that has significantly myasthenic weakness increased with time. It reached a plateau from week seven onwards after the engraftment, when 40 of the 62 mice (65%) engrafted with BMC from MG patients had myasthenic weakness. Reprinted with permission from Z.Y. Wang, P.I. Karachunski, J.F. Howard, Jr. and B.M. Conti-Fine. Transfer of myasthenic symptoms in SCID mice engrafted with lymphocytes from Myasthenia Gravis patients. Role of CD4⁺ and CD8⁺ cells. *Neurology*, 52:484-497, 1999. Copyright American Academy of Neurology, 1999.**

subjects. One week after engraftment the average holding times of mice engrafted with BMC from healthy subjects or MG patients were identical. During the following weeks, mice engrafted with BMC from healthy subjects did not develop any strength deficit, whereas the average holding time of mice engrafted with BMC from MG patients decreased moderately but steadily during the observation period. From week three onwards the average holding times of the mice engrafted with BMC from MG patients were significantly lower than those of mice engrafted with BMC from normal subjects. Figure 1B shows the frequency of muscle weakness in mice engrafted with BMC from MG patients, revealed by the hanging grid test. From week seven onwards after the engraftment two thirds of the mice engrafted with BMC from MG patients had myasthenic weakness.

The ability of the engrafted BMC to induce passive transfer of the symptoms was in general donor dependent: engraftment of BMC from certain patients caused weakness in most or all the engrafted mice, whereas the BMC from other patients, of from the same patients but at other stages of their disease (see below) did not cause weakness in any mice. Yet engraftment of BMC from a few other patients caused weakness only in some of the engrafted mice: this is likely due to the variable rate of survival of engrafted BMC and the resulting variations in the amount of antibodies produced [13-14].

For several patients we determined the effect of engraftment into the SCID mice of BMC obtained at different times. In some of those patients the severity of their symptoms was the same; in others it was changed. We observed a striking correlation between the severity of the patients' symptoms, and the ability of their BMC to transfer myasthenic weakness in the SCID mice. For example, the BMC from some patients did not cause weakness in any of the engrafted mice when the patients had class II symptoms, while they cause myasthenic symptoms in all the engrafted mice when the same patients had class IV symptoms. When we used BMC obtained at times when the patient had symptoms of similar severity, the engrafted mice developed myasthenic weakness with similar frequency. For one of these patients, the engrafted BMC did not cause MG weakness in any SCID mice, irrespective of the disease class at the time of the blood drawing.

The good correlation between severity of the patients' symptoms and ability of their BMC to transfer the disease suggests that activated anti-AChR T and B cells are especially abundant in the blood during acute phases of the disease. This agrees with the results of previous longitudinal studies on the response of T cells from MG patients to AChR antigens: the extent of the T cell response correlated with the severity of the disease [22-23]. Also longitudinal studies on the changes over several years in the serum anti-AChR antibody concentration of the same MG patients found a correlation with the changes in the disease severity, in spite of the lack of correlation between antibody concentration and disease severity among different patients [24].

SCID Mice Engrafted with BMC from MG Patients have Human Anti-AChR Antibodies in their Serum and Muscle

Human IgG and IgM appeared in the sera of mice engrafted with human BMC starting one week after the engraftment [5]: their levels reached a plateau five-six weeks after the engraftment. The human immunoglobulins in the mouse sera reached average concentrations of 5-25% of their concentration in normal human serum. The average concentrations of IgG and IgM in mice engrafted with BMC from MG patients were significantly higher than those observed in the mice engrafted with BMC from healthy subjects. This finding indicates the presence of more abundant activated immune cells in MG patients than in normal humans. This might be related to the presence of activated autoimmune T and B cells, either directly or indirectly, through the action of secreted cytokines on non-autoimmune B cells.

Human anti-AChR antibodies appeared in the serum of 52% of the mice injected with BMC from MG patients, and their concentration increased during the first five weeks after the engraftment, whereas none of mice engrafted with BMC from healthy controls had detectable human anti-AChR antibodies in the serum [5]. Fig. 2 shows the anti-AChR antibody concentrations we observed in the sera of individual mice engrafted with BMC from MG patients or healthy subjects.

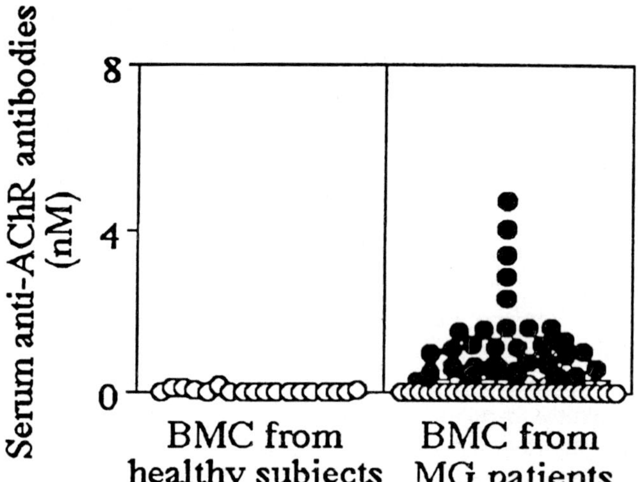

Fig. 2. Serum concentrations of human anti-AChR antibodies in individual SCID mice engrafted with BMC from MG patients and healthy subjects, measured by radioimmunoprecipitation assay. Sera were obtained 7 to 10 weeks after the engraftment from 62 mice engrafted with BMC from 17 MG patients, and 18 mice engrafted with BMC from four healthy subjects. Black symbols indicate the presence of a significant antibody concentration, and white symbols indicate that no antibodies was detected. Reprinted with permission from Z.Y. Wang, P.I. Karachunski, J.F. Howard, Jr. and B.M. Conti-Fine. Transfer of myasthenic symptoms in SCID mice engrafted with lymphocytes from Myasthenia Gravis patients. Role of CD4⁺ and CD8⁺ cells. *Neurology*, 52:484-497, 1999. Copyright American Academy of Neurology, 1999.

At the end of the experiment, we measured the concentration of mouse muscle AChR bound to human antibodies, using a radioimmunoprecipitation assay of the solubilized AChR/antibody complexes extracted from the mouse muscle [5]. Fig. 3 shows the results we obtained in individual mice engrafted with BMC from MG patients or healthy subjects, and in untreated SCID mice. Two thirds of the mice engrafted with BMC from MG patients and none of the mice engrafted with BMC from healthy subjects had significant amounts of AChR complexed by human antibodies, as compared to the background values determined in the untreated SCID mice. All SCID mice that tested positive in the solubilized AChR/antibody assay of muscle extract had human IgG at the neuromuscular junctions, as determined by imunohistochemistry of muscle sections.

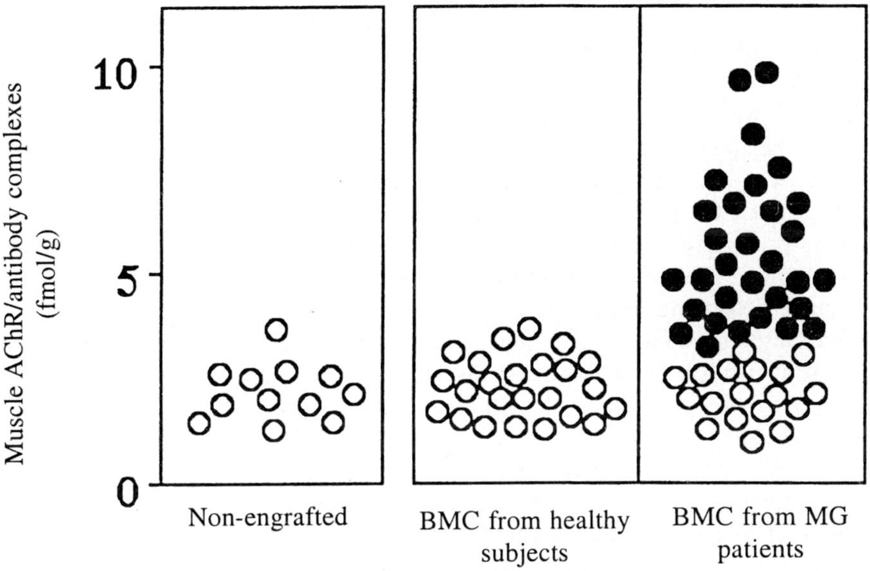

Fig. 3. Concentration of AChR bound by human anti-AChR antibodies in the muscle of SCID mice engrafted with BMC from MG patients or healthy subjects, measured by radioimmunoprecipitation assay. Muscle tissue was harvested from 51 mice engrafted with BMC from 17 MG patients and 20 mice engrafted with BMC from four healthy subjects, as indicated below the plots. Mice were sacrificed 7 to 18 weeks after the engraftment. We used also, as a negative control, muscle tissue from 12 untreated SCID mice (plot "non-engrafted"). Black symbols indicate the presence of a significant concentration of AChR/antibody complexes, and white symbols indicate that no complexes were detected. Reprinted with permission from Z.Y. Wang, P.I. Karachunski, J.F. Howard, Jr. and B.M. Conti-Fine. Transfer of myasthenic symptoms in SCID mice engrafted with lymphocytes from Myasthenia Gravis patients. Role of CD4$^+$ and CD8$^+$ cells. *Neurology*, 52:484-497, 1999. Copyright American Academy of Neurology, 1999.

One of the patients we studied was "anti-AChR antibody negative." Yet, of seven mice engrafted with her BMC, three had detectable anti-AChR antibodies in the serum, six mice developed EMG symptoms, and three of them died of respiratory failure (patient #13 in Table 1) [5]. These observations agree with those reported in another study [20], and suggest that transfer of human immune cells into SCID mice might reveal immunologic features that escape detention in more conventional assays.

Appearance of Muscle Weakness in the SCID Mice did not Correlate with the Presence of Anti-AChR Antibodies in the Serum and in the Muscle

Table 1 summarizes the frequency of serum anti-AChR antibody, muscle AChR/antibody complexes and muscle weakness after engraftment of BMC from individual MG patients. The presence of anti-AChR antibodies in the serum and even in muscle was not always predictive of reduction in the muscle strength. This agrees with the lack of correlation between anti-AChR antibody titer in the serum of MG patients and the severity of their symptoms (rev. in [2]). For example, mice engrafted with BMC from patients #7 and #14 did not develop weakness, yet all of them had human anti-AChR antibodies in the serum, and all but one had human antibody bound to muscle AChR. This suggests that patients #7 and #14 synthesize anti-AChR antibodies with low pathogenic potential. Furthermore, the presence of anti-AChR antibody in the mouse serum was not always predictive of the presence of AChR/antibody complexes in the muscle. For example, most mice engrafted with BMC from patients #2, #3 and #10 did not have detectable serum anti-AChR antibody, yet they had measurable anti-AChR/antibody complexes in the muscle. Furthermore, SCID mice engrafted with BMC from all these three patients had comparable concentrations of muscle AChR/antibody complexes. Yet, all mice engrafted with BMC from patients #3 and #10, and none of those engrafted with BMC from patient #2, developed myasthenic symptoms. These data are reconciled in a model in which the BMC from patients #2, #3 and #10 secreted small amounts of high affinity anti-AChR antibodies that all bound to the muscle AChR, leaving no anti-AChR antibodies in the sera. However, the antibodies from patients #3 and #10 impaired the neuromuscular transmission, whereas those from patient #2 did not, and must have been much less pathogenic.

We observed a different pattern in the mice engrafted with BMC from patients #5, #6 and #9 (Table 1). All mice developed significant myasthenic weakness, yet they did not have measurable concentrations of human anti-AChR antibodies in their sera, or complexed to their muscle AChR. This discrepancy is reconciled considering that the main pathogenic mechanisms of anti-AChR antibodies are accelerated destruction of AChR molecules crosslinked by the antibody, and complement-mediated destruction of the post-synaptic membrane to which the anti-AChR antibodies bind (rev. in [2]). In either case, the binding of pathogenic antibodies causes disappearance of the AChR/antibody complexes. Thus, the BMC from these patients must have synthesized small amounts of highly pathogenic, high affinity antibodies, that bound to the muscle AChR and were removed from the serum. Further, their binding to the muscle AChR must have effectively caused destruction and disappearance of the AChR/antibody complexes, resulting in the paradoxical absence of measurable muscle complexes in mice that had myasthenic weakness. In agreement with this model, one of these patients had class IV disease, yet he had extremely low serum concentrations of anti-AChR antibodies.

Table 1. Summary of the effects of engraftment into SCID mice with BMC from MG patients

Subject #	Number of engrafted mice	Mice with significant weakness¶	Mice with serum anti-AChR antibodies†	Mice with muscle AChR/ antibody complexes†	Mice with human Ig at the neuromuscular junction‡
1	4	1/4	4/4	4/4	nd
2	2	0/2	0/2	2/2	nd
3	2	2/2	0/2	2/2	2/2
4	2	0/2	1/2	0/2	nd
5	5	5/5	0/5	0/2*	0/2
6	2	2/2	0/2	0/2	0/2
7	2	0/2	2/2	2/2	1/1
8	8	4/8	5/8	4/5**	4/4
9	2	2/2	0/2	0/2	0/2
10	4	4/4	1/4	3/4	2/2
11	3	3/3	1/3	1/3	1/2
12	3	2/3	1/3	2/2**	1/1
13	7	6/7	3/7	1/4**	1/1
14	4	0/4	4/4	3/4	nd
15	4	2/4	3/4	3/4	nd
16	4	3/4	4/4	4/4	nd
17	4	4/4	3/4	2/3**	2/2
Total	62	40/62 (64.5%)	32/62 (51.6%)	33/51 (64.7%)	

¶Measured by the pancuronium-sensitized inverted grid test.
†Measured by radioimmuno precipitation assay.
‡Assessed by double immunofluorescence with α-BTX and anti-human IgG antibody.
*The carcasses of three mice engrafted with the BMC from this patient were not available.
**Some mice died overnight of respiratory failure and the carcasses were not assayed.
Reprinted with permission from Z.Y. Wang, P.I. Karachunski, J.F. Howard, Jr. and B.M. Conti-Fine. Transfer of myasthenic symptoms in SCID mice engrafted with lymphocytes from Myasthenia Gravis patients. Role of CD4⁺ and CD8⁺ cells. *Neurology*, 52: 484–497, 1999. Copyright American Academy of Neurology, 1999.

Thus, the appearance of a significant deficit of muscle strength, rather than the appearance of anti-AChR antibodies or their concentration, seems to provide the most reliable assessment of the pathogenic potential of the engrafted BMC.

$CD4^+$ Cells are Necessary for Synthesis of Anti-AChR Antibodies and Transfer of MG Symptoms, $CD8^+$ Cells are Not

The demonstration that engraftment of SCID mice with BMC from MG patients reproduces the essential clinical and immunological characteristics of MG made this chimeric system suitable to investigate whether $CD4^+$ or $CD8^+$ cells or both play an essential role as helper T cell in the synthesis of pathogenic anti-AChR antibodies.

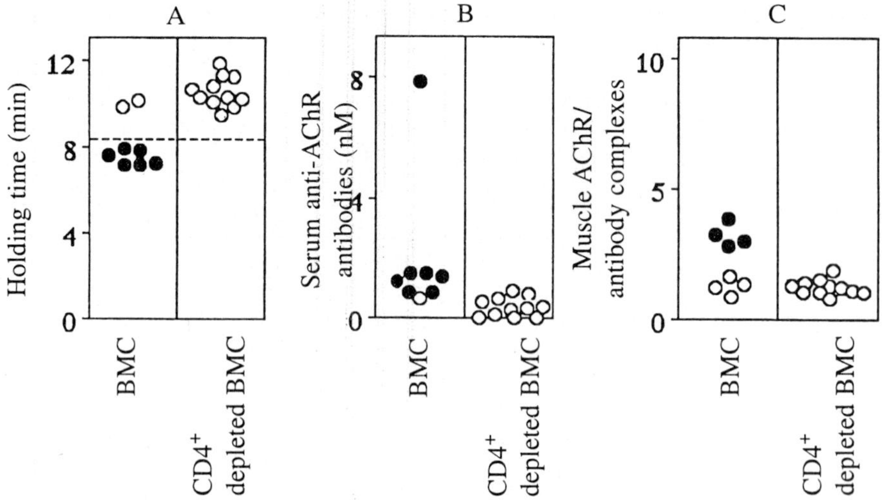

Fig. 4. CD4$^+$ cells are necessary for transfer of MG symptoms and synthesis of human anti-AChR antibodies. We engrafted eight SCID mice with BMC from patients #16-#19, and 11 mice with CD4$^+$ depleted BMC, obtained at the same time from the same patients. A: Measurement of mouse strength by pancuronium sensitized inverted grid test. Dotted line indicates the time below which we considered the mice to have significant reduction of holding time (average holding time of SCID mice engrafted with BMC from normal controls minus two SD). Black symbols indicate mice with a significantly shorter holding time as compared to the holding time of control mice engrafted with BMC from healthy subjects. None of the mice engrafted with CD4$^+$ depleted BMC developed myasthenic weakness, as measured by the holding time in pancuronium sensitized inverted grid test. Six of the mice engrafted with BMC from these patients had significantly reduced holding time. B: Serum concentration of human anti-AChR antibodies in SCID mice engrafted with BMC or CD4$^+$ depleted BMC measured by radioimmuno precipitation assay. Black symbols indicate the presence of a significant antibody concentration, and white symbols indicate that no antibodies were detected. All but one of the mice engrafted with BMC and none of the mice engrafted with CD4$^+$ depleted BMC had significant amounts of human anti-AChR antibodies in the serum. C: Concentration of AChR/human antibody complexes in the muscle of SCID mice engrafted with BMC or CD4$^+$ depleted BMC. Mice were killed 11 weeks after the engraftment. Black symbols indicate the presence of a significant concentration of AChR/antibody complexes and white symbols indicate that no AChR/antibody complexes were detected. Four of the mice engrafted with BMC and none of the mice engrafted with CD4$^+$ depleted BMC had significant amounts of AChR/ antibody complexes in the muscle. Reprinted with permission from Z.Y. Wang, P.I. Karachunski, J.F. Howard, Jr. and B.M. Conti-Fine. Transfer of myasthenic symptoms in SCID mice engrafted with lymphocytes from Myasthenia Gravis patients. Role of CD4$^+$ and CD8$^+$ cells. *Neurology*, 52:484-497, 1999. Copyright American Academy of Neurology, 1999.

To determine whether CD4$^+$ cells are necessary for induction of myasthenic weakness, we engrafted SCID mice with BMC, or BMC depleted in CD4$^+$ T cells from the same MG patients, and we investigated in these mice the appearance of myasthenic symptoms, and of human anti-AChR antibody in the serum and muscle (Fig. 4) [5]. Most mice engrafted with BMC from these patients, and none of those engrafted with their CD4$^+$ depleted BMC, developed significant muscle weakness. All but one of the mice engrafted with BMC had significant concentrations of anti-AChR antibodies in the serum, and half of them had measurable amounts of anti-AChR antibody bound to the muscle AChR. Mice engrafted with CD4$^+$ depleted BMC never had anti-AChR antibody in the serum or muscle.

Previous studies demonstrated the pivotal role of AChR-specific CD4$^+$ cells in rat EMG, using an *in vivo* cell transfer model: adoptive transfer into sublethally irradiated, thymectomized rats of a mixture of B cells and CD4$^+$ T cells from rats immunized with AChR caused synthesis of anti-AChR antibodies and EMG symptoms, while transfer of B cells alone did not [25]. The findings reviewed here prove that also in human MG CD4$^+$ cells are necessary for persistent production of pathogenic anti-AChR antibodies.

To determine whether induction of myasthenic weakness in SCID mice required CD8$^+$ cells, we used BMC and BMC depleted in CD8$^+$ T cells from an MG patient who had class IV MG symptoms, and whose BMC consistently transferred myasthenic weakness in the engrafted SCID mice. All mice engrafted with either BMC or CD8$^+$ depleted BMC developed myasthenic weakness of comparable severity [5]. Also, the mice engrafted with CD8$^+$ depleted BMC had concentrations of anti-AChR antibody that compared with or exceeded those observed in the mice engrafted with the total BMC from this patient [5]. These results support the prevailing notion that CD8$^+$ cells are not crucial for pathogenesis of MG. However, since we carried out experiments with CD8$^+$ depleted BMC with one patient only, these results do not exclude that in some MG patients CD8$^+$ cells might also have a pathogenic role.

CD4$^+$ Cells Specific for "Universal" Epitopes of the AChR α Subunit Drive Synthesis of Pathogenic Antibodies and Permit Transfer of MG Symptoms

The results reported above demonstrate that CD4$^+$ cells are necessary for persistent synthesis of anti-AChR antibodies, but do not give clues as to whether any CD4$^+$ cells would suffice for that purpose, irrespective of the antigenic specificity, or whether anti-AChR CD4$^+$ cells are uniquely effective in cooperating with the anti-AChR B cells, and helping the synthesis of pathogenic antibodies.

Furthermore, we demonstrated previously the human AChR α subunit contains four short (20 residues or less) sequence regions that are recognized by CD4$^+$ cells, and by Th1 CD4$^+$ cells, from most or all MG patients [22, 26-28]. Those sequence segments appear to be recognized by abundant populations of CD4$^+$ cells [22, 28]. The CD4$^+$ cells of MG patients always recognize a complex repertoire on the AChR sequence, on the α and the other subunits (rev. in [2]), making it difficult to devise specific immunsuppressive therapies targeted on the "rogue" autoimmune CD4$^+$ cells. However, the presence of universal α subunit epitopes, that dominate the anti-AChR CD4$^+$ response in all patients, might facilitate that task. Also in rodent EMG a few sequence regions of the AChR α subunit dominate the sensitization of pathogenic CD4$^+$ cells (rev. in [2]), and nasal or subcutaneous "tolerization" procedure using even just one of those immunodominant CD4$^+$ epitopes successfully protected mice from development of EMG [29-31]. To demonstrate that in human MG the CD4$^+$ cells that recognize "universal" epitopes of the AChR α subunit can drive the synthesis of pathogenic anti-AChR antibodies would legitimize their use for development of similar procedure for the management of human MG.

We used the chimeric SCID/human model [5] to test whether anti-AChR CD4$^+$ cells are especially effective in driving the synthesis of pathogenic antibodies, as compared to CD4$^+$ cells specific for unrelated antigens, and whether the CD4$^+$ cells that recognize universal a subunit epitopes drive the synthesis of pathogenic anti-AChR antibodies. Towards those goals, we engrafted SCID mice with CD4$^+$ depleted BMC from a myasthenic patient, and with CD4$^+$ depleted BMC supplemented with individual CD4$^+$ T cell lines propagated from this patient, and specific for the universal AChR epitope sequences, α48-67, α304-322 and α419-437. Other SCID mice were engrafted with CD4$^+$ depleted BMC from this patient supplemented with CD4$^+$ lines specific for TTD or DTD, to determine the ability of activated CD4$^+$ cells specific for other antigens to help synthesis of anti-AChR antibodies. Mice engrafted with the total BMC from this patient served as positive controls for the effectiveness of the transfer of myasthenic weakness, and of the synthesis of human anti-AChR antibodies.

Most mice engrafted with BMC have significant weakness, serum anti-AChR antibodies and muscle AChR/human antibody complexes, that were located at the neuromuscular junctions. None of the mice engrafted with CD4$^+$ depleted BMC, or engrafted with CD4$^+$ depleted BMC supplemented with CD4$^+$ cells specific for TTD or DTD developed weakness or serum anti-AChR antibodies.

Several mice engrafted with CD4$^+$ depleted BMC plus CD4$^+$ cells specific for one of the universal, immunodominant α subunit epitopes developed muscle weakness and had human anti-AChR antibodies in the serum and bound to its muscle AChR. Other mice did not develop detectable weakness, but had serum anti-AChR antibodies, and/or AChR/antibody complexes in the muscle. The frequency of muscle weakness and anti-AChR antibodies in mice engrafted with CD4$^+$ depleted BMC plus the AChR specific CD4$^+$ lines was lower than that in mice engrafted with the BMC from the same patient: this might be because the BMC include a variety of anti-AChR CD4$^+$ cells, specific for a broad repertoire, and able to help a broad repertoire of B cells. On the other hand, the CD4$^+$ depleted BMC reconstituted with an anti-AChR cell line included CD4$^+$ cells specific for a single epitope sequence.

The experiments reviewed above indicate that anti-AChR CD4$^+$ cells are uniquely effective in helping the synthesis of pathogenic anti-AChR antibodies, to an extent that cannot be matched by activated CD4$^+$ cells specific for unrelated antigens. Also, they indicate that the previously identified universal α subunit epitopes must be produced *in vivo*, and are relevant for the pathogenesis of MG, because they are recognized by CD4$^+$ that drive the synthesis of disease-inducing anti-AChR antibodies.

The existence of universal, immunodominant epitopes on the AChR α subunit had been deduced from the response of $CD4^+$ cells *in vitro* to synthetic peptides [22, 26-28]. In principle, a proliferative response *in vitro* of $CD4^+$ cells to AChR sequences might not indicate a pathogenic role *in vivo* of the cells recognizing those epitopes. Also, synthetic AChR peptides might be processed differently than the native AChR molecule, and yield epitopes which are not representative of those recognized *in vivo* by the autoimmune anti-AChR $CD4^+$ cells involved in anti-AChR synthesis. The experiments reviewed above, and reported in detail in reference 5, dispel the above concerns.

Conclusions

Transfer into SCID mice of immune cells from myasthenic patients reproduces the clinical and immunological characteristics of MG [5, 19-20]. Most mice engrafted with BMC from MG patients, but none of those engrafted with BMC from healthy controls, developed a reduction of the muscle strength, which could be reversed transiently by a cholinesterase inhibitor, as it occurs in human MG. Most of those mice, but none of the mice engrafted with BMC from healthy subjects, developed human anti-AChR antibodies in the serum and had muscle AChR complexed by human antibodies at the neuromuscular junction. Detailed examination of the effects resulting from engraftment of BMC from individual patients revealed different patterns, that are consistent with the observed lack of correlation between anti-AChR antibody titer and symptom severity in MG patients, with the complex repertoire of anti-AChR antibodies, and with the mechanisms of their pathogenic effects.

The relationships that existed between appearance of muscle weakness and presence of anti-AChR antibodies in the sera and muscle of the engrafted mice were complex and varied. Yet, we observed a close correlation between the severity of the patient's symptoms, and the ability of the engrafted BMC to cause muscle weakness, suggesting that activated anti-AChR T and B cells are especially abundant in the blood during acute phases of the disease.

These studies [5] prove that in human MG $CD4^+$ cells, and specifically anti-AChR $CD4^+$ cells, are necessary for production of pathogenic anti-AChR antibodies: SCID mice engrafted with immune cells depleted in $CD4^+$ cells, even if they were supplemented with $CD4^+$ cells specific for antigens other than the AChR, never developed anti-AChR antibodies or reduction of the muscle strength. The finding that SCID mice engrafted with $CD4^+$ depleted BMC supplemented with $CD4^+$ cells specific for universal AChR epitopes verifies that synthesis of pathogenic anti-AChR antibodies involves primarily AChR-specific $CD4^+$ cells, and demonstrates that the previously identified "universal" α subunit epitopes are relevant for the pathogenesis of MG, since they sensitize $CD4^+$ cells able to drive the synthesis of disease-inducing anti-AChR antibodies.

The results obtained in SCID mice engrafted with BMC from MG patients clearly indicates the feasibility of transferring MG symptoms and ability to synthesize human anti-AChR antibodies. Thus, this chimeric system will be useful to study the effects of manipulations of the engrafted human cells on the transferred myasthenic syndrome. Also, this system can be used to study the ability of autoimmune $CD4^+$ cells of defined epitope specificity to drive the synthesis of autoAg-specific antibodies, and therefore quantify their pathogenic potential.

Acknowledgement

This work was partially supported by the NINDS Grant NS23919 and by a Research Grant from the Muscular Dystrophy Association (to B.M. C.-F.). Dr. Wang was a recipient of a Muscular Disease Research Fellowship from the Muscular Dystrophy Association.

References

1. Toyka, K.V., D.B. Drachman, A. Pestronk and I. Kao. 1975. Myasthenia gravis: passive transfer from man to mouse. *Science* 190: 397.
2. Conti-Fine, B.M., M. Bellone, J.F. Howard Jr and M.P. Protti. 1997. Myasthenia Gravis. The Immunobiology of an Autoimmune Disease. Neuroscience Intelligence Unit. R.G. Landes. Austin, TX:1-230.
3. Hohlfeld R., I. Kalies, B. Kohleisen, K. Heininger, B.M. Conti-Tronconi and K.V. Toyka. 1986. Myasthenia gravis: Stimulation of antireceptor autoantibodies by autoreactive T cell lines. *Neurology* 36: 618.
4. Hohlfeld R., K.V. Toyka, K. Heininger, H. Grosse-Wilde and I. Kalies. 1984. Autoimmune human T lymphocytes specific for acetylcholine receptor. *Nature* 310: 244.
5. Wang, Z.-Y., P.I. Karachunski, J.F. Howard Jr. and B.M. Conti-Fine. 1999. Myasthenia in SCID mice grafted with myasthenic patient lymphocytes. Role of $CD4^+$ and $CD8^+$ cells. *Neurology* 52: 484.
6. Yuen, M.-H., M.P. Protti, B. Diethelm-Okita, L Moiola, J.F. Howard Jr. and B.M. Conti-Fine. 1995. Immunoregulatory $CD8^+$ cells recognize antigen-activated $CD4^+$ cells in myasthenia gravis patients and in healthy controls. *J. Immunol.* 154: 1508.
7. Zhang, G.-X., C.-G. Ma, B.-G. Xiao, M. Bakhiet, H. Link and T. Olsson. 1995. Depletion of $CD8^+$ T cells suppresses the development of experimental autoimmune myasthenia gravis in Lewis rats. *Eur. J. Immunol.* 25: 1191.
8. Zhang, G-X, Xiao B-G, Bakhiet M, et al. 1996. Both $CD4^+$ and $CD8^+$ T cells are essential to induce experimental autoimmune myasthenia gravis. *J. Exp. Med.* 184: 349.
9. Shenoy, M., R. Kaul, E. Goluszko, C. David and C. Christadoss. 1994. Effect of MHC class I and CD8 cell deficiency on experimental autoimmune myasthenia gravis pathogenesis. *J. Immunol.* 153: 5330.
10. Raju, R., W.-Z. Zhan, P.I. Karachunski, B.M. Conti-Fine, G.S. Siek and C. David. 1998. Polymorphism at the HLA DQ locus determines susceptibility to experimental autoimmune myasthenia gravis. *J. Immunol.* 160: 4169.
11. Raju, R., W.-Z. Zhan, P.I. Karachunski, G. Sieck, B.M. Conti-Fine and C. David. 1998. Susceptibility of HLA DR3 transgenic mice to experimental autoimmune myasthenia gravis. *Ann. N.Y. Acad. Sci.* 841: 360.
12. Bosma, G.C., M.R. Davisson, M.R. Ruetsch, H.O. Sweet, L.D. Schultz and M. J. Bosma. 1989. The mouse mutation severe combined immune deficiency (SCID) is on chromosome 16. *Immunogenetics* 29: 54.

13. Simpson, E., J. Farrant, and P. Chandler. 1991. Phenotypic and functional studies of human peripheral blood lymphocytes engrafted in scid mice. *Immunol. Rev.* 124: 97.
14. Smith, C.I.E., M.R. Abedi, K.B. Islam, M.E.B. Johansson, B. Christensson and L. Hammarstrom. 1991. Humoral immunity in scid mice reconstituted with cells from immunoglobulin-deficient or normal humans. *Immunol. Rev.* 124: 113.
15. Mima, T., Y. Saeki, S. Ohshima, et al. 1995. Transfer of rheumatoid arthritis into severe combined immunodeficient mice. The pathogenetic implications of T cell populations oligoclonally expanding in the rheumatoid joints. *J. Clin. Invest.* 96: 1746.
16. Gilhar, A., Y. Ullmann, T. Berkutzki, B. Assy and R.S. Kallish. 1998. Autoimmune hair loss (alopecia areata) transferred by T lymphocytes to human scalp explants on SCID mice. *J. Clin. Invest.* 101: 62.
17. Lafaille, J.J., F. Van de Keere, A.L. Hsu, et al. 1997. Myelin basic protein-specific T helper 2 (Th2) cells cause experimental autoimmune encephalomyelitis in immunodeficient hosts rather than protect them from the disease. *J. Exp. Med.* 186: 307.
18. Pakala, S.V., M.O. Kurrer and J.D. Katz. 1997. T helper 2 (Th2) T cells induce acute pancreatitis and diabetes in immune-compromised nonobese diabetic (NOD) mice. *J. Exp. Med.* 186: 299.
19. Schonbeck, S., F. Padberg, R Hohlfeld and H. Wekerle. 1992. Transplantation of thymic autoimmune microenvironment to severe combined immunodeficiency mice. *J. Clin. Invest.* 90: 245.
20. Martino, G., B.L. DuPont, R.L. Wollmann, et al. 1993. The human-SCID myasthenic mouse; a new approach for study of myasthenia gravis. *Ann. Neurol.* 34: 48.
21. Karachunski, P.I., N. Ostlie, M. Bellone, A.J. Infante and B. M. Conti-Fine. 1995. Mechanisms by which the I-A^{bm12} mutation influences susceptibility to experimental myasthenia gravis. A study in homozygous and heterozygous mice. Scand. *J. Immunol.* 42: 215.
22. Manfredi, A.A., M.P. Protti, X.D. Wu, J.F. Howard Jr and B.M. Conti-Tronconi. 1992. CD4$^+$ T-epitope repertoire on the human acetylcholine receptor α subunit in severe myasthenia gravis. A study with synthetic peptides. *Neurology* 42: 1092.
23. Manfredi, A.A., M.P. Protti, M.W.M. Dalton, J.F. Howard Jr. and B.M. Conti-Tronconi. 1993. T helper cell recognition of muscle acetylcholine receptor in myasthenia gravis: epitopes on the γ and δ subunits. *J. Clin. Invest.* 92: 1055.
24. Besinger, U.A., K.V. Toyka, M. Hömberg, K. Heininger, R. Hohlfeld and A. Fateh-Moghadam. 1983. Myasthenia gravis: Long-term correlation of binding and bungarotoxin blocking antibodies against acetylcholine receptors with changes in disease severity. *Neurology* 33: 1316.
25. Hohlfeld, R., I Kalies, M. Ernst, U.-P. Ketelsen and H. Wekerle. 1982. T-lymphocytes in experimental myasthenia gravis: Isolation of T-helper cell lines. *J. Neurol. Sci.* 57: 265.
26. Protti, M.P., A.A. Manfredi, C. Straub, J.F. Howard Jr. and B.M. Conti-Tronconi. 1990. Immunodominant regions for T helper sensitization on the human nicotinic receptor a subunit in myasthenia gravis. *Proc. Natl. Acad. Sci. U.S.A.* 87: 7792.
27. Moiola, L., M.P. Protti, J.F. Howard and B.M. Conti-Tronconi. 1994. Myasthenia Gravis: Residues of the a and g subunits of muscle acetylcholine receptor involved in formation of immunodominant CD4$^+$ epitopes. *J. Immunol.* 152: 4686.
28. Wang, Z.-Y., D.K. Okita, J.F. Howard Jr. and B.M. Conti-Fine. 1997. Th1 epitope repertoire on the a subunit of human muscle acetylcholine receptor in myasthenia gravis. *Neurology* 48: 1643.

29. Karachunski, P.I., N. Ostlie, D. Okita and B.M. Conti-Fine 1997. Protection from experimental myasthenia gravis in C57Bl/6 mice by sniffing of synthetic $CD4^+$ T cells epitopes. *J. Clin. Invest.* 100: 3027.
30. Wu, B., C. Deng, E. Goluszko and P. Christadoss. 1997. Tolerance to a dominant T cell epitope in the acetylcholine receptor molecule induces epitope spread and suppresses murine myasthenia gravis. *J. Immunol.* 159: 3016.
31. Karachunski, P.I., N. Ostlie, D. Okita, R. Garman and B.M. Conti-Fine. 1999. Subcutaneous administration of T epitope sequences of the acetylcholine receptor prevents experimental myasthenia gravis. *J. Neuroimmunol.* 93: 108.

Myasthenia Gravis: Disease mechanisms and immunointervention
P. Christadoss (Ed)

13. Evidence for an Upregulation of Acetylcholine Receptor Messenger Subunits Triggered by Antibody-Mediated Receptor Internalization in Human Myasthenia Gravis Muscles

Thierry Guyon[1], Abdelilah Wakkach[1], Sandrine Poea[1], Vincent Mouly[2], Isabelle Klingel-Schmitt[1], Philippe Levasseur[3], David Beeson[4], Orna Asher[5], Socrates Tzartos[6] and Sonia Berrih-Aknin[1]

[1]CNRS ESA 8078 and [3]Départment de Chirurgie Thoracique Hôpital Marie Lannelongue, 92350 Le Plessis-Robinson, France

[2]CNRS URA 1448, UFR Biomédical des Saints Pères, 75720 Paris Cedex 06

[4]Neurosciences Group, Institute of Molecular Medicine, Department of Clinical Neurology, John Radcliffe Hospital, University of Oxford, Oxford OX3 9DU, UK

[5]Department of Chemical Immunology, The Weizmann Institute of Science, Rehovot 76100, Israel

[6]The Hellenic Pasteur Institute, Athens, Greece

Introduction

The muscle nicotinic acetylcholine receptor (nAChR) is a well-characterized, ligand-gated ion channel of 270 kD that forms a pentameric complex of four homologous subunits with a molar stoichiometry of α_2, β, ε, δ [1, 2]. In mammalian muscle, regulation of nAChR subunit mRNAs and the distribution of nAChRs along the fiber are developmentally regulated. Transcript levels increase during myogenic differentiation and are repressed during muscle innervation; denervation results in re-accumulation [3]. The nAChR ε and γ-subunits are also under developmental control, with expression of two types of channels in mammals. In early embryonic stages and upon denervation, a low-conductance, long-open-time channel composed of α, β, δ and γ-subunits and distributed throughout the fiber length predominates [4], whereas in adult fibers, a high-conductance, brief-open-time channel containing α, β, δ and ε-subunits is expressed exclusively at the motor-endplate [5].

Nicotinic AChR is the main autoantigen target in myasthenia gravis (MG), a human disorder of neuromuscular transmission in which autoantibodies directed against nAChR at the neuromuscular junction are found in 85% of patient's sera and cause functional nAChR loss at the endplate post-synaptic membrane, leading to muscle weakness and fatigability of voluntary muscle [6]. The pathogenicity of anti-nAChR antibodies has been clearly demonstrated by their ability to transfer disease to normal animals [7], and to cause loss of nAChR expression in a myotube culture system [8]. Several studies failed to show any correlations between the severity of the disease and either antibody titers and the functional activity of anti-nAChR antibodies in myotube cultures, whereas the ability of patient sera to degrade nAChR does correlate with antibody titers [8, 9]. The pathogenic mechanisms of anti-nAChR antibodies directed against the endplate nAChR are well established [10], but little is known of the capacity of muscle cells to regulate nAChR expression after autoimmune attack. The α-subunit contains the main immunogenic region (MIR) recognized by autoantibodies in MG [11]. To elucidate the regulation of nAChR gene expression in human MG, we studied by quantitative RT-PCR using an internal standard for each subunit, the transcriptional regulation of nAChR subunit genes in muscle biopsy specimens from MG patients and controls. We observed an up-regulation of nAChR α, β, δ and ε mRNA levels in muscle samples from severely affected MG patients, suggesting the existence of a compensatory mechanism that attenuates the loss of nAChR in human MG endplates. We analyzed the compensatory mechanism of regulation triggered after nAChR loss by monoclonal anti-nAChR antibodies in both the TE671 muscle cell line showing no spontaneous electrical activity and cultured normal human myotubes. A similar increase in β and δ-subunit mRNA levels was observed in response to nicotinic AchR loss mediated by monoclonal anti-nAChR antibodies, suggesting the existence of a new muscular signaling pathway system coupled to nAChR internalization and independent of muscle electrical activity.

Results and Discussion

We investigated, in patients with myasthenia gravis, whether changes in the level of the affected autoantigen (nAChR) may alter the regulation of nAChR subunit gene transcription.

nAChR mRNA are Increased in MG Patient Muscles, but the Mechanism Involved is Different from Denervation

Quantitative RT-PCR studies were performed on total RNA extracted from representative muscle samples of myasthenic and non-myasthenic patients to measure the steady state level of nAChR mRNA α, β, δ and ε-subunit. Our data show an up-regulation of nAChR α, β, δ and ε subunit transcripts in MG muscles compared to normal muscles and correlated with the severity of the disease. The mean number of nAChR β-subunit molecules was $5.3 \pm 1.1 \times 10^5$/µg of total RNA in control samples, and $12 \pm 2.4 \times 10^5$ ($p < 0.02$ versus controls) and 21.5 $\pm$ 6.4×10^5/µg of total RNA ($p < 0.002$ versus controls) in MG patients with moderate and severe forms, respectively. The mean number of nAChR δ-subunit molecules was $4.4 \pm 0.5 \times 10^5$/µg of total RNA in control samples and 6.7 ± 1.1

$\times 10^5$ (not significantly different from controls) and $9.5 \pm 1.9 \times 10^5$ ($p < 0.01$ versus controls) in patients with moderate and severe forms, respectively. Similarly, the mean number of nAChR ε-subunit molecules was $0.06 \pm 0.01 \times 10^5$/μg of total RNA in control samples and $0.15 \pm 0.03 \times 10^5$ (not significantly different from controls) and $0.25 \pm 0.07 \times 10^5$ ($p < 0.006$ vs controls) in patients with moderate and severe forms, respectively. These results are in accordance with data obtained in denervation models and in muscles of MG animal models where a clear increase in nAChR messengers was observed by in situ experiments in all the muscle fibers [12, 13]. However, we have analyzed by Northern blot the level of myogenic factor transcripts in muscle biopsies of total muscle RNA from 8 MG patients and 4 control muscle samples (data not shown). We observed no increase in myogenic transcript levels in MG muscles compared to healthy muscles, whereas myogenin, MyoD and MRF4 mRNA levels are up-regulated in denervated models [13, 14]. In addition, we performed RT-PCR with primers specific for the γ subunit on total muscle RNA from 6 MG patients (3 severely and 3 moderately affected) and 3 controls. Total RNA extracted from the TE671 muscular cell line (mainly expressing the fetal form of nAChR; [15]) was used as a positive control for γ-subunit expression. The γ-subunit was not amplified by PCR in MG or control muscle, by contrast to the TE671 muscular cell line. Southern blotting of PCR amplification products showed a faint band in a few samples, indicating that the fetal subunit is hardly expressed in the human adult sternocleidomastoid muscle explored in this study, whereas a strong increase in γ-subunit mRNA levels is observed in denervation models [16]. Similarly, we observed ε-subunit mRNA up-regulation in MG muscles, whereas minor modifications of ε-subunit mRNA levels are observed in denervation models [17]. All of these findings suggest that the mechanism involved in the regulation of nAChR expression in human MG differs from that underlying the denervation process. It is important to underline that MG is not generally associated with denervation or morphological modifications of motoneuron endings [18], and acetylcholine release at muscle endplates from MG patients is increased [19]. Although a decrease in miniature endplate potential amplitude is generally observed in MG muscles, as in denervation models, our observation is compatible with data showing that blockade of electrical activity does not necessarily modify γ-subunit gene expression. Indeed, γ-subunit mRNA expression is virtually unmodified in tetrodotoxin (TTX) and α-BgT-blocked motoneuron models [17]. Alternatively, the observed changes in myasthenic muscle could be explained by adaptation to long-term muscle inactivity. Indeed, Adams et al. found an adaptive response in long-term denervated rat muscles, in which nAChR γ-subunit mRNA levels are decreased while nAChR ε-subunit mRNA levels are increased [20]. However, this is unlikely, as no expression of the fetal subunit was observed in EAMG rodent muscles after early exploration [13].

Interestingly, in control muscles, the mean ε-subunit mRNA level was much lower than that of the other subunits ($0.06 \pm 0.01 \times 10^5$ molecules/μg of total RNA), raising the possibility that ε-subunit mRNA expression is limiting in control muscle. The same pattern of relative expression between the ε-subunit and the other subunit mRNA levels was observed in muscle from MG patients with moderate disease and severe disease, raising the hypothesis that in both normal and MG muscles, ε-subunit mRNA is expressed in limited amounts compared to the other subunits. However, we cannot exclude that ε-subunit mRNA are more efficiently translated than those of the other subunit.

To determine which nAChR subunit is most sensitive to regulation, the increase in mRNA expression for each subunit was calculated for all MG muscle samples as the ratio of the mRNA molecule number to the mean mRNA molecule number in control muscle (Table 1). Median values indicated that the increase in ε-subunit mRNA was greater than that in the other subunit mRNAs, both in MG patients with a severe form of the disease (3.l-fold for ε-subunit versus 2.5-fold for β-subunit, 2. 1-fold for α-subunit and 1.7-fold for δ-subunit mRNA) and those with a moderate form (2.8-fold for ε-subunit versus 1.8-fold for β-subunit, 1.3-fold for δ-subunit and 0.6-fold for α-subunit mRNA). In addition, the maximum increase in transcripts coding for each nAChR subunit was about 18-, 16- and 13.9-fold for α, β and ε-subunit mRNA, whereas the maximum increase in δ-subunit mRNA was only about 5-fold. Thus, the δ-subunit appeared to be less sensitive to regulation in both moderately and severely affected MG patients (Table 1).

Table 1. AChR subunit increase ratio in MG patients compared to healthy controls

			AChR subunit increase rate			
			α	β	δ	ε
MG	Mild form	Seronegative	0.9 (3)*	1.7 (3)	1.8 (2)	2.2 (2)
		Seropositive	0.7 (4)	2.5 (7)	1.4 (5)	2.8 (4)
	Severe form	Seronegative	4.6 (5)	6.8 (3)	1.4 (3)	6.5 (3)
		Seropositive	4.4 (8)	3.1 (9)	2.4 (8)	3.4 (8)
	Max. increase		18	16	5	13.9

α, β, δ and ε-subunit mRNA expression was studied in 20 MG patients and 6 controls, in 22 MG patients and 7 controls, in 18 MG patients and 7 controls and in 17 MG patients and 5 controls, respectively.
Results are expressed as the mean ratio between the number of molecules in the patient muscle and the mean number of molecules in the control muscle. The increase is more clearly observed in severely affected patients. The δ subunit is less compensated compared to the other ones.
*Number of patients studied.

Evidence of an Anti-nAChR Antibody-Dependent Regulatory Mechanism
It is interesting that muscle from seronegative patients also showed an increase in α, β as well as δ or ε-subunit mRNA (Table 1). These data demonstrate that the increase in nAChR subunit mRNA observed in muscle from most MG patients does not correlate with the anti-nAChR autoantibody titer. It has been established that altered nAChR function can modulate the electrical activity of muscle cells

and could, in turn, increase nAChR gene expression via activation of second messengers such as Ca^{2+} [21]. As the impairment of electrical activity is clear in seronegative patients [22], the most likely hypothesis is that a muscle activity pathway is involved in the compensatory mechanism induced in seronegative MG muscles. To further study this hypothesis, we analyzed the effect of anti-nAChR monoclonal antibodies (MAb35 and MAb192) on both surface nAChR expression (by ^{125}I-α-Bgt binding studies) and nAChR α, δ and β-subunit mRNA levels (by quantitative PCR assays) in the TE671 muscle cell line (Table 2), which expresses nAChR [15]. We used MAb35 and MAb192, directed against the extracellular MIR region of nAChR to induce surface nAChR internalization by antigenic modulation in muscle cells [23]. Incubation of TE671 cells for 16 hours with MAb35 or Mab192 induced a loss of nAChR expression at the TE671 cell surface, which was then compensated for by an up-regulation of β and δ-subunit messenger levels. Of note, in the same conditions, no modification of α-subunit messenger levels was observed (Table 2), possibly due to the strong expression of a partially mature form of the nAChR α-subunit found in the cytoplasm of TE671 cells [24]. The specificity of the antibody effect on nAChR expression was checked by incubating the TE671 cells for 16 hours with two monoclonal antibodies (MAb164 and MAbI55) directed against the intracellular part of nAChR. No effect on messenger up-regulation and nAChR expression was observed with these monoclonal antibodies (Table 2).

Table 2. Effect of monoclonal anti-nAChR antibodies and *a*-Bgt on nAChR mRNA and protein levels in TE671 cell line

		% of expression after treatment			
		AChR subunit mRNA			AChR protein
		α	β	δ	
Anti-cytoplasmic epitope	Mab 155	106	100	100	100 ± 2
	Mab 164	79	104	114	97 ± 3
Anti-MIR epitope	Mab 35	97	192	285	25 ± 2
	α-Bgt	100	108	107	–

Results are expressed as the percentage of expression of α, β, and δ AChR subunits mRNAs compared to untreated cultures. RNA was extracted from α-Bgt, MAb164/ Mab155 (anti-cytoplasmic epitopes) and MAb35 (anti-MIR)-treated cells, as well as from untreated cells. A clear increase in β- and δ-subunit mRNA levels was observed in MAb35-treated cells, whereas α-Bgt and Mab164/Mab155 had no effect on messenger levels. The loss of nAChR is indicated in each set of conditions (right column).

As there is no spontaneous electrical activity in our culture system, these findings suggest an original anti-nAChR antibody-dependent regulatory mechanism in addition to the muscular activity pathway that could be involved in seropositive MG muscles. It is not clear, however, how nAChR loss at the cell surface triggers such a compensatory mechanism, as nAChR is not directly coupled to second messenger generation.

We showed that blockade of nAChR function by α-Bgt, which does not induce nAChR internalization in TE671 cells, did not induce an increase in the nAChR β- and δ-subunit mRNA level (Table 2). The loss of surface nAChR after anti-nAChR antibody exposure is essentially due to antigenic modulation requiring antibody-dependent cross-linking of membrane-bound receptors [23], resulting in nAChR internalization and in an increased degradation rate, as well as to complement-mediated membrane lysis [25]. Thus, our findings suggest the involvement of nAChR internalization and/or membrane lysis in the up-regulation of mRNA expression. As regards the regulatory signaling pathway triggered by nAChR antibody-mediated loss, there are two main possibilities:

1. The synaptic junction forms a superstructure characterized by an extraordinarily dense clustering of receptors for nerve-derived signals and colocalized with nAChR. Some receptors, such as ErbB3/ErbB2 for heregulin (ARIA), which display intrinsic tyrosine kinase activity, have been studied. These receptors accumulate densely at the neuromuscular junction and are involved in nAChR expression [26]. Heregulin stimulates nAChR gene expression in muscle via an independent electrical activity signaling pathway [27]. Thus, in the case of seropositive MG patients, internalization of nAChR at the muscle endplate and/or post-synaptic membrane lysis could locally modify the structure of the postsynaptic membrane and the ultrastructural conformation of these receptors, which could then activate transducer signals and a tyrosine kinase-signaling pathway, which could in turn trigger transcription of nAChR gene subunits.

2. Disruption of actin networks by cytochalasin has been reported to up-regulate nAChR expression in TE671 cells, suggesting the involvement of the cytoskeleton in membrane receptor regulation [28]. Some physical interactions between nAChR and other cytoskeletal proteins have been reported, namely interactions between the nAChR β-subunit and rapsyn involved in phosphorylation of the receptor and its clustering [29]. Recently, an association between nAChR, src and fyn (a member of the tyrosine kinase src family) was also observed [30]. Evidence for an interaction between the src SH3 domain and an actin-associated protein of 110 KDa has been described [31]. Thus, co-internalization of nAChR and the attached protein and/or post-synaptic membrane lysis could modulate the stability of the neighboring proteins and/or modulate the activity of tyrosine kinase-coupled proteins, which could in turn trigger up-regulation of nAChR messengers.

Conclusion

Taken together, our data show that the mechanism regulating the expression of nAChR genes in muscle from patients with MG differs from that of denervation models. We demonstrate that blockade of electrical activity, is not the only regulatory pathway involved in nAChR mRNA regulation. Monoclonal anti-nAChR antibodies are able to up-regulate nAChR mRNA expression via an nAChR-coupled signaling pathway triggered by receptor internalization. The compensatory mechanism triggered by nAChR loss demonstrates that the target muscle is not passively attacked by the autoantibodies; this mechanism of compensation could be one factor contributing to the mildness of the disease.

Acknowledgments

This work was supported by grants from AFM (Association Francaise Contre Les Myopathies), AFIRST (Association Franco-Israélienne pour la Recherche Scientifique et Technique), CNRS (Centre National de la Recherche Scientifique), CNAMTS (Caisse Nationale d'Assurance Maladie des Travailleurs Salariés), the Myasthenia Gravis Association and the BIOMED-1 program of EU (CT93-1100).

References

1. Raftery, M., M. Hunkapillar, C. Strader and L. Hood. 1980. Acetylcholine Receptor: Complex of Homologous Subunits. *Science* 208: 1454–1457.
2. Popot, J.L. and J.P. Changeux. 1984. The Nicotinic Receptor of Acetylcholine: Structure of an Oligomeric Integral Membrane Protein. *Physiol. Rev.* 64: 1162–1239.
3. Buonanno, A. and J.P. Merlie. 1986. Transcription Regulation of the Nicotinic Acetylcholine Receptor Gene During Muscle Development. *J. Biol. Chem.* 261: 11452–11455.
4. Mishina, M., T. Takai. K. Imoto, M, Noda, T. Takahashi and S. Numa. 1986. Molecular Distinction Between Fetal and Adult Forms of Muscle Acetylcholine Receptor. *Nature* 321: 406–411.
5. Shieh, B.H., M. Ballivet and J. Schmidt. 1988. Acetylcholine Receptors Synthesis Rate and Levels of Receptor Subunit Messengers RNAs in Chick Muscle. *Neuroscience* 24: 175–187.
6. Fambrough, D.M., D.B. Drachman and S. Satyamurti. 1973. Neuromuscular Junction in MG: Decreased Acetylcholine Receptor. *Science* 182: 293–295.
7. Toyka, K.V., D.R. Drachman, A. Pestronk and I. Kao. 1975. Myasthenia Gravis: Passive Transfer From Man to Mouse. *Science* (Wash. DC). 190: 397–399.
8. Eymard, B., S. de la Porte, C. Pannier, S. Berrih Aknin, E. Morel, M. Fardeau, J.F. Bach and J, Koenig. 1988. Effect of Myasthenic Patient Sera on the Number and Distribution of Acetylcholine Receptors in Muscle and Nerve–Muscle Cultures from Rat. Correlations with Clinical State. *J. Neurol. Sci.* 86: 41–59.
9. Tzartos, S.J. D. Sophianos, K. Zimmerman and A. Starzinski Powitz. 1986. Antigenic Modulation of Human Myotube Acetylcholine Receptor by Myasthenic Sera. Serum Titer Determines Receptor Internalization Rate. *J. Immunol.* 136: 3231–3238.
10. Richman, D.P., R.L. Wollmann, R.A. Maselli, C.M. Gomez, A.L. Corey, M.A. Agius and R.H. Fairclough. 1993. Effector Mechanisms of Myasthenic Antibodies. *Ann. N .Y. Acad. Sci.* 681: 264–273.
11. Tzartos, S., Kokla, S.L. Walgrave and B.M. Conti-Tronconi. 1988. Localization of the Main Immunogenic Region of Human Muscle Acetylcholine Receptor to Residues 67–76 of the α Subunit. *Proc. Natl. Acad. Sci.* USA 85: 2899.
12. Brenner, H.R., V. Witzemann and B. Sakmann. 1990. Imprinting of Acetylcholine Receptor Messenger RNA Accumulation in Mammalian Neuromuscular Synapses. *Nature* 344: 544–547.

13. Asher, O., W.A. Kues, V. Witzemann, S.J. Tzartos, S. Fuchs and M.C. Souroujon. 1993. Increased Gene Expression of Acetylcholine Receptor and Myogenic Factors in Passively Transferred Experimental Autoimmune Myasthenia Gravis. *J. Immunol.* 151: 6442–6450.
14. Asher, O., S. Fuchs, D. Zuk, D. Rapaport and A. Buonanno. 1992. Changes in the Expression of mRNA for Myogenic Factors and Other Muscles Specific Proteins in Experimental Autoimmune Myasthenia Gravis. *FEBS (Fed. Eur. Biochem. Soc.) Letters* 299: 15–18.
15. Luther, M.A., R. Schoepfer, P. Whiting, B. Casey, Y. Blatt, M.S. Montal, M. Montal and J. Lindstrom. 1989. A Muscle Acetylcholine Receptor is Expressed in the Human Cerebellar Medulloblastoma Cell Line TE671. *J. Neurosci.* 9: 1082–1096.
16. Goldman, D., H.R. Brenner, and S. Heinemann. 1988. Acetylcholine Receptor α, β, γ and δ subunit mRNA levels are regulated by muscle activity. *Neuron.* 1: 329–333.
17. Witzemann, V., H.R. Brenner and B. Sakmann. 1991. Neural Factors Regulate nAChR Subunit mRNAs at Rat Neuromuscular Synapses. *J. Cell. Biol.* 114: 125–141.
18. Drachman, D.B. 1994. Myasthenia Gravis. *N. Engl. J. Med.* 330: 1797–1810.
19. Plomp, J.J., G.Th.H. Van Kempen, M. De Baets, Y.M.F. Graus, J.B.M. Kuks, and P.C. Molenaar. 1995. Acetylcholine Release in Myasthenia Gravis: Regulation at Single End-Plate Level. *Ann. Neurol.* 37; 627–636.
20. Adams, L., B.M. Carlson, L. Henderson and D. Goldman. 1995. Adaptation of Nicotinic Acetylcholine Receptor, Myogenin and MRF4 Gene Expression to Long-Term Muscle Denervation. *J. Cell. Biol.* 131: 1341–1349.
21. Laufer, R. and J.P. Changertx, 1989. Activity-Dependent Regulation of Gene Expression in Muscle and Neuronal Cells. *Mol. Neurobiol.* 3: 1–53.
22. Mossman, S., A. Vincent and J. Newsom-Davis. 1986. Myasthenia Gravis Without Acetylcholine-Receptor Antibody: A Distinct Disease Entity. *The Lancet* i: 116–119.
23. Sophianos, D. and S.J. Tzartos. 1989. Fab Fragments of Monoclonal Antibodies Protect the Human Acetylcholine Receptor Against Antigenic Modulation Caused by Myasthenia Gravis. *J. Autoimm.* 2: 777–789.
24. Conroy, W.G., M.S. Saedi and J. Lindstrom. 1990. TE671 Cells Express an Abundance of a Partially Mature Acetylcholine Receptor α Subunit Which has Characteristics of an Assembly Intermediate. *J. Biol. Chem.* 265: 21642–21651.
25. Engel, A.G. and G. Fumagalli. 1982. Mechanisms of Aetylcholine Receptor Loss from the Neuromuscular Junction. *Ciba Found. Symp.* 90: 197–224.
26. Altiok, N., J.L. Bessereau and J.P. Changeux. 1995. ErbB3 and ErbB2/neu Mediate the Effect of Heregulin on Acetylcholine Receptor Gene Expression in Muscle: Differential Expression at the Endplate. *EMBO (Eur. Mol. Biol. Organ.) J.* 14: 4258–4266.
27. Altiok, N., S. Altiok and J.P. Changeux. 1997. Heregulin-Stimulated Acetylcholine Receptor Gene Expression in Muscle: Requirement for MAP Kinase and Evidence for a Parallel Inhibitory Pathway Independent of Electrical Activity. *EMBO J.* 16: 717–725.
28. Bencherif, M. and R.J. Lukas. 1993. Cytochalasin Modulation of Nicotinic Cholinergic Receptor Expression and Muscarinic Receptor Function in Human TE671/RD Cells: A Possible Functional Role of the Cytoskeleton. *J. Neurochem.* 61: 852–864.
29. Hill, J.A., Jr. 1992. Nicotinic Receptor-Associated 43K Protein and Progressive Stabilization of the Postsynaptic Membrane. *Mol. Neurobiol.* 6: 1–17.

30. Fuhrer, C., and Z.W. Hall. 1996. Functional Interaction of Src Family Kinases with the Acetylcholine Receptor in C2 Myotubes. *J. Biol. Chem.* 13: 32474–32481.

31. Flynn, D.C., T.H. Leu, A.B. Reynolds and J.T. Parsons. 1993. Identification and Sequence Analysis of cDNAs encoding a 110–Kilodalton Actin Filament-Associated pp60src Substrate. *Mol. Cell. Biol.* 13: 7892–7900.

Myasthenia Gravis: Disease mechanisms and immunointervention
P. Christadoss (Ed)

14. Oral Administration of Peptide Tα146-162 Prevents EAMG in Mice

F. Baggi, F. Andreetta, E. Caspani, M. Milani, O. Simonicini, R. Longhi*, F. Cornelio, R. Mantegazza and C. Antozzi

Department of Neuromuscular Diseases,
National Neurological Institute "Carlo Besta", Milan, Italy

*Institute of Biocatalysis and Molecular Recognition, Milan, Italy

Introduction

Myasthenia gravis (MG) is an autoimmune disorder of the neuromuscular junction in which antibodies to the acetylcholine receptor (anti-AChR Ab) lead to muscle weakness and fatigability [1]. MG is treated with corticosteroids and immunosuppressive drugs which exert a non-specific action on the immune system. Moreover, their efficacy is frequently limited, and sometimes overwhelmed, by drug toxicity [2]. Experimental autoimmune MG (EAMG), the animal model of human myasthenia, is a T cell-dependent, B cell-mediated disorder suitable for the investigation of new therapeutic strategies. Indeed, data available on the structure and immunological recognition of the nicotinic AChR allow the design of antigen-specific approaches potentially able to modulate the autoimmune response to the AChR.

Considerable lines of evidence have shown that antigen-specific T cells can be tolerized by the oral administration of antigens. This promising approach has been extensively investigated in T cell-mediated animal models, particularly those dealing with experimental autoimmune encephalomyelitis (EAE), but data on antibody mediated animal models are still limited [3]. EAMG offers the unique opportunity to investigate a similar approach in a prototypical antibody-mediated disorder in which AChR epitopes recognized by T lymphocytes have been well characterized in both mice and rats. CD4+ T cells from C57Bl/6 (B6) mice immunized with TAChR recognize three different regions of the extracellular domain of the TAChR α-subunit (sequences Tα111-126, Tα146-162 and Tα 182-198) and one within the cytoplasmic domain (Tα 360-368) [4-6]. The immunodominance of the epitope Tα146-162 in B6 mice was further confirmed in the EAMG-resistant bm12 strain of mice (B6.C-H-2bm12), which carries three amino acid substitutions in the I-A^b subunit of MHC class II molecules [7]. Indeed, T cells from TAChR-primed bm12 mice showed very low proliferative responses to peptides Tα146-162 compared to B6 mice. Therefore, the characterization of immunodominant T cell epitopes on AChR suggests their potential use for tolerization studies. EAMG has been prevented by the oral and nasal administration of the whole TAChR [8-12], but the process of antigen purification as well as its high immunogenicity may limit its use for treatment purposes. Single immunodominant epitopes represented by synthetic peptides can be potentially used as substitutes for the native antigen to induce tolerance to the AChR. Thus far, EAMG has been prevented by the subcutaneous administration of peptide Tα146-162 [13] and by the nasal delivery of a pool of TAChR α-subunit synthetic peptides [14]. To our knowledge, no data are yet available on the oral administration of the immunodominant epitope Tα146-162 in EAMG in mice.

We investigated the immunological and clinical effects of the oral administration of peptide Tα146-162 in B6 mice. We report here that the oral administration of this peptide suppressed T cell responses to the immunodominant (Tα146-162) and to a subdominant (Tα182-198) epitope as well as to the whole TAChR, and prevented the clinical manifestations of the disease. Peptide treatment significantly reduced antibody titers to mouse AChR as well as AChR loss in muscle of tolerized mice. The tolerogenic effect induced by peptide Tα146-162 was mediated by downregulation of Th1- and Th2-associated cytokines.

Methods

Animals

Female C57Bl/6 (B6) mice, 6-7 weeks of age, were purchased from Charles River (Calco, Italy) and housed at the animal facility of the Neurological Institute.

Antigens

AChR was purified from Torpedo Californica electroplax tissue (Aquatic Research Consultants, San Pedro, CA) by affinity chromatography on Naja-naja siamensis toxin coupled to Sepharose 4B as reported [15]. Peptides corresponding to sequences Tα146-162 (LGIWTYDGTKVSISPES) and Tα182-198 (RGWKHWVYYTCCPDTPY) of the Torpedo AChR α-subunit, as well as a control peptide (sequence 751-765 of human complement factor H, KEFDHNSNIRYRCRG, Swiss-Prot P08603), were synthesized using f-moc chemistry on an Applied Biosystems, Inc. 431A automated peptide synthesizer.

Immunization and treatment protocols

Two groups of experiments were performed to investigate: (a) the effect of oral feeding with peptide Tα146-162 on primary antigen-specific responses of lymph node cells (T cell tolerance) and (b) the induction of tolerance to TAChR by feeding B6 mice with Tα146-162 before TAChR immunizations and two subsequent boosts for the induction of clinical EAMG. Tα146-162 peptide was administered by gavage under light anesthesia with ether, in 400 μl of PBS. Mice were fed 1 mg of Tα146-162 four times every other day before immunization; control animals received PBS or the control peptide. Two days after the last feeding, mice were immunized by injection in the hind foot pads with 20 μg of TAChR emulsified in complete Freund's adjuvant (CFA) for T cell tolerance studies. EAMG was induced in animals with the same amount of TAChR injected at time 0, + 30 and +75 days [16].

Lymphocyte proliferation assay

Primary antigen-specific responses were studied from T cells isolated from lymph nodes (LN) of treated and untreated mice. Ten days after immunization, popliteal and inguinal LN were removed and processed into single cell suspensions. T cell proliferations from EAMG mice were measured in the spleens obtained from animals sacrified one month after the second boost (day 105). T cells from each mice were cultured in RPMI1640 medium containing 100 μg/ml streptomycin, 100 μg/ml penicillin, 2 mM L-glutamine, 1 mM sodium pyruvate (GibcoBRL-Life Technology Italia, Milan, Italy) and 10% fetal calf serum (Sigma Italia, Milan, Italy). Concanavalin A was used at 4 μg/ml as a positive control for the T cell response; antigen-specific T cell proliferation was tested with different concentrations of TAChR (2.5, 0.25 and 0.025 μg/ml) and peptide (50, 10 and 1 μg/ml). [^{3}H]-thymidine (Amersham Italia, Milan, Italy) at 1 μCi/well was added to triplicate wells after three days of culture; cells were harvested after a further 16 hours and [^{3}H]-thymidine uptake was measured by liquid scintillation counting. Results are expressed either as Stimulation Index (S.I.: ratio between the mean of c.p.m. from antigen-stimulated culture and the mean of c.p.m. from unstimulated culture) or as mean c.p.m. of triplicates.

Clinical evaluation of EAMG

B6 mice were evaluated for signs of EAMG according to an EAMG score as follows: grade 0: normal strength; grade 1: normal appearance at rest, fatigability induced by repetitive paw grips on the cage grid; grade 2: signs of weakness at rest; grade 3: moribund; and grade 4: dead. After the second boost, we quantified muscle strength by measuring the holding time from an inverted grid (time taken for each mouse to release the hold). The test was arbitrarily stopped when the holding time exceeded 12 min. Results are expressed in minutes as the mean of three different evaluations for each animal (adapted from [14]). The clinical evaluations were performed blindly.

Anti-AChR antibody assay

Anti-TAChR and anti-mouse AChR Ab were assayed by radioimmunoprecipitation. Serial dilutions of experimental and control sera were incubated overnight with 0.5 pmol [^{125}I]α-bungarotoxin (α-BTX) labeled TAChR. Rabbit anti-mouse IgG (Dako, Denmark) was added and incubated for 4 h at room temperature. The pellets were washed twice with cold PBS 1% Triton X-100 and counted in a γ-counter (Canberra Packard). Results are expressed as pmol of α-BTX binding sites per milliliter of mouse serum. For the mouse-AChR Ab assay, mouse muscle AChR was incubated with [^{125}I]α-BTX for 2 h. Mouse serum (0.5 μl) was added to the labeled antigen and incubated overnight. Antibody-AChR complexes were precipitated by incubating for 2.5 h with 30 μl of rabbit anti-mouse IgG. Pellets were washed with 1 ml cold PBS buffer 1% Triton X-100. Specific binding was determined using mouse AChR preincubated in an excess of unlabelled α-BTX. Radioactivity was determined by γ-counting and specific binding values were subtracted from test samples. The antibody titers were expressed as pmol of toxin binding sites per milliliter of mouse serum.

AChR Content in Mouse Muscle

Mouse AChR was extracted from the whole mouse carcass. Each carcass was weighed and homogenized for 1 min at high speed in 4 volumes of 0.01M TRIS-HCl (pH 7.5), 0.001 M EDTA. AChR from pellets was solubilized with 10% Triton X-100 in TRIS-EDTA buffer overnight at 4°C. Muscle AChR preparations were centrifuged at 100,000 xg for 30 min at 4°C. Aliquots of muscle AChR extract, labeled with $[^{125}I]\alpha$-bungarotoxin, were transferred to DE-81 DEAE Disk (Whatman), washed with cold buffer, and radioactivity was determined by γ-counting. Specific binding (from parallel tubes pre-incubated with unlabelled α-BTX) was subtracted from each sample. Results were expressed as pmol of toxin binding sites per gram of carcass.

Cytokine Assay

Capture ELISAs for the detection of mouse IL-2, IFN-γ, IL-4, and IL-10 were performed according to manufacturer's recommendation (Genzyme Corp., Cambridge, MA). Popliteal and inguinal lymph nodes (LN) or splenic T cells were cultured in the presence of 2.5 μg/ml TAChR in 24-well plates at a cell density of 1.5×10^6/ml in complete RPMI1640 medium supplemented with 10% fetal calf serum. Supernatants were harvested at appropriate times for each cytokine and stored at –80°C.

Statistical analysis

Results from treated and control groups were compared by two-tailed Student's t-test using Statview 4.5 (Abacus Concepts Inc., Berkeley, CA).

Results

We first verified whether the feeding of peptide Tα146-162 was able to induce T cell tolerance to the peptide itself and hence to the whole antigen in mice immunized with TAChR. Four doses of 1 mg of peptide were administered every other day before immunization. Ten days later, animals were killed and the reactivity of LNC was measured in vitro against different concentrations of Tα146-162 and TAChR. Peptide feeding reduced significantly antigen-specific T cell proliferations to both the peptide and to TAChR (Fig. 1A, B). In a different set of experiments performed according to the same protocol, we observed that peptide feeding suppressed antigen-specific T cell proliferation also to the subdominant peptide Tα182-198 as shown in Fig. 2B. A similar observation of epitope spread has been reported by Wu and coworkers in B6 mice tolerized by the subcutaneous administration of peptide Tα146-162 [13]. The ability of a single immunodominant epitope to induce antigen-specific T cell tolerance was a prerequisite to subsequent studies on oral tolerization of EAMG with peptides.

On the basis of the above results, we verified the hypothesis that Tα146-162 feeding could improve the clinical manifestations of the disease. B6 mice were

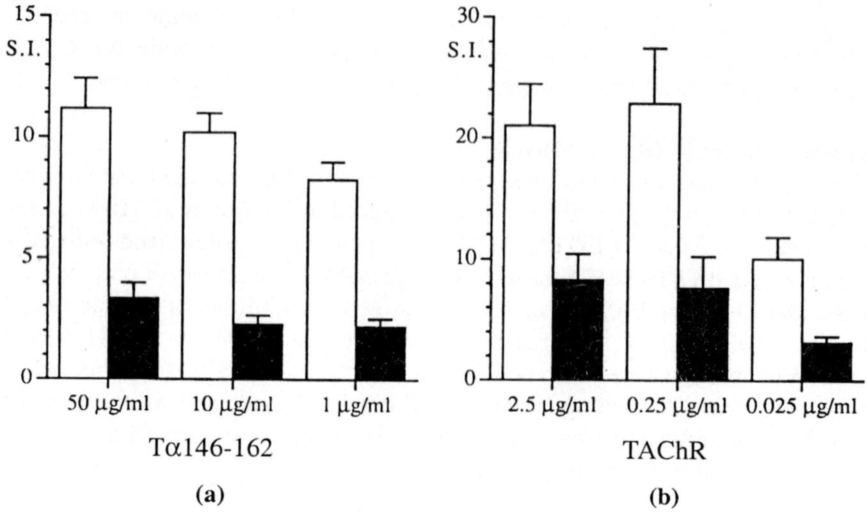

Fig. 1. Oral administration of peptide Tα146-162 suppresses T cell responses to the peptide itself and to TAChR (panel A: $p < 0.001$; panel B: $p < 0.02$).

treated with 1 mg per dose of peptide Tα146-162 four times every other day and immunized with TAChR two days after the last feeding; subsequently, animals were boosted twice at +30 and +75 days from the first immunization. Each boost with TAChR was preceded by the same schedule of Tα146-162, PBS or control peptide administration. We first compared the protective effect of peptide Tα146-162 versus PBS. No deaths due to EAMG occurred in peptide-fed (n = 12) compared to 3 in PBS-fed animals (n = 10). No overt clinical sign of EAMG was observed in peptide-treated animals, while the mean clinical score (± SEM) of PBS-treated mice was 1.9 ± 0.53. To confirm the specificity of the protective

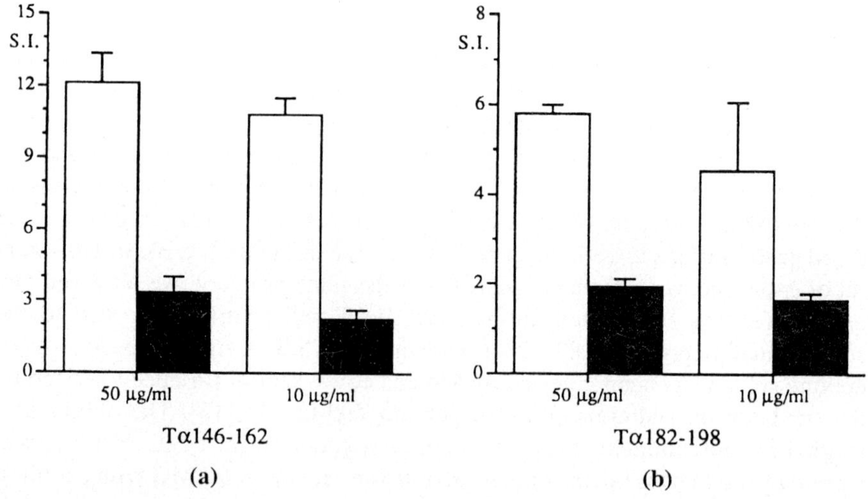

Fig. 2. Oral administration of peptide Tα146-162 suppresses T cell proliferation to the subdominant epitope Tα182-198 (panel A, $p < 0.05$; panel B, $p < 0.001$).

effect of our peptide, we compared its effect to that of an unrelated control peptide administered in a subsequent experiment performed according to the same schedule. Again, no deaths occurred in Tα146-162-treated ($n = 12$) compared to 2 in the control peptide group ($n = 12$). The mean clinical score was 0.42 ± 0.15 in Tα146-162-treated animals and 1.5 ± 0.4 in control peptide-fed mice ($p = 0.014$). We also evaluated the degree of fatigability in normal mice, PBS-fed and peptide-treated animals expressed as the holding time from an inverted grid. As shown in Fig. 3A, peptide-treated mice were protected from EAMG fatigability compared to PBS-fed animals. The mean holding time of peptide-fed mice was comparable to that of normal mice. The same observation was reproduced when treatment with Tα146-162 was compared to the control peptide. As shown in Fig. 3B, mice fed the control peptide were not protected against clinical EAMG.

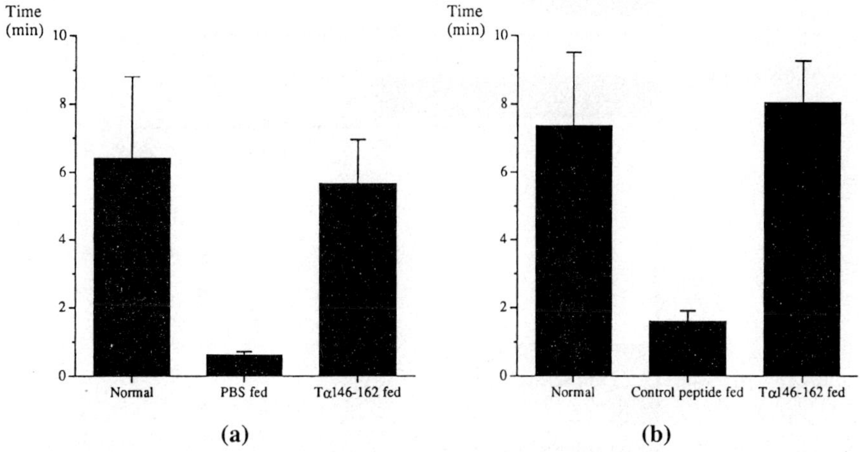

Fig. 3. Oral administration of peptide Tα146-162 improves EAMG fatigability (panel A, $p = 0.009$; panel B, $p < 0.001$).

At the end of the clinical evaluation period, mice from each treatment group (peptide Tα146-162 vs. PBS and peptide Tα146-162 vs. control peptide) were sacrified, and spleen cells were challenged in vitro with different concentrations of peptide Tα146-162 and TAChR for T cell proliferation studies. Proliferative responses of splenic T cell from peptide treated animals were significantly reduced at all the concentrations of antigens used compared to PBS-treated animals (Fig. 4A). These findings were reproduced when Tα146-162-fed animals were compared to control peptide-fed mice, confirming again the specificity of the tolerogenic effect of peptide Tα146-162 at the T cell level (Fig. 4B).

Then, we evaluated the levels of pathogenic autoantibodies and AChR content in muscle of animals from our different treatment groups. Serum levels of anti-AChR antibodies were evaluated in blood samples collected at the time of killing. We measured the level of pathogenic anti-mouse AChR antibodies in the serum of Tα146-162 treated mice and control groups. Peptide treatment induced a statistically significant reduction of anti-mouse AChR Ab in Tα146-162-treated mice compared with PBS-fed (Fig. 5A, upper panel, $p = 0.01$) and control-

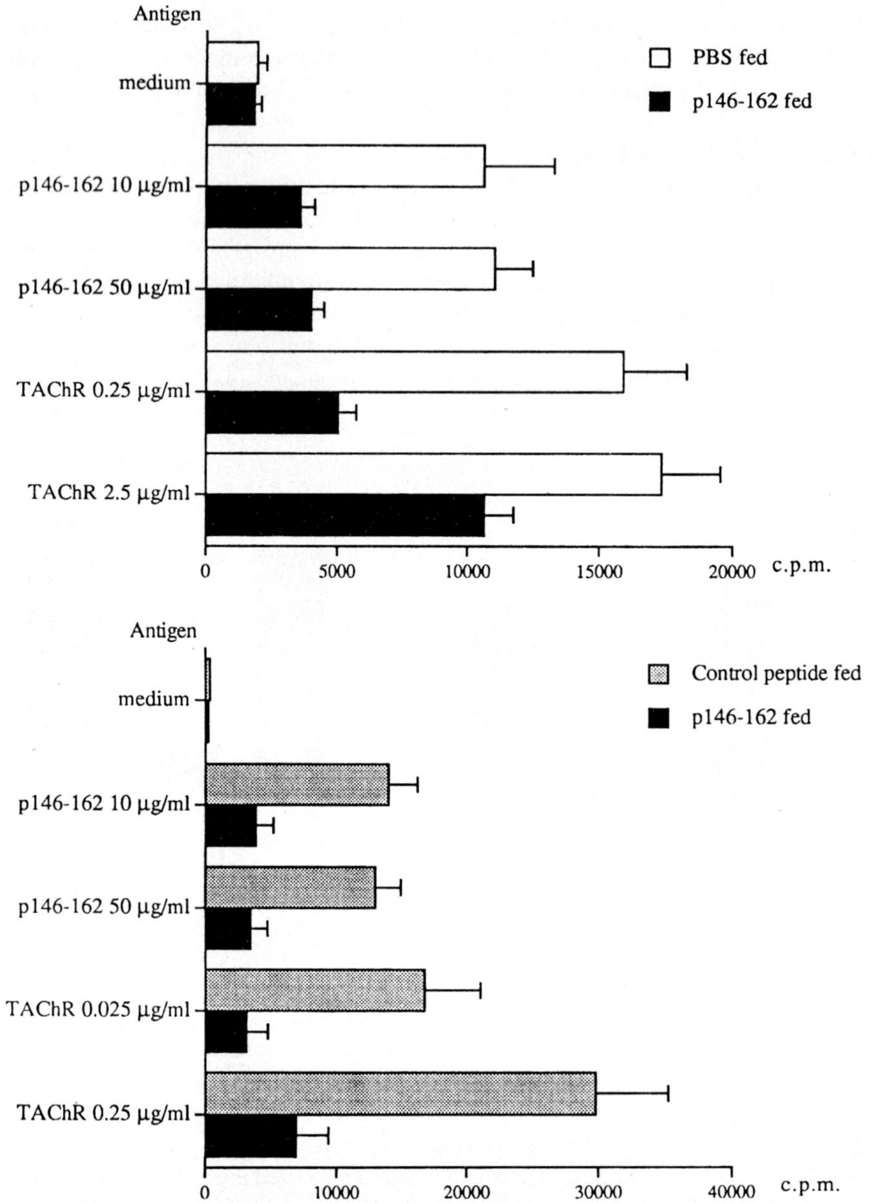

Fig. 4. Oral administration of peptide Tα146-162 inhibits antigen-specific T cell responses from spleen cells (panel A: Tα146-162-fed vs. PBS-fed mice, panel B: Tα146-162-fed vs. control peptide-fed mice; $p < 0.01$ for both experiments).

peptide-fed animals (Fig. 5A, lower panel, $p = 0.03$). As a further objective measure of the protective effect of peptide Tα146-162 treatment, we measured the AChR content in muscle from treated and control animals. As shown in Fig. 5B, muscle AChR content was statistically higher in peptide-fed compared to PBS-fed mice (upper panel, $p = 0.014$). These results were again confirmed when the experiment was repeated with the control peptide as the control group (lower panel, $p = 0.026$). A slight difference of AChR content between normal and Tα146-162 treated mice was in keeping with the observation that peptide treatment did not completely abrogate anti-mouse AChR Abs; however such a difference was not statistically significant ($p = 0.06$, Fig. 5B, upper panel; $p = 0.1$, Fig. 5B lower panel).

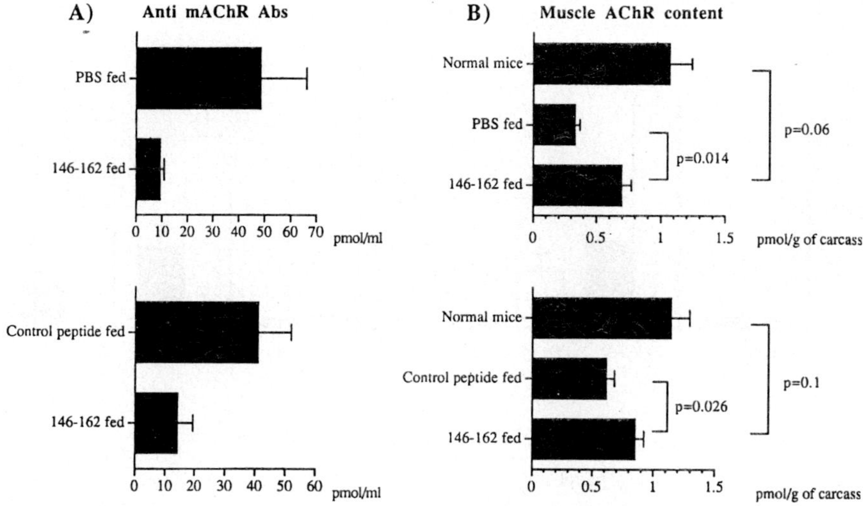

Fig. 5. Effect of the oral administration of peptide Tα146-162 on antimouse AChR antibodies (panel A) and AChR content in muscle (panel B).

To further elucidate the mechanisms associated with peptide treatment, we measured Th1- and Th2-associated cytokines in culture supernatants from spleen cells from mice treated with Tα146-162 and compared the findings to those in animals treated with the control peptide. As shown in Fig. 6, both IFNγ and IL-2 (Th1-type cytokines) were significantly reduced in supernatants from spleen cells cultured with either TAChR or Tα146-162 compared to results from animals treated with the control peptide; IL-10 (Th2-type) was reduced in supernatants from cells stimulated with TAChR. We also investigated IL-4 (Th2-type), however this cytokine was undetectable in all culture supernatants. These findings confirm the importance of Th1 down-regulation as one of the crucial mechanisms underlying the tolerogenic effect induced via the oral route. It is interesting to note that the same pattern of cytokine behavior was observed in B6 mice tolerized by the subcutaneous administration of peptide Tα146-162 [13]. These findings are in keeping with the observation that IFNγ is involved in the regulation of the humoral immune response to the AChR as shown by studies on EAMG in IFNγ knockout mice [16], and that tolerance can be reversed by the administration of IFNγ [17]. On the contrary, both anergy of AChR-specific T cells and activation of AChR-specific regulatory Th2 cells have been reported to occur in B6 mice tolerized by the nasal route [14]. Differences in protocols used for induction of EAMG and treatments (oral vs nasal vs subcutaneous) can partially explain these findings and indicate that further studies of the immunological mechanisms associated with mucosal tolerization are still needed. However, it is worth noting that we did not observe a shift from Th1 to a Th2 cytokine profile associated with our treatment. In this regard, the effect of immune deviation in an antibody-mediated disease such as EAMG should be better addressed.

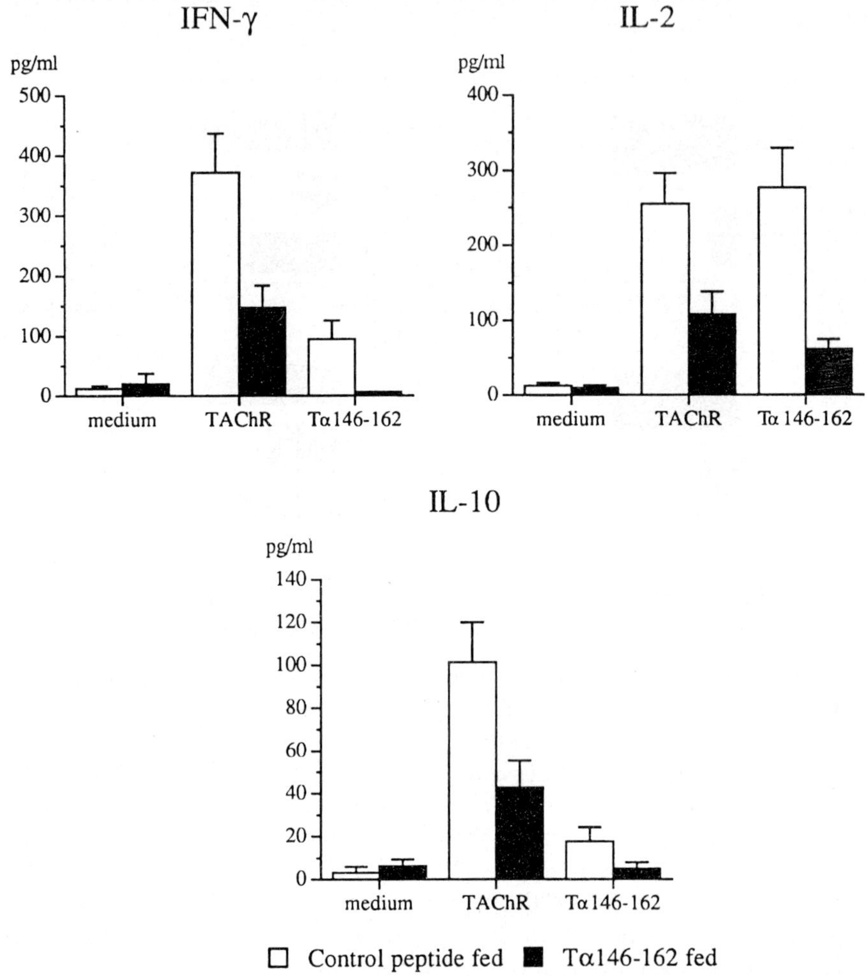

Fig. 6. IFN-γ, IL-2 and IL-10 levels in culture supernatants of spleen cells from Tα146-162-fed compared to control peptide-fed animals.

Conclusions

We report in this paper that EAMG, a T cell-dependent, antibody-mediated disease, can be prevented by the administration of a single synthetic peptide corresponding to an immunodominant T cell epitope of the AChR α subunit. Oral tolerization with native antigens or their synthetic peptide fragments has been investigated in several T cell-dependent models of autoimmune disease but data on antibody mediated disorders such as EAMG are still lacking. We report here that the oral administration of the immunodominant T cell epitope Tα146-

162 of the AChR α-subunit suppressed T cell responses to the native antigen and to the subdominant epitope Tα182-198, and improved the clinical manifestations of the disease. The protective effect induced by feeding peptide Tα146-162 was associated with reduced levels of pathogenic antibodies to mouse AChR and with increased AChR content in the muscles of treated animals compared to PBS-fed controls. The specificity of peptide Tα146-162 treatment was confirmed by comparison with an unrelated control peptide that did not exert any inhibitory effect on clinical features, and on cellular and humoral responses to the AChR. Prevention of EAMG by feeding peptide Tα146-162 was mediated by down-regulation of IFN-γ, IL-2 and IL-10 production by TAChR-reactive T cells. We therefore demonstrate here that oral feeding with a single immunodominant epitope can prevent an antibody-mediated disease, and these findings further support the feasibility of antigen-specific immunotherapy of EAMG. Recent results on the use of synthetic peptides, as well as on recombinant fragments of the AChR α subunit [18], are likely to open new perspective in this field of research.

Acknowledgements

This work was partially supported by a Telethon Grant #1051 to C.A.

References

1. Drachman, D.B. 1994. Myasthenia gravis. *N. Engl. J. Med.,* 330, 1797–1810.
2. Drachman, D.B. 1996. Immunotherapy in neuromuscular disorders: current and future strategies. *Muscle & Nerve,* 19, 1239–1251.
3. Weiner, H.L. 1997. Oral tolerance: immune mechanisms and treatment of autoimmune diseases. *Immunology Today,* 18, 335–343.
4. Shenoy, M., E. Goluzsko and P. Christadoss. 1994. The pathogenic role of acetylcholine receptor a chain epitope within α146–162 in the development of experimental autoimmune myasthenia gravis in C57BL6 mice. *Clin. Immunol. Immunopathol.* 73: 338-343.
5. Bellone, M., N. Ostlie, S. Lei and B.M. Conti-Tronconi. 1991. Experimental myasthenia gravis in congenic mice: sequence mapping and H-2 restriction of T helper epitopes on the α subunits of Torpedo Californica and murine acetylcholine receptor. *Eur. J. Immunol.,* 21: 2303-2310.
6. Fujii, Y. and J. Lindstrom. 1988. Specificity of the T cell immune response to acetylcholine receptor in experimental autoimmune myasthenia gravis. Response to subunits and synthetic peptides. *J. Immunol.,* 140: 1830-1837.
7. Chistadoss, P., J.M. Lindstrom, R.W. Melvold and N. Talal. 1985. Mutation at I-A beta chain prevents experimental autoimmune myasthenia gravis. *Immunogenetics,* 21, 33-38.
8. Wang, Z.-Y., J. Qiao and H. Link. 1993. Suppression of experimental autoimmune myasthenia gravis by oral administration of acetylcholine receptor. *J. Neuroimmunol.,* 44, 209–214.
9. Okumura, S., K. McIntosh and D.B. Drachman. 1994. Oral administration of acetylcholine receptor: effects on experimental autoimmune myasthenia gravis. *Ann. Neurol.,* 36, 704–713.

10. Drachman, D.B., S. Okumura, R.N. Adams and K. McIntosh. 1996. Oral tolerance in myasthenia gravis. *In* Oral tolerance: mechanism and applications, eds. Weiner, H.L., Mayer, L.F., Ann. NY. Acad. Sci., 778, 258–272.
11. Ma, C.-G., G.X. Zhang, B.-G. Xiao, J. Link, T. Olsson and H. Link. 1995. Suppression of experimental autoimmune myasthenia gravis by nasal administration of acetylcholine receptor. *J. Neuroimmunol.* 58, 51–60.
12. Shi, F.D., X. F. Bai, H.L. Li, Y.M. Huang, P.H. Van der Meide and H. Link. 1998. Nasal tolerance in experimental autoimmune myasthenia gravis (EAMG): induction of protective tolerance in primed animals. *Clin. Exp. Immunol.,* 111, 506–512.
13. Wu, B., C. Deng, E. Goluszko and P. Christadoss. 1997. Tolerance to a dominant T cell epitope in the acetylcholine receptor molecule induces epitope spread and suppresses murine myasthenia gravis. *J. Immunol.,* 159, 3016–3023.
14. Karachunski, P.I., N.S. Ostlie, D.K. Okita and B.M. Conti-Fine. 1997. Prevention of experimental myasthenia gravis by nasal administration of synthetic acetylcholine receptor T epitope sequences. *J. Clin. Invest.,* 100, 3027–3035.
15. Aharonov, A., R. Tarrab-Hazdai, I. Silman and S. Fuchs. 1977. Immunochemical studies on acetylcholine receptor from Torpedo californica. *Immunochemistry,* 14, 129–137.
16. Balasa B., C. Deng, J. Lee, L.M. Bradley, D.K. Dalton, P. Christadoss and N. Sarvetnick, 1997. Interferon γ (IFN-γ) is necessary for the genesis of acetylcholine receptor-induced clinical experimental autoimmune myasthenia gravis in mice. *J Exp. Med.,* 186, 385–391.
17. Li, H.L., F.D. Shi, X.F. Bai, Y.M. Huang, P.H. van der Meide, B.G. Xiao and H. Link. 1998. Nasal tolerance to experimental autoimmune myasthenia gravis: tolerance reversal by nasal administration of minute amounts of interferon-gamma. *Clin. Immunol. Immunpathol.* 87, 15–22
18. Barchan, D., O. Asher, S. Tzartos, S. Fuchs and M.C. Souroujon. 1998. Modulation of the anti-acetylcholine receptor response and experimental autoimmune myasthenia gravis by recombinant fragments of the acetylcholine receptor. *Eur. J. Immunol.,* 28: 616–624.

Myasthenia Gravis: Disease mechanisms and immunointervention
P. Christadoss (Ed)

15. Protective Role of Th2 Cells in Mouse Experimental Myasthenia Gravis

Peter I. Karachunski[1], Norma S. Ostlie[1], David K. Okita[1,2] and Bianca M. Conti-Fine*[1,2]

[1]Department of Biochemistry, Molecular Biology and Biophysics, University of Minnesota, St. Paul, MN 55108.

[2]Department of Pharmacology, School of Medicine, University of Minnesota, Minneapolis, MN 55455.

*Previously known as Binaca M. Conti-Tronconi.

Introduction

CD4$^+$ cells comprise Th1 and Th2 cells that differ in their function and in the cytokines they secrete [1-3]. Th1 cells mediate effector functions of the immune system: they secrete pro-inflammatory cytokines and can be cytotoxic. Also, they help the synthesis of IgG subclasses that bind complement, and therefore are most effective in causing cell and tissue damage. Th2 cells modulate immune responses by secreting anti-inflammatory cytokines, like IL-4 and IL-10, that down-regulate the function of antigen-presenting cells and Th1 cells. Th2 cells are not cytotoxic and help synthesis of antibodies that do not bind complement, such as IgE, IgG4 in humans and its homologue in mice, IgG1.

Th1 cells may be effectors of T cell-mediated autoimmune diseases, whereas Th2 cells have been implicated in their down regulation [1-4]. However, Th2 cells may also cause T cell-mediated autoimmune diseases [5-8]. The many studies on the role of Th2 and Th1 cells in T cell mediated autoimmune diseases suggest that both subsets may have both effector and down regulatory functions.

Both Th1 and Th2 cells may be implicated in antibody-mediated autoimmune diseases. Antibodies able to activate complement are likely to be especially effective in causing tissue damage, pointing to an important role of Th1 cells in the pathogenesis of antibody-mediated autoimmune lesions [1-4]. Because Th2 cells have effective helper function, they may also be involved in antibody-mediated autoimmune diseases. This has been shown in certain human and experimental autoimmune conditions [9-12]. However, Th2-induced antibodies do not fix complement or bind the phagocyte Fc receptor [1-4], and are unlikely to cause severe tissue injury.

Myasthenia gravis (MG) and its animal model, experimental MG (EMG), are caused by antibodies against the muscle acetylcholine receptor (AChR) [13]. EMG is induced by immunization with purified AChR [13]. Th1 cells may have a pathogenic role in both MG and EMG. AChR-specific Th1 cell lines could be propagated from MG patients [14-15]. All MG patients had in their blood abundant AChR-specific Th1 cells that recognize a rich epitope repertoire, which included, at least for the AChR subunit tested (the α subunit), all the epitopes previously identified by several independent studies as recognized by T cells in MG patients [13]. Transgenic mice that produced IFN-γ at the neuromuscular junction developed functional disruption of the junction and a syndrome reminiscent of MG [18]. Mice deficient in IL-12, a cytokine crucial for development of Th1 cells, were resistant to EMG, whereas administration of IL-12 at the time of the immunization with AChR facilitated EMG development [19].

Circumstantial evidence suggests that anti-AChR Th2 cells may protect from, rather than cause, EMG. C57Bl/6 (B6) mice develop EMG after immunization with AChR purified from *Torpedo* electric tissue (TAChR) [20]. Nasal or subcutaneous administration to B6 mice of synthetic TAChR peptides forming $CD4^+$ epitopes activated Th2 cells specific for the peptides administered, caused reduced synthesis of anti-AChR antibodies and prevented EMG [21-23].

IL-4 is essential for generation of Th2 responses [24-25], and IL-4 knock out (KO) mice have effective Th1 function, but severely impaired Th2 function [26]. Their $CD4^+$ cells do not express other Th2 cytokines, and they have very low amounts of Th2-driven IgG1 in the serum [26-28]. IL-4 KO B6 mice are an excellent model system to investigate the role of IL-4, and indirectly that of Th1 and Th2 cells, in the pathogenesis and prevention of EMG. Induction of EMG in B6 mice requires multiple AChR injections, and the frequency of EMG is 20-70% even after prolonged AChR immunization [13]. Thus, the B6 background is a good readout system to reveal both increases and decreases in susceptibility to EMG.

To obtain direct evidence about the protective or pathogenic role of Th2 cells in EMG, we investigated the appearance of anti-AChR antibodies and of EMG in wild-type and IL-4 KO B6 mice, immunized with TAChR [29]. Also, we determined whether nasal administration to the IL-4 KO mutants of immunodominant $CD4^+$ epitopes of the TAChR affected the anti-TAChR antibody synthesis and prevented EMG, as it does in wild-type B6 mice [21, 29]. We will review and discuss below the results of those studies, which we have reported in detail previously [21, 24, 29].

IL-4 KO mice had increased susceptibility to EMG, and were not protected from EMG by nasal treatment with TAChR $CD4^+$ epitopes

We immunized wild-type and IL-4 KO B6 mice with three subcutaneous injections, one month apart, of purified TAChR in Freund's adjuvant. All IL-4 KO mice, but only 58% of the wild-type B6 mice developed EMG (Fig. 1). IL-4 KO mice developed a more severe form of disease, as indicated by their shorter holding times in the strength test we used [21, 30].

Thus, absence of Th2 cells appear to remove an important protective mechanism

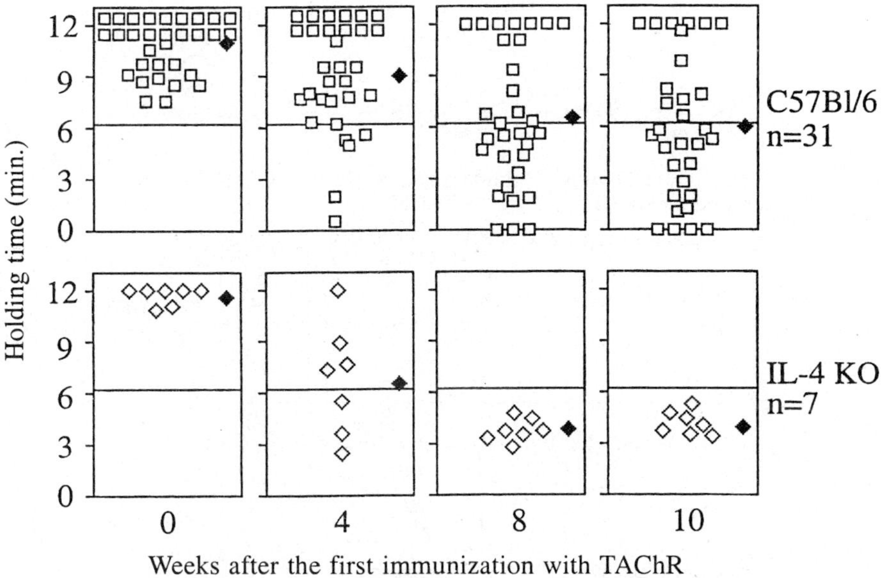

Fig. 1. Strength of wild-type and IL-4 KO B6 mice immunized with TAChR 3 times, one month apart. We report results obtained 4, 8 and 10 weeks after the first immunizing injection. For each group we report the results obtained for the same mice before the TAChR immunization (panels "0 weeks"). Results at 8 and 10 weeks were consistent, and reflect the maximum observed frequency of EMG symptoms. Black symbols represent the average holding time of the groups of mice used in these experiments: wild-type B6 mice had significantly longer holding time than the IL-4 KO mice at 8 ($P > 0.001$) and 10 ($P > 0.03$) weeks. Reproduced with permission from P.I. Karachunski et al (1999), *J. Neuroimmunol.* 95: 73-84. Copyright Elsevier Science B.V., 1999.

in EMG. To directly test this possibility, we investigated the effect in IL-4 KO B6 mice of a nasal 'tolerization' procedure that in wild-type B6 mice sensitizes TAChR-specific Th2 cells, effectively reduces the synthesis of anti-AChR antibody, and protects them from EMG [21]. The procedure involves nasal instillation, before and during the TAChR immunization, of a pool of three 20-residue synthetic sequences of the TAChR α subunit, that form epitopes that dominate the sensitization of anti-TAChR $CD4^+$ cells in B6 mice [20] (referred to as 'α epitope pool').

Nasal administration of the α epitope pool to the IL-4 KO mutants did not prevent EMG, or affect the severity of the symptoms (Fig. 2). Most peptide-treated and all sham-treated IL-4 KO mice developed EMG, and the average holding time of peptide-treated and sham-treated mice was the same. Nasal treatment with peptides prevented EMG in wild-type B6 mice: only 4-8% of the peptide-treated mice developed EMG symptoms, as compared to 58% of the sham-treated mice.

IL-4 KO mice have functional Th1 cells [26]. Thus, these results indicate that sensitization of Th1 cells is sufficient to cause EMG. This agrees with the

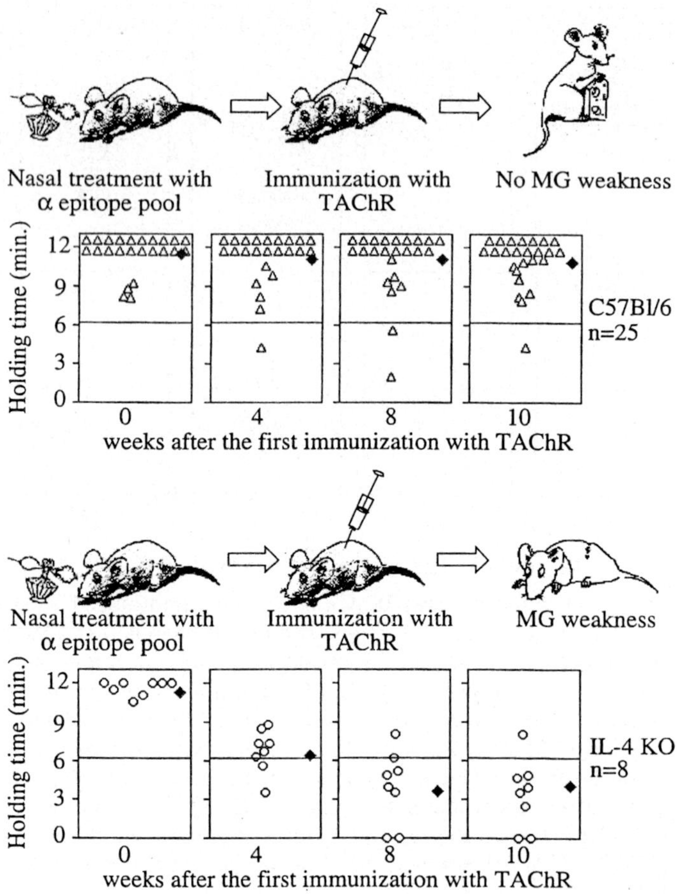

Fig. 2. Strength of wild-type and IL-4 KO B6 mice treated nasally with the α epitope pool and immunized with TAChR. We show results obtained 4, 8 and 10 weeks after beginning of the immunization. Panels '0 weeks' report results obtained for the same mice before TAChR immunization. Black symbols represent the average holding time of the groups of mice used in these experiments. Average holding time of peptide-treated IL-4 KO mice was the same as the sham-treated group that inhaled clean PBS, whereas wild-type B6 mice that inhaled the α epitope pool had significantly ($P >$ 0.001) longer holding time than the sham-treated mice. Reproduced with permission from P.I. Karachunski et al (1999), *J. Neuroimmunol.* 95: 73-84. Copyright Elsevier Science B.V., 1999.

conclusion of another study that demonstrated that IL-12 is necessary in induction of EMG [19]. Also, these results demonstrate that Th2 cells are not necessary for EMG development, and suggest that IL-4, and therefore Th2 cells, may down-regulate the anti-TAChR antibody response and prevent the resulting EMG symptoms. Finally, they indicate that sensitization of modulatory anti-TAChR Th2 cells is an important mechanism of the protection from EMG that results from nasal 'tolerization' procedures.

Nasal treatment of IL-4 KO mice with a pool of TAChR CD4$^+$ epitopes did not cause reduced synthesis of anti-TAChR antibodies, or Th1-induced anti-TAChR antibodies

To directly demonstrate a role of IL-4 on the modulation of the anti-TAChR antibody response, we measured the anti-TAChR antibody concentration in the sera of wild-type and IL-4 KO B6 mice treated nasally with the α epitope pool or sham-treated with clean PBS, and immunized with TAChR [21, 29].

Nasal treatment of wild-type B6 mice with the synthetic TAChR CD4$^+$ epitopes reduced substantially their synthesis of anti-TAChR antibodies (Fig. 3A, top panel), whereas peptide treated and sham-treated IL-4 KO mice had similar serum concentrations of anti-AChR antibodies, that were comparable to those of sham-treated wild-type B6 mice (Fig. 3A, bottom panel).

We investigated the effect of nasal treatment with the α epitope pool on the synthesis of Th1-dependent anti-TAChR antibodies in IL-4 KO B6 mice, and as

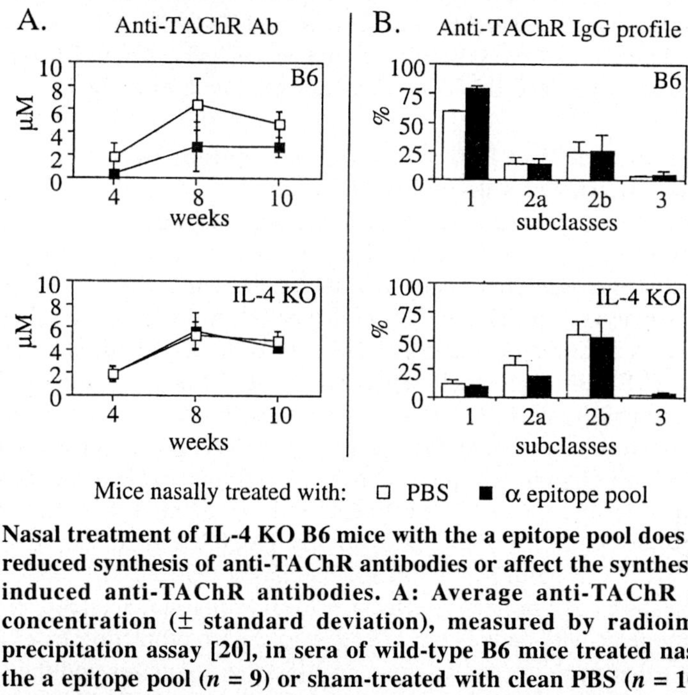

Fig. 3. Nasal treatment of IL-4 KO B6 mice with the a epitope pool does not cause reduced synthesis of anti-TAChR antibodies or affect the synthesis of Th1-induced anti-TAChR antibodies. A: Average anti-TAChR antibody concentration (± standard deviation), measured by radioimmmuno-precipitation assay [20], in sera of wild-type B6 mice treated nasally with the a epitope pool (*n* = 9) or sham-treated with clean PBS (*n* = 10), and of IL-4 KO B6 mice treated nasally with the a epitope pool (*n* = 8) or sham-treated with clean PBS (*n* = 7). Sera were obtained 4, 8 and 10 weeks after beginning of the immunization with TAChR, as indicated along the abscissa of plots. B: Relative amounts of anti-TAChR IgG of different subclasses, as indicated below the plots, expressed as percent of the total anti-TAChR IgG, in sera from wild-type and IL-4 KO B6 mice, as indicated inside the plots. Mice had been treated nasally with the α epitope pool (black columns), or had been sham-treated with clean PBS (white columns). Sera were obtained 10 weeks after beginning of the immunization with TAChR. Reprinted with permission from P.I. Karachunski, et al (1999), *J. Neuroimmunol.* 95: 73-84. Copyright Elsevier Science B.V., 1999.

a control in wild-type B6 mice. We used sera of peptide-treated and sham-treated IL-4 KO and wild-type B6 mice immunized with TAChR, and determined by ELISA [23] the relative concentrations of different anti-TAChR IgG subclasses synthesized with the help of Th1 cells (IgG2a and IgG2b, IgG3) or Th2 cells (IgG1) (Fig. 3B). Peptide- and sham-treated mice wild-type B6 mice had similar relative concentrations of Th1-dependent IgG subclasses, whereas the relative concentration of the Th2-driven anti-TAChR IgG1 was significantly ($P < 0.001$) increased in the peptide-treated mice. This is likely due to synthesis of antibodies to the peptides administered. Anti-peptide antibodies may cross-react with TAChR in ELISA because of the partial denaturation of the TAChR when absorbed onto the plastic ELISA plates [31]. Peptide- and sham-treated IL-4 KO mice had the same relative concentrations of all IgG subclasses. They had substantial amounts of anti-TAChR IgG2a and IgG2b, that were lower than but comparable to the amount of total anti-TAChR IgG: therefore in IL-4 KO mice the anti-TAChR IgG are mostly IgG2a and IgG2b. IL-4 KO mice had minimal amounts of anti-TAChR IgG3, and measurable amounts of anti-TAChR IgG1, although less ($P < 0.0001$) than wild-type B6 mice. Synthesis of IgG1 is both IL-4- and IL-2-dependent, and therefore IL-4 KO mice may still synthesize IgG1.

Nasal treatment of IL-4 KO mice with the α epitope pool reduced the activity of anti-AChR Th1 cells

Tolerance induced by nasal, oral or systemic administration of an antigen or of epitope sequences can result from several mechanisms, that include: anergy or deletion of antigen-specific T cells and induction of antigen specific regulatory Th2 cells (reviewed in [21-23]). In wild-type B6 mice nasal or subcutaneous treatment with TAChR peptide sequences that form CD4$^+$ epitopes caused both anergy of Th1 cells and sensitization of Th2 cells specific for the peptides administered nasally [21-23]. Thus, it was impossible to discern which of those mechanisms was responsible for the protective effects. To determine which mechanisms best explained the protection resulting from nasal tolerance procedures, we assessed the effect of nasal treatment of IL-4 KO mice with the α epitope pool, on sensitization of CD4$^+$ cells to the TAChR and to the administered epitopes [21, 29]: if nasal peptide treatment caused reduced Th1 cell activity, in spite of the absence of protective effects, it would suggest that anergy or deletion of the pathogenic Th1 cells is not effective to ensure protection from EMG.

Towards that goal, we assessed the proliferative responses and the secretion of Th1 cytokines evoked by challenge *in vitro* with the TAChR or with the peptides administered nasally, of spleen CD4$^+$ cells from IL-4 KO B6 mice that had been treated nasally with the α epitope pool or sham treated with PBS, and immunized with TAChR.

We tested the proliferative responses to the TAChR, the different TAChR subunits (α, β, γ and δ), and the individual peptides screening the α subunit sequence. We used as representative antigens of the TAChR subunits, equimolar pools of overlapping synthetic peptides spanning the sequence of each subunit: the responses to those peptide pools of CD4$^+$ cells from TAChR-immunized mice compare well with the responses to purified TAChR subunits [20]. Fig. 4

reports the results of a typical experiment. The cells from sham-treated mice responded vigorously to the TAChR and to the α subunit, whereas they responded minimally or not at all to the other subunits. This agrees with the results of our previous studies [20, 30, 32], that demonstrated that the α subunit dominated the sensitization of anti-TAChR CD4$^+$ cells in B6 mice. The cells from peptide-treated mice responded well to the TAChR and to the α subunit, but significantly less than the cells of sham-treated mice. Like wild-type B6 mice [20, 30, 32-34], CD4$^+$ cells from sham-treated IL-4 KO B6 mice recognized strongly peptides Tα150-169, Tα181-200, Tα360-378 and Tα146-162, that overlaps Tα150-169. The CD4$^+$ cells from peptide-treated mice responded minimally or not at all to the peptides we administered nasally, although they still recognized Tα146-162 strongly.

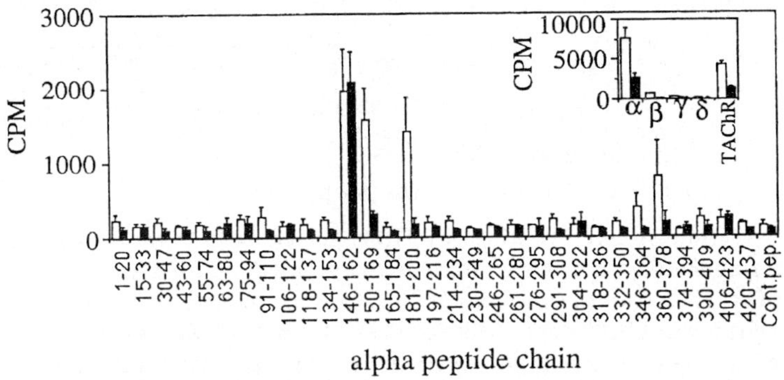

Fig. 4. CD4$^+$ spleen cells from IL-4 KO mice treated nasally with the α epitope pool and immunized with TAChR have a reduced proliferative response to TAChR, and to the peptides administered nasally. Responses of CD8$^+$ depleted spleen cells from mice treated nasally with the α epitope pool (black columns) or sham-treated with clean PBS (white columns) to TAChR and to pools of overlapping synthetic peptides spanning the sequence of each TAChR subunits (inset), and to individual overlapping synthetic peptides screening the TAChR α subunit sequence, as indicated at the bottom of the panel. Columns represent average cpm ± standard deviation of triplicate cultures. Columns showing "Cont. pep." are average cpm ± standard deviation of triplicate cultures cultivated in the presence of a 20-residue peptide synthesized by the same method, unrelated to TAChR sequence. Reprinted with permission from P.I. Karachunski, et al (1999), *J. Neuroimmunol.* 95: 73-84. Copyright Elsevier Science B.V., 1999.

We tested the secretion of IL-2, IFN-γ, IL-4 and IL-10 by CD4$^+$ spleen cells from peptide-treated and sham-treated IL-4 KO B6 mice immunized with TAChR, after challenge *in vitro* with TAChR or with the α epitope pool. Fig. 5 reports the results of a typical experiment that assessed the secretion of IL-2 and IFN-γ of cultures challenged with TAChR or the α epitope pool. The cells from peptide- and sham-treated mice, after challenge with TAChR or the α epitope pool, secreted similar levels of IL-2. The cells from peptide-treated mice secreted significantly less ($P < 0.005$) IFN-γ than the cells from sham-treated mice, both after challenge with TAChR or with the α epitope pool. CD4$^+$ spleen cells from IL-4 KO mice did not secrete any IL-4 and IL-10.

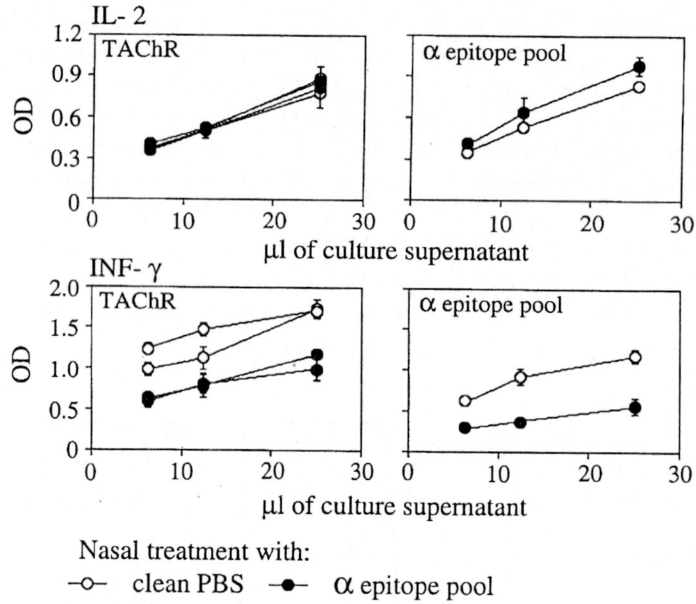

Fig. 5. Secretion of Th1 cytokines by CD4$^+$ spleen cells from IL-4 KO B6 mice immunized with TAChR, after challenge *in vitro* with TAChR or α epitopes pool. IL-2 (top panels) and IFN-g (bottom panels) in the supernatant of cultures of CD8$^+$ depleted spleen cells from IL-4 KO mice treated nasally with α epitope pool (black symbols) or sham-treated with clean PBS (white symbols), and immunized with TAChR. Two independent cell cultures were cultivated in the presence of TAChR, and one culture in presence of α epitope pool, as indicated inside the plots. Symbols represent the average ± standard deviation of duplicate ELISA determinations, using increasing amounts of the supernatant of each culture, as indicates below the plots, after 72 h of incubation with the antigen. Spontaneous secretion of IL-2 and IFN-γ by cells cultivated in the absence of any stimulus has been subtracted from these data. Reprinted with permission from P.I. Karachunski, et al (1999), *J. Neuroimmunol.* 95: 73-84. Copyright Elsevier Science B.V., 1999.

These results indicate that anergy or deletion of Th1 cells had occurred in the peptide-treated IL-4 KO mice, because their CD4$^+$ spleen cells had a reduced proliferative response to the TAChR, to the TAChR α subunit and to the individual peptides administered nasally, and synthesized less IFN-γ after challenge *in vitro* with TAChR or the α epitope pool. However, the reduced anti-TAChR Th1 response did not suffice to protect from EMG or to reduce the synthesis of anti-TAChR antibodies. Consequently, the strong reduction in synthesis of anti-TAChR antibodies observed in wild-type B6 mice after nasal or subcutaneous administration of TAChR peptides forming CD4$^+$ epitopes [21–23] must be mediated by activation of regulatory Th2 cells. Perhaps anergy of anti-TAChR Th1 cells might result in protection from EMG if one could use a full complement of the TAChR epitope sequences recognized by the pathogenic Th1 clones, in doses adequate to cause anergy or deletion of all the specific Th1 clones.

The finding that CD4$^+$ spleen cells from IL-4 KO mice that sniffed the α epitope pool responded to peptide Tα150-169 much less than the sham-treated mice, but still responded strongly to the overlapping peptide Tα146-162 (Fig. 5) indicates that the sequence region α146-169 contains overlapping epitopes that sensitize different pathogenic CD4$^+$ clones. The residual population of Th1 cells that recognized epitopes within the amino terminal part of the sequence region α146-169 (i.e. those that responded to Tα146-162, not to Tα150-169) sufficed to cause EMG in the peptide-treated IL-4 KO mice. This verifies the importance of this sequence for sensitization of pathogenic Th1 cells [20, 30, 32-35].

Conclusions

The studies reviewed here indicate that IL-4, and therefore Th2 cells, are not necessary for EMG development, and may down-regulate the synthesis of anti-TAChR antibodies and the resulting EMG symptoms; and that sensitization of Th1 cells is sufficient to cause EMG. Also, they indicate that sensitization of protective antigen-specific Th2 cells, rather that anergy or deletion of pathogenic Th1 cells, is a crucial mechanism mediating the protective effects of nasal "tolerization" procedures.

This conclusion explains why nasal or subcutaneous administration of a single TAChR CD4$^+$ epitope peptide protected from EMG [21-23]. Regulatory Th2 cells against one epitope can down-regulate the Th1 response to the whole cognate antigen through secretion of cytokine that act on all Th1 cells in topographic proximity, irrespective of their specificity (antigen-driven bystander suppression) [32]. Furthermore, Th2 determinant spreading [36] may also explain how sensitization of Th2 cells to an individual epitope protects from an autoimmune disease that involves the whole cognate autoantigen.

The main pathogenic mechanisms of anti-AChR antibodies in MG and EMG are activation of complement and accelerated degradation of AChR molecules cross linked by the antibodies [13]. The conclusion that Th1, rather than Th2 cells, are involved in causing EMG underlines the importance of complement in EMG pathogenesis, since Th1-dependent antibodies are most effective at binding complement. One of the protective mechanisms of IL-4 and of anti-TAChR Th2 cells might be stimulation of synthesis of anti-TAChR IgG that do not bind complement, and may compete for AChR binding with the Th1-induced, complement activating antibodies. The finding that IL-4 KO and wild-type B6 mice develop similar levels of anti-AChR antibodies in spite of their different susceptibility to EMG, but in B6 mice the anti-TAChR IgG include a substantial fraction of IgG1 is consistent with this possibility.

Th2 cells might have a pathogenic role in certain circumstances. Anti-AChR antibodies may cause accelerated degradation of the AChR without the need of complement [13]. Th2-induced anti-AChR antibodies may be pathogenic in muscle groups that are especially susceptible to myasthenic weakness when the concentration of AChR at the synapses is reduced, even in the absence of complement-mediated damage of the neuromuscular junction. The functional properties of extrinsic ocular muscles make them especially susceptible to weakness when a reduction of the AChR function occurs [13]. Thus, Th2 cells might be pathogenic in ocular MG. Further studies will be necessary to exclude a pathogenic role of Th2 cells in the pathogenesis of mouse EMG, and especially of human MG.

Acknowledgement

This work was partially supported by the NINDS grant NS23919 (to B.M.C.-F.).

References

1. Abbas, A., K. Murphy and A. Sher. 1996. Functional diversity of helper T lymphocytes. *Nature* 383: 787.
2. Romagnani, S. 1997. The Th1/Th2 paradigm. *Immunol. Today.* 18: 263.
3. Weigle, W.O. and C.G. Romball. 1997. $CD4^+$ T-cell subsets and cytokines involved in peripheral tolerance. *Immunol. Today.* 18: 533.
4. O'Garra, A. 1998. Cytokine induce the development of functionally heterogeneous T helper cell subsets. *Immunity* 8: 275.
5. Pakala, S.V., M.O. Kurrer and J.D. Katz. 1997. T helper 2 (Th2) T cells induce acute pancreatitis and diabetes in immune-compromised nonobese diabetic (NOD) mice. *J. Exp. Med.* 186: 299.
6. Lafaille, J.J., F. Van de Keere, A.L. Hsu, J.L. Baron, W. Haas, C.S. Raine and S. Tonegawa. 1997. Myelin basic protein-specific T helper 2 (Th2) cells cause experimental autoimmune encephalomyelitis in immunodeficient hosts rather than protect them from the disease. *J. Exp. Med.* 186: 307.
7. Manoury-Schwartz, B., G. Chiocchia, N. Bessis, O. Abehsira-Amar, F. Batteux, S. Muller, S. Huang, M..C. Boissier and C. Fournier. 1997. High susceptibility to collagen-induce arthritis in mice lacking IFN-γ receptors. *J. Immunol.* 158: 5501.
8. Vermeire, K., H. Heremans, M. Vandeputte, S. Huang, A. Billiau, and P. Matthys. 1997. Accelerated collagen-induced arthritis in IFN-γ receptor-deficient mice. *J. Immunol.* 158: 5507.
9. Erb, K.J., B. Ruger, M. von Brevern, B. Ryffel, A. Schimpl and K. Rivett. 1997. Constitutive expression of Interleukin (IL-4) in vivo causes autoimmune-type disorders in mice. *J. Exp. Med.* 185: 329.
10. Fuss, I.J., W. Strober, J.K. Dale, S. Fritz, G.R. Pearlstein, J.M. Puck, M.J. Lenardo and S.E. Strauss. 1997. Characteristic T helper 2 T cell cytokine abnormalities in autoimmune lymphoproliferative syndrome, a syndrome marked by defective apoptosis and humoral autoimmunity. *J. Immunol.* 158: 1912.
11. Nakajima, A., S. Hirose H. Yagita and K. Okumura. 1997. Roles of IL-4 and IL-12 in the development of lupus in NZB/W F_1 mice. *J. Immunol.* 158: 1466.
12. Peng, S.L., J. Mosiehi and J. Craft. 1997. Roles of interferon-g and interleukin-4 in murine lupus. *J. Clin. Invest.* 99: 1936.
13. Conti-Fine, B.M., M. Bellone, J.F. Howard Jr. and M.P. Protti. 1997. Myasthenia Gravis. The Immunobiology of an Autoimmune Disease. R.G. Landes. Chapman & Hall, Springer.
14. Moiola, L., P. Karachunski, M.P. Protti, J.F. Howard and B.M. Conti-Tronconi. 1994. Epitopes on the β subunit of human muscle acetylcholine receptor recognized by $CD4^+$ cells of Myasthenia Gravis patients and healthy subjects. *J. Clin. Invest.* 93: 1020.
15. Moiola, L., M.P. Protti, J.F. Howard and B.M. Conti-Tronconi. 1994. Myasthenia Gravis: Residues of the a and g subunits of muscle acetylcholine receptor involved in formation of immunodominant $CD4^+$ epitopes. *J. Immunol.* 152: 4686.

16. Wang, Z-Y., D. Okita, J.F. Howard Jr. and B.M. Conti-Fine. 1997. Thl epitope repertoire on the α subunit of human muscle acetylcholine receptor in myasthenia gravis. *Neurology.* 48: 1643.
17. Wang, Z-Y., D. Okita, J.F. Howard Jr. and B.M. Conti-Fine. 1998. T-cell recognition of muscle acetylcholine receptor subunits in generalized and ocular myasthenia gravis. *Neurology.* 50: 1045.
18. Gu, D., L. Wogensen, N.A. Calcutt, C. Xia, S. Zhu, J.P. Merlie, H.S. Fox, J. Lindstrom, H.C. Powell and N. Sarvetnick. 1995. Myasthenia gravis-like syndrome induced expression of interferon-γ in neuromuscular junction. *J. Exp. Med.* 181: 547.
19. Moiola, L., F. Galbiati, G. Martino, S. Amadio, E. Brambilla, G. Comi, A. Vincent, L.M.E. Grimaldi and L. Adorini. 1998. IL-12 is involved in the induction of experimental autoimmune myasthenia gravis, an antibody-mediated diseases. *Eur. J. Immunol.* 28: 2487.
20. Bellone, M., N. Ostlie, S. Lei and B. Conti-Tronconi. 1991. Experimental myasthenia gravis in congenic mice. Sequence mapping and H-2 restriction of T helper epitopes on the a subunits of *Torpedo californica* and murine acetylcholine receptors. *Eur. J. Immunol.* 21: 2303.
21. Karachunski, P., N. Ostlie, D. Okita and B.M. Conti-Fine. 1997. Protection from experimental myasthenia gravis in C57Bl/6 mice by sniffing of synthetic CD4$^+$ T cells epitopes. *J. Clin. Invest.* 100: 3027.
22. Wu, B., C. Deng, E. Goluszko and P. Christadoss. 1997. Tolerance to a dominant T cell epitope in the acetylcholine receptor molecule induces epitope spread and suppresses murine myasthenia gravis. *J.Immunol.* 159: 3016.
23. Karachunski, P.I., N.S. Ostlie, D. Okita, R. Garman and B.M. Conti-Fine. 1999. Subcutaneous administration of T epitope sequences of the acetylcholine receptor prevents experimental Myasthenia Gravis. *J. Neuroimmunol.*, 93: 108.
24. Le Gros, G., S.Z. Ben-Sasson, R. Seder, F.D. Finkelman and W.E. Paul. 1990. Generation of interleukin 4 (IL-4)-producing cells *in vivo* and *in vitro*: IL-2 and IL-4 are required for *in vitro* generation of IL-4-producing cells. *J. Exp. Med.* 172: 921.
25. Swain, S.L., A.D. Weinberg, M. English and G. Huston. 1990. IL-4 directs the development of different subsets of helper T cells. *J. Immunol.* 145: 3796.
26. Kühn, R., K. Rajewsky and W. Müller. 1991. Generation and analysis of interleukin-4 deficient mice. *Science* 254: 707.
27. Kopf, M., G. Le Gros, M. Bachmann, M.C. Lamers, H. Bluethmann and G. Kohler. 1993. Disruption of the murine IL-4 gene blocks Th2 cytokine responses. *Nature.* 362: 245.
28. Lawrence, R.A., J.E. Allen, W.F. Gregory, M. Kopf and R.M. Maizels. 1995. Infection of IL-4-deficient mice with the parasitic nematode Brugia malayi demonstrates that host resistance is not dependent on a T helper 2-dominated immune response. *J. Immunol.* 154: 5995.
29. Karachunski, P.I., N.S. Ostlie, D. Okita and B.M. Conti-Fine. 1999. Interleukin-4 deficiency facilitates development of experimental myasthenia gravis and precludes its prevention by nasal administration of CD4$^+$ epitope sequences of the acetylcholine receptor. *J. Neuroimmunol.* 95: 73.
30. Karachunski, P., N. Ostlie, M. Bellone, A.J. Infante and B.M. Conti-Fine. 1995. Mechanisms by which the I-A^{bm12} mutation influences susceptibility to Experimental Myasthenia Gravis. A study in homozygous and heterozygous mice. *Scand. J. Immunol.* 42: 215.
31. Conti-Fine, B.M., K.E. McLane and S. Lei. 1996. Antibodies as tools to study the

structure of membrane proteins the case of the nicotinic acetylcholine receptor. *Ann. Rev. Biophys. Biomol. Struct.* 25: 197.

32. Bellone M., N. Ostlie, P. Karachunski and B.M. Conti-Tronconi. 1993. Cryptic epitopes on nicotinic acetylcholine receptor are recognized by autoreactive $CD4^{+}$cells. *J. Immunol.* 151: 1025.
33. Bellone, M., N. Ostlie, S. Lei, X-D. Wu and B.M. Conti-Tronconi. 1991. The I-A^{bm12} mutation, which confers resistance to Experimental Myasthenia Gravis, drastically affects their epitope repertoire of murine $CD4^{+}$ cells sensitized to nicotinic acetylcholine receptor. *J. Immunol.* 146: 2253.
34. Wall, K.A., J-Y. Hu, P. Currier, S. Southwood, A. Sette and A.J. Infante. 1994. A disease-related epitope of *Torpedo* acetylcholine receptor. Residues involved in I-A^{b} binding, self-nonself discrimination, and TCR antagonism. *J. Immunol.* 152: 4526.
35. Infante, A.J., P.A. Thompson, K.A. Krolick, and K.A. Wall. 1991. Determinant selection in murine experimental autoimmune myasthenia gravis: Effect of the bm12 mutation on T cell recognition of acetylcholine receptor epitopes. *J. Immunol.* 146: 2977.
36. Tian, J., M.A. Atkinson, M. Clare-Salzler, A. Herschenfeld, T. Forsthuber, P.V. Lehmann and D.L. Kaufman. 1996. Nasal administration of glutamate decarboxylase (GAD65) peptides induces Th2 responses and prevents murine insulin-dependent diabetes. *J. Exp. Med.* 183: 1561.

Myasthenia Gravis: Disease mechanisms and immunointervention
P. Christadoss (Ed)

16. Antigen-Specific Therapy of Experimental Autoimmune Myasthenia Gravis: Mucosal tolerance with recombinant fragments of the human acetylcholine receptor

Sara Fuchs[1], Sin-Heyog Im[1], Dora Barchan[1] and Miriam C. Souroujon[1,2]

[1]Department of Immunology, The Weizmann Institute of Science, Rehovot 76100, Israel

[2]The Open University of Israel, Tel-Aviv, Israel

Introduction

Two important observations in 1973 resulted in a breakthrough in Myasthenia Gravis (MG) research. The first by Fambrough et al [1] showed reduced levels of acetylcholine receptor (AChR) at the neuromuscular junction of patients with MG and the second, by Patrick and Lindstrom [2], demonstrated that rabbits immunized with AChR develop an autoimmune response to AChR, resulting in muscle weakness, and a decremental electromyogram response to repeated nerve stimulation, which are characteristic to MG. These two pivotal observations were seminal for elucidating and understanding the autoimmune nature of MG, and prompted a vast amount of research into both MG and its experimental animal model, experimental autoimmune myasthenia gravis (EAMG).

EAMG has been an excellent model for investigating physiological, histological, immunological and genetic aspects of human MG, as well as for examining various approaches for its treatment. The availability of an experimental model disease for MG, induced by a well-defined antigen (AChR), provides a valuable tool for attempting regulation and suppression of the disease. We have employed both *non-specific* and *specific* immunosuppressive treatment modalities for EAMG. For non-specific treatment we have used corticosteroids and the antimetabolite azathioprine which were empirically found to be effective in the treatment of MG. We employed these drugs (hydrocortisone and azathioprine) in order to suppress or rather to prevent the onset of EAMG in rabbits and to follow the mechanism of suppression [3, 4].

Although immunosuppressive drugs have been useful in the treatment of both MG and EAMG, there are disadvantages in using such agents which may suppress the entire immune system and may have adverse side effects. The ideal treatment of choice should be a *specific* one, namely, a drug that will affect selectively the immunological reactivity which leads to the neuromuscular disorder, leaving the overall immune response intact [5]. Several approaches to specifically suppress EAMG by antigen-specific means have been reported. These include the use of modified derivatives of AChR [6, 7], recombinant AChR fragments [8], anti-idiotypes [9, 10], synthetic peptides [11-13], and oral [14, 15] or nasal [16] administration of AChR.

Denatured AChR

The first attempt for specific immunosuppression of EAMG has been achieved in our laboratory, by employing denatured AChR as an immunomodulating reagent [4, 6]. We have first observed that a denatured Torpedo AChR preparation that was prepared by reduction and carboxymethylation in 6M guanidine hydrochloride and designated reduced-carboxymethylated AChR, or RCM-AChR, was devoid of myasthenogenic activity as well as of α-bungarotoxin (α-BTX) binding activity. Rabbits immunized repeatedly with RCM-AChR did not develop any clinical signs of EAMG, although they developed high titers of antibodies which cross-react with AChR. Differences between the antigenic specificities of AChR and denatured AChR were observed. AChR and RCM-AChR bound to anti-RCM-AChR in an identical manner, whereas there was only a partial cross reactivity between anti-AChR and RCM-AChR, suggesting the presence in this antiserum of antibodies against some antigenic determinants which do not exist on the denatured receptor. Thus, the major difference between AChR and RCM-AChR leading to their different pathogenicity, resides in their different antigenic specificity. The difference in specificity between anti-AChR and anti-RCM-AChR was reflected also by their effects on the binding of α-BTX to AChR: whereas anti-AChR antibodies block the *in vitro* binding of α-BTX to AChR very effectively, anti-RCM-AChR antibodies block this binding only to a very limited extent [17].

The immunological, pharmacological and pathological properties of RCM-AChR made it an appropriate potential candidate for attempting specific immunosuppression of EAMG. Indeed, RCM-AChR, which by itself was devoid of myasthenogenic activity, was shown to have both preventive and therapeutic effects on the experimental neuromuscular block induced by the intact receptor [6]. The onset of EAMG was either delayed or completely prevented in rabbits preimmunized with RCM-AChR. In addition to the protective potential of RCM-AChR, its therapeutic effect on an ongoing disease was observed as well. A single administration of RCM-AChR in complete Freund's adjuvant to myasthenic rabbits during the initial stages of clinical development of EAMG, led to a suppression of EAMG in about 50% of myasthenic rabbits.

Although successful in immunosuppression of EAMG in rabbits, RCM-AChR could not be considered for treatment of MG as it would not be possible to use derivatives of Torpedo AChR in humans, and human AChR could not be available in the large amounts needed for therapy.

From Denatured Torpedo AChR to Human AChR Recombinant Fragments

On the basis of our experience in regulating rabbit EAMG by denatured AChR, it was concluded that the optimal reagent for developing specific therapy of human MG, should be nonpathogenic by itself, should be derived from, and cross react with self receptor, and should be available in large quantities. The cloning of human AChR and the detailed analysis of the specificity of the immune response in MG led us to investigate the potential of recombinant fragments of *human* AChR for the treatment of MG.

The antibody response towards AChR in myasthenia is heterogeneous, and possibly only part of the anti-AChR antibodies present in the sera of MG patients are actually involved in the pathogenesis of the disease. Therefore, the identification of immunopathogenic regions in AChR, and especially those that react with sera from a variety of MG patients, is important for devising strategies for antigen-specific immunotherapeutic procedures. Such a strategy could involve the administration of derivatives of AChR which do not induce myasthenia but are capable of specific suppression (or tolerization) of the autoimmune attack on muscle AChR.

The extracellular portion of the AChR-subunit is the target for the majority of the anti-AChR antibodies in MG sera. Recombinant proteins corresponding to this region have therefore the potential for developing antigen-directed therapy for MG. These fragments are larger than selected peptide epitopes and may therefore have a broader specificity, and hence an advantage for the modulation of the heterogeneous anti-AChR response in myasthenia. With this in mind, we have prepared recombinant fragments of the human AChR α-subunit, corresponding to the entire extracellular domain (Hα1-210), and to segments of it, that encompass either the main immunogenic region (MIR) (Hα1-121) or the ligand binding site (Hα122-210) [8], and we are employing them for examining their immunomodulatory potential for rat EAMG. We chose to work with recombinant fragments corresponding to the *human* AChR sequence for modulation of *rat* EAMG, as they are highly homologous to rat AChR sequence (> 95%) and if beneficial in the rat model, could be considered later for human MG.

The immunomodulatory potential of the human recombinant fragments was first tested *in vitro* in TE671 cells, and *in vivo,* in EAMG passively transferred by an anti-AChR monoclonal antibody [8]. The recombinant proteins Hα1-121 and Hα1-210 were shown to interfere with the antigenic modulation of AChR in TE671 cells by anti-AChR antibodies. The fragments had an effect on the antigenic modulation caused by the MIR-specific mAb198 [18]. Preincubation of mAb 198 as well as of two other anti-MIR mAbs with increasing concentrations of the fragments, had a dose-dependent protective activity. Moreover, these fragments protected AChR in TE671 cells against antigenic modulation induced by polyclonal anti-AChR sera from myasthenic rats.

In addition, Hα1-121 and Hα1-210 were capable of modulating *in vivo* the course of EAMG, induced by passive transfer of mAb 198. Myasthenic symptoms were observed 24-48 hrs following the administration of mAb 198 alone, and were accompanied by a reduction in the muscle AChR content (48% of normal controls). Preincubation of mAb 198 with fragment Hα1-121 prevented the appearance of myasthenic symptoms and the reduction in muscle AChR content [8]. Similar results were obtained with the Hα1-210 recombinant fragment, but not with either Hα122-210, which does not contain the MIR, or BSA. Administration of the recombinant fragments alone did not result in any myasthenic symptoms in the rats.

Mucosal Tolerance with Recombinant Fragments

The observation that mucosal delivery of antigens can induce a state of peripheral immunological tolerance opens new opportunities to investigate antigen-specific immunomodulation of autoimmune diseases. This observation has been tested as an approach to modulate autoimmune diseases [19] such as experimental autoimmune encephalomyelitis (EAE) [20], uvetis (EAU) [21], arthritis [22], diabetes [23], thyroiditis [24] and also EAMG.

As mentioned above, there have been recent reports on modulation of EAMG induction in rats by oral or nasal administration of the entire AChR molecule purified from the Torpedo electric organ [14-16]. However, Torpedo AChR, being a highly immunogenic and a xenogeneic protein, and available in limited amounts, is less likely to be considered for therapeutic purposes in humans [25, 26]. In some of the modulation experiments by mucosal administration of Torpedo AChR, antibodies to Torpedo and rat self-AChR were markedly increased and antigen-specific T cell responses were not suppressed. The potential expansion of activated autoreactive T cells by the antigen used for tolerization of an ongoing disease must not be underestimated. We therefore propose that treatment of an ongoing autoimmune disease may require a *modified* syngeneic antigen with reduced immunogenic potential, like the recombinant fragments employed in this study. We have embarked recently on a study to investigate the immunomodulatory potential of recombinant fragments of the *human* AChR to regulate EAMG, following their nasal or oral administration [27, 28]. As mentioned above, such human-derived fragments, if also effective in regulating human MG, can be available in large amounts needed for the long -term treatment of MG patients.

Nasal Tolerization

The nasal route for administration of a tolerogen might be especially attractive as it is effective in very low doses and avoids gastric proteolytic degradation of the antigen. In recent studies we have employed recombinant fragments of the extracellular domain of human AChR α-subunit and demonstrated that nasal administration of such fragments prevents the onset of EAMG in rats and immunosuppresses an already existing disease [5, 27, 28].

For prevention of EAMG by nasal pretreatment with recombinant fragments we have employed the three different fragments mentioned above [8]. The fragments were expressed as fusion proteins with glutathione S-transferase (GST). The fragments were administered intranasally for 12 consecutive days (5 µg/rat/day). Control rats were administered with GST. Two days following the last intranasal application, rats were immunized with Torpedo AChR, for induction of EAMG. Significant protection against EAMG was observed in rats pretreated with either of the AChR fragments. Eight weeks after induction of EAMG, all 10 rats in the control GST-pretreated group, had clinical symptoms of EAMG (two died), whereas 67, 56 and 33% of rats in the groups pretreated with Hα1-210, Hα1-121 and Hα122-210, respectively, were completely protected and did not exhibit any symptoms of EAMG.

The analysis of body weight and of AChR content verified the protective effect of the nasal pretreatment, as evaluated by clinical symptoms of EAMG. Rats in the control GST-treated group lost 12.8 ± 9.2 gr. per rat, between 3 and 7 weeks following induction of EAMG, whereas rats in the groups pretreated intranasally with Hα1-210, Hα1-121 or Hα122-210 gained 15.0 ± 6.3, 13.6 ± 2.5 and 9.2 ± 8.6 gr. per rat, respectively, during this period. Rats with EAMG, in the control GST-treated group, lost about 56% of their muscle AChR content, whereas there was only a small loss in AChR content in rats pretreated with Hα1-210 or Hα1-121 (11 and 25%, respectively). The protective effect in the pretreated rats was accompanied by reduced proliferative T-cell response to AChR, reduced levels of IL-2 (a Th1 cytokine) and reduced levels of anti-self AChR antibodies. Adoptive transfer experiments in which spleen cells from intranasally treated rats were injected i.p. into naive rats (100×10^6 spleen cells per rat), before injection of Torpedo AChR for induction of EAMG, indicated that protection from EAMG could be passively transferred. This suggests the involvement of active suppression in the protective effect of nasal tolerance, induced by the recombinant fragments [28].

The ultimate goal is to treat an ongoing EAMG rather than preventing its onset. To that end we studied the immunomodulatory effect of intranasal treatment with Hα1-210, when given 3 or 7 days after induction of EAMG. It should be noted that on day 7 following AChR immunization, rats usually display clinical symptoms associated with the first, acute phase of EAMG. A therapeutic effect on EAMG, albeit lower in extent than in pretreatment experiments, was observed following treatment at the acute phase of EAMG. Among the rats treated at the acute phase of EAMG 30% remained healthy for at least 8 weeks following AChR administration. The effect on clinical manifestation was also corroborated by AChR content and change in body weight, as well as by a marked decrease in lymphoproliferative responses to AChR. The therapeutic effect of the nasal treatments resulted in a switch in the IgG isotypes, from IgG2b and IgG2c to IgG1, which may indicate a shift from a Th1 to a Th2 T-cell type activity [28].

Oral Tolerization

In parallel with studies on *nasal* tolerization we are also investigating the potential of an *orally* administered recombinant fragment of human AChR, to prevent EAMG and to suppress an already existing disease in rats. The recombinant fragment employed in this study corresponds to residues 1-205 of the human AChR α-subunit (Hα1-205) and has been expressed without any fusion partner. Such a fragment may be more suitable for treatment of MG patients than fragments with fusion partners. Even though oral administration requires higher doses of tolerizing protein, it is more convenient for application in humans and may be safer than nasal administration [29, 30].

For prevention of EAMG by oral pretreatment, rats were fed with Hα1-205 (0.6 mg/dose) or ovalbumin (OVA) as control, three times a week for two weeks. Two days after the last feeding, rats were immunized with Torpedo AChR for induction of EAMG. Significant protection against EAMG was observed in rats pretreated with Hα1-205. Eight weeks after induction of EAMG, all 10 rats in the control group were sick (mean clinical score: 2.8), whereas among rats pretreated with Hα1-205, 70% were completely protected and the remaining 30% showed mild symptoms as compared to the control group. The mean clinical score in the Hα1-205-treated rats was 0.5. Quantitative parameters of disease included assessment of body weight and muscle AChR content of the rats. Rats in the control group lost 8.8 ± 9.2 gr. per rat, between 3 and 8 weeks following induction of EAMG, while rats in the Hα1-205-orally pretreated group gained at the same time 9.8 ± 5.3 gr. per rat. The analysis of AChR content verified the observations of clinical symptoms. Myasthenic rats in the control OVA-pretreated group, lost about 60% of their muscle AChR content. On the other hand, there was only 8.5% loss in the AChR content in rats from the Hα1-205-pretreated group. The protective effect of the oral pretreatment was accompanied by a marked reduction in AChR-specific proliferative T-cell response and IL-2 production, as well as by a decrease in anti-rat AChR antibodies. Delayed type hypersensitivity (DTH) to Torpedo AChR, a known Th1-regulated response was also reduced in Hα1-205-treated rats, indicating that pretreatment with AChR-specific fragments induces a suppressed T-cell response to AChR.

Oral administration with Hα1-205 was also employed to treat an already ongoing EAMG, either in the acute or chronic phase of the disease. For treatment at the *acute* phase of EAMG, oral administration with Hα1-205 (0.6 mg/dose) was initiated on day 8 after induction of EAMG and continued with three days intervals for 9 weeks. For treatment of chronic EAMG, rats presenting a clinical score of 1 were selected 8 weeks after EAMG induction and were given 7 oral administrations of Hα1-205 with three days intervals. In both treatments, oral administration of Hα1-205 had a suppressive effect on EAMG, as assessed by clinical evaluation, body weight, receptor content, as well as by various immunological parameters. When treated at the acute phase of EAMG, all 10 rats in the control OVA-treated group got sick and at 10 weeks after disease induction 6/10 died of EAMG. On the other hand, in the Hα1-205-treated group, 6/10 were completely healthy and none of them died. Likewise, there was a significant suppression on EAMG in rats treated with Hα1-205, at the chronic phase of EAMG. Suppression of EAMG following treatment at the acute or chronic EAMG was accompanied by a marked reduction in AChR-specific T cell responses and IL-2 production, as well as in anti-self AChR antibody titers.

Clonal anergy, active suppression, and clonal deletion have been proposed as potential mechanisms involved in oral tolerance induction. It seems that clonal anergy is not involved in the tolerance induced by feeding with AChR-derived fragments, as preincubation of lymph node cells from Hα1-205-treated rats with exogenous IL-2 did not restore the reduction in AChR-specific T-cell proliferative responses in these cells. On the other hand, active suppression appeared to be involved in the oral tolerance induced, as it was in nasal tolerance, since some protection was adoptively transferred to recipient rats by splenocytes from rats fed with Hα1-205. In addition, active suppression was also demonstrated by changes in cytokine profile. Oral treatment of acute EAMG with Hα1-205 resulted in suppression of Th1 type (IL-2 and IFN-γ) cytokine mRNA levels and up-regulation of Th2 type (IL-10) and Th3 type (TGF-b) cytokine mRNA levels, indicating that oral treatment of Hα1-205 induced a shift from a Th1 towards a Th2/Th3 cytokine profile. Such a shift was also observed by measuring AChR-specific IgG isotypes in rats following oral administration of Hα1-205, in protection or treatment experiments of EAMG. The relative levels of IgG1 in Hα1-205-treated rats were higher than in control OVA-treated rats, whereas IgG2 subtypes (in particular IgG2b, and IgG2c) were lower in the Hα1-205-treated rats as compared to controls. The correlation of IgG2b and IgG2c levels with severity of disease, may suggest that these isotypes are involved in the pathogenesis of EAMG.

Conclusions

Developing a specific treatment for an autoimmune disease depends on knowing the autoantigen(s) involved. This is the case with myasthenia gravis where the nature, structure and specificity of the autoantigen, AChR, is known and extensively studied. The approach of using recombinant fragments of AChR for handling myasthenia is based on our previous studies demonstrating the suppressive effect on EAMG, of a denatured derivative of Torpedo AChR, which by itself is nonpathogenic. The application of recombinant fragments of *human* AChR is a step forward towards the possible application for MG. We employ fragments corresponding to the extracellular domain of the AChR α-subunit, as it is considered to be immunologically most relevant to myasthenia. However, the recombinant approach employed to synthesize the fragments allows us to easily prepare additional fragments of the AChR α-subunit, or of other subunits, if they are found to be more efficient.

The mucosal application of AChR fragments to suppress EAMG is another advantage of our approach. Either nasal or oral application of the fragments for the treatment of EAMG in rats proves to lead to significant protective and/or therapeutic effects and to be safe and convenient. In our hands the suppression by the recombinant AChR fragments has been, by far, more beneficial than that by any short peptides. Finally, the potential of the described therapeutic approach for human MG is yet to be investigated. Even if it does not replace the present treatment modalities, it may be employed in combination with them, which may give better results and lower side effects.

Acknowledgments

The work described in this manuscript was supported in part by the Muscular Dystrophy Association of America (MDA), the Association Français Contre le Myopathies (AFM), The Robert Koch-Minerva Center for Research in Autoimmune Diseases and The Leo and Julia Forchheimer Center for Molecular Genetics at The Weizmann Institute of Science.

References

1. Fambrough, D.M., D.B. Drachman and S. Satyamurti, S. 1973. Neuromuscular junction in myasthenia gravis: decreased acetylcholine receptors *Science* 182, 293.
2. Patrick, J. and J.M. Lindstrom. 1973. Autoimmune response to acetylcholine receptor. *Science* 180, 871.
3. Abramsky, O., R. Tarrab-Hazdai, A. Aharonov and S. Fuchs. 1976. Immunosuppression of experimental autoimmune myasthenia gravis by hydrocortisone and azathioprine. *J. Immunol.* 117, 225.
4. Fuchs, S., D. Bartfeld, Z. Eshhar, C. Feingold, D. Mochly-Rosen, D. Novick, M. Schwartz and R. Tarrab-Hazdai. 1980. Immune regulation of experimental myasthenia. *J. Neurol. Neurosurg. and Psych.* 43, 634.
5. S. Fuchs. 1999. Antigen-specific immunomodulation of experimental auto-immune myasthenia gravis. *In*: The Decade of Autoimmunity. Y. Shoenfeld, ed., Elsevier Sci. Publishers, Amsterdam, p. 255.
6. Bartfeld, D. and S. Fuchs. 1978. Specific immunosuppression of experimental autoimmune myasthenia gravis by denatured acetylcholine receptor. *Proc. Natl. Acad. Sci.* USA. 75, 4006.
7. Krolick, K.A., T.-M. Yeh and A. Edlund. 1996. Lewis rats given antibodies against denatured acetylcholine receptor become resistant to induction of experimental autoimmune myasthenia gravis. *Cell. Immunol.* 172, 10.
8. Barchan, D., O. Asher, S. Tzartos, S. Fuchs and M.C. Souroujon. 1998. Modulation of the anti-acetylcholine receptor response and experimental autoimmune myasthenia gravis by recombinant fragments of the acetylcholine receptor. *Eur. J. Immunol.* 28, 616.
9. Souroujon, M.C., A.R. Pachner and S. Fuchs. 1986. The treatment of passively transferred experimental myasthenia with anti-idiotypic antibodies. *Neurology* 35, 622.
10. Souroujon, M.C. and S. Fuchs. 1987. Anti-idiotypic antibodies in the regulation of experimental autoimmune myasthenia gravis. *Ann. N.Y. Acad. Sci.,* 505, 676.
11. Souroujon, M.C., S. Carmon and S. Fuchs. 1992. Modulation of anti-acetylcholine receptor antibody specificities and of experimental autoimmune myasthenia gravis by synthetic peptides. *Immunol. Lett.* 34, 19.
12. Atassi, M.Z., K.H. Ruan, K. Jinnai, M. Oshima and T. Ashizawa. 1992. Epitope-specific suppression of antibody response in experimental autoimmune myasthenia gravis by a monomethoxypolyethylene glycol conjugate of a myasthenogenic synthetic peptide. *Proc. Natl. Acad. Sci.* USA 89, 5852.
13. Shenoy, M., Oshima, M., Atassi, M.Z. and Christadoss, P. 1993. Suppression of experimental autoimmune myasthenia gravis by epitope- specific neonatal tolerance to synthetic region alpha 146-162 of acetylcholine receptor. *Clin. Immunol. Immunopathol.* 66, 230.
14. Wang, Z.-Y., J. Qiao and H. Link. 1993. Suppression of experimental autoimmune myasthenia gravis by oral administration of acetylcholine receptor. *J. Neuroimmunol* 44, 209.
15. Okumura, S., K. McIntosh and D.B. Drachman. 1994. Oral administration of acetylcholine receptor: effects on experimental autoimmune myasthenia gravis. *Ann. Neurol.* 36, 704.
16. Ma, C.-G., G.-X. Zhang, B.-G. Xiao, J. Link, T. Olsson and H. Link. 1995. Suppression of experimental autoimmune myasthenia gravis by nasal administration of acetylcholine receptor. *J. Neuroimmunol.* 58, 51.

17. D. Bartfeld and S. Fuchs. 1977. Immunological characterization of an irreversibly denatured acetylcholine receptor. *FEBS Lett.* 77, 214.
18. Sophianos, D. and S.J. Tzartos. 1989. Fab fragments of monoclonal antibodies protect the human acetylcholine receptor against antigenic modulation caused by myasthenic sera. *J. Autoimmunity* 2, 777.
19. Weiner, H. L. 1997. Oral tolerance for the treatment of autoimmune diseases. *Annu. Rev. Med.* 48: 341.
20. Higgins, P.J. and H.L. Weiner. 1988. Suppression of experimental autoimmune encephalomyelitis by oral administration of myelin basic protein and its fragments. *J. Immunol.* 140: 440.
21. Nussenblatt, R.B., R.R. Caspi, R. Mahdi, C.C. Chan, F. Roberge, O. Lider and H.L. Weiner. 1990. Inhibition of S-antigen induced experimental autoimmune uveoretinitis by oral induction of tolerance with S-antigen. *J. Immunol.* 144: 1689.
22. Thompson, H., and N. Staines. 1990. Could specific oral tolerance be a therapy for autoimmune disease? *Immunol today* 11:396.
23. Zhang, Z.J., L. Davidson, G. Eisenbarth and H.L. Weiner. 1991. Suppression of diabetes in nonobese diabetic mice by oral administration of porcine insulin. *Proc. Natl. Acad. Sci.* USA 88: 10252.
24. Peterson, K.E. and H. Braley Mullen. 1995. Suppression of murine experimental autoimmune thyroiditis by oral administration of porcine thyroglobulin. *Cell. Immunol.* 166:123.
25. Drachman, D.B., S. Okumura, R.N. Adams and K. McIntosh. 1996. Oral tolerance in myasthenia gravis. *In*: Oral tolerance: mechanism and applications, eds. Weiner, H.L., Mayer, L.F., *Ann. N Y. Acad. Sci.* 778, 258.
26. Shi, F.D., X.F. Bai, H.L. Li, Y.M. Huang, P.H. Van der Meide and H. Link. 1998. Nasal tolerance in experimental autoimmune myasthenia gravis (EAMG): induction of protective tolerance in primed animals. *Clin. Exp. Immunol.* 111: 506.
27. Barchan, D., S.-H. Im, M.C. Souroujon and S. Fuchs. 1998. Antigen-specific therapy of experimental autoimmune myasthenia gravis: mucosal tolerance with recombinant fragments of the human acetylcholine receptor. *J. Neuroimmunol.* 92, 1.
28. Barchan, D., M.C. Souroujon, S.-H. Im, C. Antozzi and S. Fuchs. 1999. Antigen-specific immunotherapy of experimental mysthenia: nasal tolerization with recombinant fragments of the human acetylcholine receptor α-subunit. *Proc. Natl. Acad. Sci.* USA 96: 8086.
29. Heritage, P.L., B.J. Underdown, A.L. Arsenault, D.P. Snider and M.R. McDermott. 1997. Comparison of murine nasal-associated lymphoid tissue and Peyer's patches. *Am. J. Respir. Crit. Care. Med.* 156: 1256.
30. Wu, H.Y. and M.W. Russell. 1997. Nasal lymphoid tissue, intranasal immunization, and compartmentalization of the common mucosal immune system. *Immunol. Res.* 16: 187.

Myasthenia Gravis: Disease mechanisms and immunointervention
P. Christadoss (Ed)

17. Immunomodulation of Myasthenia Gravis Associated Autoimmune Responses by an Altered Peptide Ligand: Mechanisms of action

Miri Pass-Rozner, Anat Faber-Elmann, Michael Sela and Edna Mozes

Department of Immunology, The Weizmann Institute of Science, Rehovot 76100, Israel

Introduction

Myasthenia gravis (MG) and its experimental animal model, experimental autoimmune myasthenia gravis (EAMG), are immune disorders characterized by circulating antibodies and lymphocyte autoreactivity to nicotinic acetylcholine receptor (AChR). Although the production of acetylcholine receptor specific antibodies is directly attributed to B cells, there is extensive evidence that T cells have a key role in the etiopathology of the disease in humans and animals [1-4]. Since the α-subunit of the AChR was shown to be predominant for T cell epitopes [2], we have used peptides representing different sequences of the human AChR α-subunit to study the role of T cells in the initiation, development and immunomodulation of myasthenia gravis.

Myasthenogenic T Cell Epitopes of the Human AChR α-Subunit

To investigate which parts of the AChR α-subunit are associated with MG, peripheral blood lymphocytes (PBL) of patients with MG and healthy controls were tested for their ability to respond to synthetic peptides that represent different sequences of the human AChR α-subunit. Two of eight peptides representing sequences p195-212 and p257-269 of the human AChR α-subunit discriminated significantly between the group of MG patients and healthy controls in a proliferation assay on PBL. HLA-DR11 and HLA-DR3 were associated with proliferative responses to peptides p195-212 and p257-269, respectively, suggesting that certain peptides of the AChR are especially immunogenic for certain HLA-DR types [5]. The peptides also discriminated significantly between MG patients and controls based on sera antibodies that bound to them [5]. Thus, these results demonstrated T cell epitopes of the human AChR that might play a specific role in MG.

We have further demonstrated that the epitopes which were specifically recognized by T lymphocytes of patients with MG also represent specific T cell epitopes associated with autoreactivity to AChR in mice [6]. Thus, following immunization with the Torpedo AChR, lymphocytes of SJL mice proliferated to p195-212 even better than to the immunizing antigen; however, they did not proliferate to p259-271 (that triggered responses identical to p257-269). On the other hand, lymph node cells of BALB/c mice responded well to p259-271, but not to p195-212 [6].

In order to characterize the T cells that recognize the two T cell epitopes, p195-212 and p259-271, T cell lines and clones were established and characterized. The involvement of p195-212- and p259-271- specific T cells in the pathogenicity of MG was determined by the induction of EAMG in naive mice following their inoculation with activated T cells of syngeneic lines specific to the immunodominant myasthenogenic T cell epitopes. The MG-related manifestations in the inoculated mice were determined by objective parameters, namely, production of antibodies to self (murine) AChR and decremental compound muscle action potentials (CMAP) consistent with impairment of neuromuscular transmission [4]. The ability of T cell lines specific to the myasthenogenic T cell epitopes to induce experimental autoimmune myasthenia gravis supports the role of T cells in this disease.

Peptide Analogs to the Myasthenogenic T Cell Epitopes as Potential Modulators of Myasthenia Gravis

Several immunotherapeutic strategies, including the use of immunosuppressive therapy, plasmapheresis and intravenous immunoglobulin have been used for treatment of MG [3]. Ideally the goal of therapy in MG should be to eliminate the autoimmune response to the AChR specifically without interfering with immune responses to other antigens. Because T cells play a critical role in the autoimmune responses in MG and since T cells can be inactivated, or rendered "anergic," they provide a powerful target for attempting immunotherapy at the initial stages of activation, before the autoimmune responses develop. A more specific approach would be to use altered peptide ligands (APL) of the myasthenogenic peptides in an attempt to preserve and even improve their MHC binding, while distorting their interaction with the T cell antigen receptor so that they will antagonize the original antigen. To this end, single substituted analogs of the myasthenogenic peptides p195-212 and p259-271 were synthesized and characterized. Using a murine model we showed that the analog of p195-212, 207Ala, and that of p259-271, 262Lys, were able to inhibit the *in vitro* proliferative responses of the specific T cell lines and to down-regulate the *in vivo* priming of lymph node cells of mice primed to the myasthenogenic peptides [7-9]. These single substituted analogs, 207Ala and 262Lys, were found to bind to murine and to human MHC molecules as efficiently as the original peptides [8-10].

One of our goals has been to design an analog that will inhibit T cell responses to both myasthenogenic peptides p195-212 and p259-271. To this end we synthesized dual analogs composed of the tandemly arranged, two single analogs either sequentially (207Ala-262Lys) or reciprocally (262Lys-207Ala). Both dual analogs could bind to MHC class II molecules on antigen-presenting cells (APC) of SJL and BALB/c mice. However, analog 262Lys-207Ala was more efficient in its binding to MHC of both strains and was used in further experiments [11].

Similar to the single amino acid substituted analogs, the dual analog 262Lys-207Ala was tested for its ability to inhibit the proliferative responses of T cell lines specific to both myasthenogenic peptides, namely, p195-212 and p259-271. It was shown to inhibit the proliferation of both T cell lines in a dose-dependent manner with a maximum of above 90% [11]. The dual analog was also shown to be capable of inhibiting efficiently (90-100%) the in vivo priming of lymph node cells of mice to either myasthenogenic peptides [11].

We have further demonstrated that the dual analog has a potential to inhibit the *in vivo* proliferation of lymph node cells when administered at the stage that the T cells are already activated to the myasthenogenic peptides, namely 7 days following priming with either p195-212 or p259-271. The inhibitory capacity of the dual analog could be observed when the latter was administered intravenously (i.v.), intraperitoneally (i.p.), subcutaneously (s.c.) or orally [11].

For the dual analog to be considered of therapeutic potential, it must be able to treat an established disease. Indeed we have demonstrated that oral administration of the dual analog, twice a week for 4 weeks to BALB/c mice in which EAMG was induced by the pathogenic p259-271-specific T cell line, reversed EAMG manifestations in the treated mice [11].

We have demonstrated that PBL from above 80% of MG patients proliferated in response to stimulation by either of the myasthenogenic epitopes or by both [5, 10]. It was therefore of importance to test the inhibitory efficacy of the dual analog on the above responses. Indeed, the dual analog was shown to inhibit specifically T cell stimulation in above 90% of the responder patients to either myasthenogenic peptide [10]. Thus the dual analog is an efficient inhibitor of p195-212- and p259-271-specific T cell responses of MG patients and might have therapeutic potential.

Results and Discussion

Effect of the Dual Analog on EAMG Induced in C57BL/6 Mice with the Torpedo AChR

As mentioned above, the dual analog inhibited the *in vivo* priming of lymph node cells of SJL and BALB/c mice immunized with the myasthenogenic peptides p195-212 and p259-271, and it reversed EAMG manifestations in mice that were inoculated with T cell lines specific to the myasthenogenic peptides [11]. Because EAMG is routinely induced in mice using the Torpedo AChR and C57BL/6 mice are the most susceptible to disease induction using the receptor, it was of interest to follow the effect of the dual analog on EAMG induced in C57BL/6 mice with the Torpedo AChR. Mice were immunized with the Torpedo AChR in CFA. When clinical symptoms were observed mice were treated with the dual analog that was given orally 3 times a week for 8 weeks. Table 1 demonstrates results obtained to the present. As can be seen in the table, 40% of the Torpedo AChR-injected mice (22/25) developed a disease that could be diagnosed either by evaluating their muscle weakness (clinical score) or by electromyography (EMG). Six of the mice that developed EAMG died before starting treatment with the dual analog. The rest of the sick mice (16 mice) were divided into two groups. Eleven mice were treated with the dual analog for a period of 8 weeks and five mice were not treated. All of the 11 treated mice survived. The treatment had beneficial effects on 8 out of the 11 treated mice (72%), as manifested by the observed regaining of muscle strength and reversal of myasthenic decrement. Of the 5 mice that developed EAMG and were not treated, 2 mice died, 2 remained sick and one mouse underwent spontaneous remission. Thus, the dual analog ameliorates manifestations of AChR induced EAMG.

Table 1. The beneficial effects of treatment with the dual analog on EAMG induced by Torpedo AChR (TAChR)

Number of mice immunized with TAChR	EAMG Development	Dual analog administration (11 mice)	PBS administration (5 mice)
55	22/55 (40%)*	Recovery 8/11 (72%) Sick 3/11 (28%) Mortality 0/11 (0%)	Spontaneous recovery 1/5 (20%) Sick 2/5 (40%) Mortality 2/5 (40%)

*6 out of the 22 mice which developed EAMG died before treatment.

Immunomodulation of Cytokines by the Dual Analog

The maintenance of self-tolerance, at least in part, appears to depend on T cell regulation. There is evidence for a role of Th1-type and/or proinflammatory cytokines in the pathogenesis of autoimmune diseases [12, 13]. The effect of Th2-type cytokines was also investigated in these diseases. There are studies showing that Th2-type cytokines have a protective effect in autoimmune diseases like experimental autoimmune encephalomyelitis (EAE) [14, 15] and insulin-dependent diabetes mellitus (IDDM) [16, 17]. It has been shown that alternative regulatory populations exist that are somehow associated with, but distinct from Th2 cells. These regulatory CD4+ T cells subsets were shown to secrete the cytokine-transforming growth factor (TGF)-β (18). The importance of cytokines in EAMG was also demonstrated. The Th1-type cytokine IFN-γ was shown to play a pathogenic role in EAMG in mice and rats [11, 19], whereas TGF-β plays an important role in tolerance induction to EAMG [20]. Reports concerning the role of IL-4 in EAMG are controversial [20-22].

In an attempt to elucidate the mechanism of action of the dual analog we first tested whether it has an effect on the pattern of cytokines secreted by p195-212-specific T cell lines. Cells of these lines were incubated with the myasthenogenic peptide p195-212 with or without the dual analog in the presence of irradiated splenocytes which served as APC. As can be seen in Table 2, peptide p195-212 caused the cells to secrete a small amount of IFN-γ, and high doses of IL-4, IL-10 and TGF-β. The dual analog, in the presence of p195-212, caused a decrease in the secretion of all secreted cytokines mentioned above except for

TGF-β. Thus, the only cytokine that was not affected by the dual analog is the immunosuppressive cytokine TGF-β.

Table 2. The effect of the dual analog on the cytokine secretion of p195-212-specific T cell line

Cytokine	w/o p195-212	p195-212	p195-212+ 262Lys-207Ala
IFN-γ	0%	100%	47%
IL-2	–*	–	–
IL-4	1%	100%	42%
IL-10	3%	100%	76%
TGF-beta	48%	100%	102%

*IL-2 secretion was below detectable levels.
Cytokine secretion upon stimulation with p195-212 was considered as 100% (IFN-γ 100% = 2.09 ng/ml, IL-4 100% = 78.7 ng/ml, IL-10 100% = 17.36 ng/ml and TGF-beta 100% = 195.2 ng/ml).

After demonstrating that the dual analog has an effect on the cytokine secretion of p195-212-specific T cell lines, we have further tested the *in vivo* effect of the dual analog on lymph node cell priming to p195-212. To this end we have first examined whether the dual analog has an effect on lymph node cells of SJL mice primed with p195-212, when administered orally prior to immunization with the myasthenogenic peptide (pretreatment). The mice were pretreated orally with the dual analog at a dose of 500 μg/mouse every other day for a week before they were immunized with p195-212 in CFA. Pretreatment with the dual analog inhibited (up to 95%) the proliferative response to p195-212 of lymph node cells of the treated mice. These results suggest that the dual analog prevented the priming of the lymph node cells with the myasthenogenic peptide. One of the possible mechanisms by which the dual analog can exert its inhibitory effect is by inducing anergy. One of the methods used to show the latter is by restoring the proliferative capacity of the cells following their culturing with recombinant IL-2 (rIL-2). Our results showed that addition of 100 U/ml of rIL-2 led to proliferation rates of lymph node cells of pretreated mice comparable to those of lymph node cells of non-treated animals. Similar results were obtained when the dual analog was administered i.p. These results may indicate that one of the routes by which the dual analog exerts its inhibitory effect is by causing the cells to undergo anergy.

We have also determined the effect of *in vivo* pretreatment with the dual analog on the cytokine profile of the treated mice. To this end, SJL mice were pretreated orally with the dual analog or with PBS and then immunized with p195-212. Ten days post immunization, the splenocytes of the mice were stimulated with p195-212. Supernatants were collected and the levels of the various cytokines were determined. As shown in Table 3, upon stimulation with p195-212 the splenocytes of pretreated mice secreted lower amounts of IL-2 and IFN-γ in comparison to splenocytes of mice pretreated with PBS (same results were obtained when the cells were stimulated with ConA.). Thus, the oral pretreatment with the dual analog reduced the levels of both Th1-type cytokines. In contrast, pretreatment with the dual analog caused the splenocytes, upon stimulation with p195-212 (or with ConcanavalinA), to secrete higher amounts of IL-4, IL-5 and IL-10 (Th2-type cytokines) and TGF-β (Th3-type cytokine) in comparison to cells of non-treated mice. Similar results were also demonstrated when the mice were pretreated with the dual analog i.p., suggesting a common mechanism for both routes of administration. These latter results suggest that the pretreatment with the dual analog causes a shift from Th1-type cytokines (IL-2 and IFN-γ) to Th2- (IL-4, IL-5 and IL-10) and Th3-type (TGF-β) cytokines. It is noteworthy that TGF-β is considered to be a cytokine which has the ability to suppress inflammatory responses induced by proinflammatory cytokines.

Table 3. The effect of 262Lys-207Ala on the cytokine network of SJL mice pretreated orally with the dual analog

Cytokine	*In vivo* oral pretreatment	*In vitro* stimulation	
		w/o p195-212	p195-212
IL-2	PBS	0%	100%
	262Lys-207Ala	0%	81% ↓
IFN-gamma	PBS	14%	100%
	262Lys-207Ala	0%	33% ↓
IL-4	PBS	0%	100%
	262Lys-207Ala	0%	900%↑
IL-5	PBS	0%	100%
	262Lys-207Ala	0%	333%↑
IL-10	PBS	35%	100%
	262Lys-207Ala	119%	341%↑
TGF-beta	PBS	85%	100%
	262Lys-207Ala	94%	175%↑

SJL mice were pretreated orally with the dual analog (500 μg/mouse/administration for 4 times every other day) and then immunized with 10 μg/mouse p195-212 in complete Freund's adjuvant.

Cytokine secretion upon stimulation with p195-212 was considered as 100% (IL-2 100% = 192 pg/ml, IFN-γ 100% = 2502 pg/ml, IL-4 100% = 2 pg/ml, IL-5 100% = 24 pg/ml, IL-10 100% = 314 pg/ml, TGF-β 100% = 195pg/ml).

It was of interest to determine whether the effect of the cytokine network seen in the pretreated mice can be also observed when the dual analog is administered concomitantly with p195-212 immunization. SJL mice were immunized with p195-212 in CFA concomitant with an oral administration of the dual analog (500 μg/mouse). Ten days later the splenocytes of the mice were cultured with p195-212 or ConA, the supernatants were collected and cytokine levels were determined. As can be seen in Table 4, oral administration of the dual analog caused a decrease in the secretion of IL-2 and IFN-γ in comparison to the splenocytes of the non-treated mice. The levels of the Th2-type cytokines, namely IL-4, IL-5 and IL-10, were elevated upon the oral administration of the dual analog, as well as that of the Th3-type cytokine TGF-β. Thus, the effect of the dual analog on the cytokine network was similar whether it was administered concomitantly with or prior to the immunization with p195-212. Taking into consideration the reported role of IFN-γ in the pathogenicity of myasthenia gravis, the decrease in the IFN-γ secretion seen following administration of the dual analog may be an important factor in the mechanism by which the dual analog immunomodulates EAMG-associated T cell responses. It was also shown that administration of AChR orally at milligram doses or nasally at microgram doses prior to induction of EAMG effectively abrogated the disease [23, 24]. These studies showed that the number of AChR-reactive IFN-γ and IL-4 mRNA were reduced in tolerant animals, while numbers of AChR-reactive, TGF-β mRNA-expressing cells were strongly upregulated in comparison with numbers detected in non-tolerized EAMG control rats, implying that active suppression could be an important mechanism in the inhibition of EAMG induction. Our results support the importance of TGF-β, which acts via immunosuppressive mechanisms that include the downregulation of the Th1-type cytokines. The dramatic up-regulation, upon treatment with the dual analog, of the Th2/Th3 cytokines which are considered to be protective against a few diseases, may contribute another insight to the complex cytokine network in EAMG.

Table 4. The effect of the dual analog 262Lys-207Ala on the cytokine network of p195-212 immunized SJL mice when administered orally concomitant with immunization

Cytokine	*In vivo* oral administration	*In vitro* stimulation: w/o stimulation	*In vitro* stimulation: with stimulation
IL-2	–	0%	100%
	262Lys-207Ala	0%	44% ↓
IFN-gamma	–	0%	*100%
	262Lys-207Ala	3%	*59% ↓
IL-4	–	0%	100%
	262Lys-207Ala	0%	824% ↑
IL-5	–	16%	*100%
	262Lys-207Ala	50%	*158% ↑
IL-10	–	109%	100%
	262Lys-207Ala	119%	160% ↑
TGF-beta	–	13%	100%
	262Lys-207Ala	187%	433% ↑

SJL mice were immunized with 10 μg/mouse p195-212 in complete Freund's adjuvant with concomitant oral administration of the dual analog (500 μg/mouse).
All stimulations were performed with p195-212 except those indicated with * that were stimulated with ConA. Cytokine secretion upon stimulation with p195-212 or ConA was considered as 100% (IL-2 100% = 144 pg/ml, IFN-γ 100% = 15.4 ng/ml, IL-4 100% = 2 pg/ml, IL-5 100% = 24 pg/ml, IL-10 100% = 64.8 pg/ml and TGF-β 100% = 14.3 pg/ml).

Effect of the dual analog on phospholipase C (PLC) activity

Stimulation of a T cell through its antigen-specific receptor by antigen or anti-receptor antibodies initiates a series of biochemical events which result in cellular proliferation and cytokine production. TCR engagement by ligand is a complex event that may activate multiple discrete pathways [25, 26]. One of the earliest detectable events following stimulation with an antigen is the activation of a number of protein tyrosine kinases which subsequently leads to receptor autophosphorylation and increased tyrosine phosphorylation of numerous cellular proteins, including PLC [25-27]. The receptor autophosphorylation creates high-affinity binding sites for several proteins containing SH2 domains, including PLCγ1, which is the main isoform of PLC in T cells. The phosphorylation and activation of PLCγ1 results in hydrolysis of phosphatidylinositol-4,5-biphosphate (PIP_2), which in turn yields the second messengers inositol-1,4,5-triphosphate (IP_3) and diacyl glycerol. These second messengers are respectively responsible for the TCR-induced rapid and sustained increase in the concentration of intracellular calcium ions and the activation of protein kinase C.

Studies of T cell responses to altered peptide ligands have provided functional evidence that a T cell receptor can respond to small changes in its ligand, resulting in different outcomes [25, 28, 29]. Such small changes in the ligand can convert fully activating ligands into partially activating (partial agonists) or even inhibitory ones (antagonists).

One of our aims has been to gain more insight into signaling events that may be responsible for the activation of the specific T cell lines by the myasthenogenic peptides and for the inhibition of this activation by the dual analog. We decided to concentrate on one of the early enzymes participating in the signal transduction through the TCR-PLC. Therefore, we first examined whether the myasthenogenic peptides can activate PLC in the specific T cell lines. To this end we prelabeled specifically the phosphoinositides of the cells of the line with [^{3}H] inositol. Cells were then incubated with syngeneic APC and with the indicated peptides, and at the end of the reaction, the inositol phosphates were extracted, separated and radioactivity was determined by a beta counter.

Table 5 shows that both myasthenogenic peptides, p259-271 and p195-212, stimulated generation of inositol phosphates. Most of the generated inositol phosphates were IP_1 (six folds of the amount of inositol polyphosphates in the case of the p259-271 specific T cell line, and three folds in the case of p195-212). The generation of inositol phosphates by the peptide-specific T cell lines resulted because of the specific stimulation by the appropriate myasthenogenic peptide, since the T cell lines did not respond to triggering by the reversed forms of these peptides. The ability of the dual analog to inhibit the PLC activity induced by each of the myasthenogenic peptide p259-271 and p195-212 was tested. As shown in Table 5, the concomitant addition of the dual analog to the assay mixture, which included one of the myasthenogenic peptides-specific T cell lines, APC and the appropriate myasthenogenic peptide could inhibit the generation of IP_1 and IP_2+IP_3 induced by p259-271 or p195-212 by up to 51%-67%. In order to verify that the inhibition was not a mere result of MHC blockade, we performed similar assays in which the reversed dual analog at the same concentration was added to the cells concomitant with the myasthenogenic peptides. Table 5 also shows that while the dual analog inhibited the stimulation by the myasthenogenic peptides, the reversed dual analog at the same concentration did not prevent the activation of PLC by these peptides.

Table 5. The dual analog inhibits inositol phospholipid hydrolysis induced in T cell lines by the myasthenogenic peptides

	p195-212		p259-271	
	IP_1	IP_2+IP_3	IP_1	IP_2+IP_3
w/o peptide	17%	29%	7%	13%
+peptide	100%	100%	100%	100%
+peptide +dual analog	49%	49%	33%	37%
+peptide +reversed dual analog	95%	104%	113%	124%

Cells of the peptide-specific line were prelabeled with myo-[2-^{3}H]inositol, and incubated with different concentrations of the dual analog or its reversed peptide, together with the appropriate peptide p195-212 or p259-271, and with APC. The reaction was terminated after 2 hr for p259-271, or after 3.5 hr for p195-212 and the levels of the inositol phosphates were measured. The levels of inositol phosphates generated by cells that were activated by each myasthenogenic peptide in the absence of the analog were considered as 100% activation [for p195-212 100% IP_1 = 7936 cpm, 100% IP_2 + IP_3 = 3218 cpm and for p259-271 100% IP_1 = 7547 cpm, 100% IP_2 + IP_3 = 1510 cpm].

We have recently shown that the dual analog of the myasthenogenic peptides could not induce PLC activity but caused tyrosine phosphorylation of PLCγ1 [30]. Moreover, the analog could inhibit PLC activity induced by the myasthenogenic peptides, but it could not inhibit the induced tyrosine phosphorylation. Taken those results together, the dual analog, which is composed of two altered myasthenogenic peptides appears to be a partial agonist.

It is noteworthy that most of the studies reported by other researchers used anti-CD3 antibodies to activate the cells and to measure PLC activity. Studies performed using peptides and their analogs were focused on the inability of the altered peptides to activate PLC and not on the potential use of the analogs to inhibit the signal transduced by the original peptide and thus to inhibit autoreactive T cells.

The intracellular mechanisms by which the dual analog exerts its effects on the T cells *in vivo* have not been studied yet. Since we have shown *in vitro* that the myasthenogenic peptides stimulate PLC activity in the peptide-specific T cell lines, and that the dual analog inhibits this stimulation, it was of interest to find out whether the dual analog can inhibit the PLC activity of the specific T cells *in vivo* as well. For that purpose we tested the response (in terms of PLC activity) of lymph node T cells originated from p259-271-immunized mice, that were *in vivo* treated or not treated with the dual analog, to *in vitro* stimulation by p259-271. As can be seen in Table 6, *in vitro* triggering of lymph node T cells from p259-271-immunized mice (that were not treated with the dual analog) elevated the PLC activity by around 48%. However, *in vitro* presentation of p259-271 to lymph node T cells that were derived from the dual analog-treated animals, caused a reduction of about 31% in the PLC activity. Thus, according to our results, down regulation of *in vivo* autoimmune responses caused by the dual analog correlates with its inhibitory capacity of PLC activation triggered by pathogenic epitopes.

Table 6. The dual analog inhibits inositol phospholipid hydrolisis in lymph node T cells derived from mice that were immunized with the myasthenogenic peptide and treated subcutaneously with the dual analog

In vivo treatment	*In vitro* treatment		
		IP^1	IP^2+IP^3
	w/o p259-271	100%	100%
+p259-271	+p259-271	149%±10	147%±11
	w/o p259-271	100%	100%
+p259-271+dual analog	+p259-271	72%±7	66%±10

BALB/c mice were immunized with p259-271 (10 μg/mouse) and treated or not treated with the dual analog (subcutaneously, 150 μg/mouse). Lymph node T cells were isolated (using goat-anti-mouse-Ig), prelabeled with myo-[2-^{3}H]inositol, washed and incubated for 24 hr with the myasthenogenic peptide p259-271 (25-50 μM), in the presence of APC. The levels of the generated inositol phosphates were measured. The levels of inositol phosphates generated by T cells that were not activated *in vitro* by p259-271 were considered as 100% activation. Results are mean of four independent experiments. 100% for IP^1 were 3191±1568 cpm and 785±239 cpm for $IP_2 + IP_3$.

Conclusions

A dual analog composed of two single amino acid-substituted analogs was prepared and tested for its ability to down-regulate *in vitro* and *in vivo* MG-associated autoimmune responses.The dual analog inhibits both *in vitro* and *in vivo* T cell responses specific to the myasthenogenic T cell epitopes, p195-212 and p259-271. The dual analog has also beneficial effects on the clinical manifestations of EAMG, induced either by pathogenic T cell lines specific to the myasthenogenic peptides or by Torpedo AChR. The mechanisms by which the dual analog exerts its effects were investigated both *in vitro*, in T cell lines specific to the myasthenogenic peptides, and *in vivo* in mice treated with it. One of the possible mechanisms by which the dual analog down-regulates the MG-associated autoimmune responses is via anergy induction, since *in vitro* addition of rIL-2 could overcome the unresponsive state that follows administration of the dual analog. The dual analog down-regulated the cytokines secreted by p195-212-specific T cell lines (except from TGF-*β*) *in vitro*, whereas it shifted the cytokine balance in p195-212 immunized mice that were treated *in vivo* with it from the Th1-type profile to the TH2/3-type profile that was shown to have a protective effect in a few autoimune diseases. At the signal transduction level, the dual analog inhibited PLC activity both *in vitro* and *in vivo*. Based on the results presented in this study, it can be concluded that the dual analog acts as a partial agonist which delivers through the TCR a signal that is qualitatively different from the signal delivered by the myasthenogenic peptides. The different signal delivered by the dual analog may involve signal transduction pathways and proteins that are not activated when the myasthenogenic peptides bind to the TCR. These different pathways may lead to activation of different transcription factors that activate genes different from those activated upon stimulation with the myasthenogenic peptides. The latter may result for example, in the production of the different profile of cytokines observed following exposure to the dual analog. The secretion of immunosuppressive cytokines like the Th2/Th3-type cytokines may affect not only the specifically primed lymphocytes, but rather other lymphocytes in the microenviroment (bystander suppression) and lead to the effective immunomodulation of MG-related manifestations demonstrated upon treatment with the dual analog.

Acknowledgements

This research was supported by Teva Pharmaceutical Industries Limited., Israel (M.S. and E.M.). A gift of the Torpedo acetylcholine receptor from Dr. Y. Pass and Prof. J.P. Changeux is gratefully acknowledged.

References

1. Ahlberg, R., Q. Yi, R. Pirskanen, G. Matell, C. Swerup, E.P. Rieber, G. Riethmuller, G. Holm and A.K. Lefvert. 1994. Treatment of myasthenia gravis with anti-CD4 antibody: improvement correlates to decreased T cell autoreactivity. *Neurology.* 44: 1732.
2. Lindstrom, J., D. Shelton and Y. Fuji. 1988. Myasthenia gravis. *Adv. Immunol.* 42: 233.
3. Drachman, D.B. 1994. Myasthenia gravis. *N. Engl. Med.* 25: 1797.
4. Kirshner, S.L., Y. Katz-Levy, I. Wirguin, Z. Argov and E. Mozes. 1994. Fine specificity of T cell lines and clones that are capable of inducing autoimmune manifestations in mice. *Cell. Immunol.* 157: 11.
5. Brocke, S., C. Brautbar, L. Steinman, O. Abramsky, J. Rothbard, D. Newmann, S. Fuchs and E. Mozes. 1988. Proliferative responses and antibody titers specific to human acetylcholine receptor synthetic peptides in patients with myasthenia gravis and relation to HLA class II genes. *J. Clin. Invest.* 82: 1894.
6. Brocke, S., M. Dayan, J. Rothbard, S. Fuchs and E. Mozes. 1990. The autoimmune response of different mouse strains to T-cell epitopes of the human acetylcholine receptor alpha subunit. *Immunology.* 69: 495.
7. Katz-Levy, Y., S.L. Kirshner, M. Sela and E. Mozes. 1993. Inhibition of T-cell reactivity to myasthenogenic epitopes of the human acetylcholine receptor by synthetic analogs. *Proc. Natl. Acad. Sci.* USA. 90: 7000.
8. Katz-Levy, Y., M. Dayan, I. Wirguin, M. Fridkin, M. Sela and E. Mozes. 1998. Single amino acid analogs of a myasthenogenic peptide modulate specific T cell responses and prevent the induction of experimental autoimmune myasthenia gravis. *J. Neuroimmunol.* 85: 78.
9. Kirshner, S. L., E. Zisman, M. Fridkin, M. Sela and E. Mozes. 1996. Altered

peptide ligands of a myasthenogenic epitope as modulators of specific T-cell responses. *Scand. J. Immunol.* 44: 512.

10. Zisman, E., Y. Katz Levy, M. Dayan, S.L. Kirshner, M. Paas Rozner, A. Karni, O. Abramsky, C. Brautbar, M. Fridkin, M. Sela and E. Mozes. 1996. Peptide analogs to pathogenic epitopes of the human acetylcholine receptor alpha subunit as potential modulators of myasthenia gravis. *Proc. Natl. Acad. Sci. USA*. 93: 4492.
11. Katz Levy, Y., M. Paas Rozner, S. Kirshner, M. Dayan, E. Zisman, M. Fridkin, I. Wirguin, M. Sela and E. Mozes. 1997. A peptide composed of tandem analogs of two myasthenogenic T cell epitopes interferes with specific autoimmune responses. *Proc. Natl. Acad. Sci. USA*. 94: 3200.
12. Liblau, R.S., S.M. Singer and H.O. McDevitt. 1995. Th1 and Th2 CD4+ T cells in the pathogenesis of organ-specific autoimmune diseases. *Immunol. Today.* 16: 34.
13. Olsson, T. 1995. Critical influences of the cytokine orchestration or the outcome of myelin antigen-specific autoimmunity in experimental autoimmune encephalomyelitis, multiple sclerosis. *Immunol. Rev.* 144: 245.
14. Khoury, S.J., W.W. Hancock and H.L. Weiner. 1992. Oral tolerance to myelin basic protein and natural recovery from experimental autoimmune encephalomyelitis are associated with downregulation of inflammatory cytokines and differential upregulation of transforming growth factor β, interleukin 4 and prostaglandin E expression in the brain. *J. Exp. Med.* 176: 1355.
15. Kennedy, M.K., D.S. Torrance, K.S. Picha and K.M. Mohler. 1992. Analysis of cytokine mRNA expression in the central nervous system of mice with experimental autoimmune encephalomyelitis reveals that IL-10 mRNA expression correlates with recovery. *J. Immunol. 149: 2496.*
16. Shimada, A., B. Charlton, P. Rohane, C. Taylor-Edwards and C.G. Fathman. 1996. Immune regulation in type 1 diabetes. *J. Autoimmun.* 9: 263.
17. Tian, J., M.A. Atkinson, M. Clare-Salzer, A. Herschenfeld, T. Forsthuber, P.V. Lehmann and D.L. Kaufman. 1996. Nasal administration of glutamate decarboxylase (GAD65) peptides induces Th2 responses and prevents murine insulin-dependent diabetes. *J. Exp. Med.* 183: 1561.
18. Powrie, F., J. Carlino, M.W. Leach, S. Mauze and R.L. Coffman. 1996. A critical role for transforming growth factor-β but not interleukin 4 in the suppression of T helper type 1-mediated colitis by CD45RBlowCD4+T cells. *J. Exp. Med.* 183: 2669.
19. Balasa, B., C. Deng, J. Lee, L.M. Bradley, D.K. Dalton, P. Christadoss and N. Sarvetnick. 1997. Interferon γ (IFN-γ) is necessary for the genesis of acetylcholine receptor-induced clinical experimental autoimmune myasthenia gravis. *J. Exp. Med.* 186: 385.
20. Ma, C.G., G.X. Zhang, B.G. Xiao and H. Link. 1996. Cellular mRNA expression of interferon-gamma (IFN-γ), IL-4 and transforming growth factor-beta (TGF-β) in rats nasally tolerized against experimental autoimmune myasthenia gravis (EAMG). *Clin. Exp. Immunol.* 104: 509.
21. Shi, F.D., G.X. Zhang, X.F. Bai, P.H. van Der Meide and H. Link. 1997. Cellular mRNA expression of interferon-gamma (IFN-γ), IL-4 and IL-10 relates to resistance to experimental autoimmune myasthenia gravis (EAMG) in young Lewis rats. *Clin. Exp. Immunol.* 108: 523.
22. Balasa, B., C. Deng, J. Lee, P. Christadoss and N. Sarvetnick. 1998. The Th2 cytokine IL-4 is not required for the progression of antibody-dependent autoimmune myasthenia gravis. *J. Immunol.* 161: 2856.
23. Ma, C.G., G.X. Zhang, B.G. Xiao, J. Link, T. Olsson and H. Link. 1995. Suppression

of experimental autoimmune myasthenia gravis by nasal administration of acetylcholine receptor. *J. Neuroimmunol.* 58: 51.

24. Wang, Z.Y., j. Qiao and H. Link. 1993. Suppression of experimental autoimmune myasthenia gravis by oral administration of acetylcholine receptor. *J. Neuroimmunol.* 44: 209.
25. Alberola-Ila, J., S. Takaki, J.D. Kerner and R.M. Perlmutter. 1997. Differential signaling by lymphocyte antigen receptors. *Annu. Rev. Immunol.* 15: 125.
26. Cantrell, D. 1996. T cell antigen receptor signal transduction pathways. *Annu. Rev. Immunol.* 14: 259.
27. Chan, A.C. and A.S. Shaw. 1995. Regulation of antigen receptor signal transduction by protein tyrosine kinases. *Curr. Opin. Immunol.* 8: 394.
28. Evavold, B.D., J. Sloan-Lancaster and P.M. Allen. 1993. Tickling of the TCR: selective T cell functions stimulated by altered peptide ligands. *Immunol. Today.* 14: 602.
29. Sloan-Lancaster, J. and P.M. Allen. 1996. Altered peptide ligand-induced partial T cell activation: molecular mechanisms and role in T cell biology. *Annu. Rev. Immunol.* 14: 1.
30. Faber-Elmann, A., M. Paas-Rozner, M. Sela and E. Mozes. 1998. Altered peptide ligands act as partial agonists by inhibiting phospholipase C activity induced by myasthenogenic T cell epitopes. *Proc. Natl. Acad. Sci.* USA. 95: 14320.

Myasthenia Gravis: Disease mechanisms and immunointervention
P. Christadoss (Ed)

18. Antigen-Specific Immunointervention in Experimental Myasthenia Gravis

Caishu Deng and Premkumar Christadoss
Department of Microbiology & Immunology, The University of Texas Medical Branch, Galveston, TX 77555-1070

Introduction

Myasthenia gravis (MG) and its animal model experimental autoimmune myasthenia gravis (EAMG) are neuromuscular junction transmission defect disorders. Both MG and EAMG are autoimmune diseases caused by antibodies attacking the nicotinic acetylcholine receptor (AChR) of the neuromuscular junctions. Conventionally, MG has been treated with immunosuppressive drugs, such as corticosteroids, azathioprine, cyclophosphamide, cyclosporine A, and symptom-relieving drugs. These medications may be effective, but the main drawback of immunosuppressive therapy is its non-specificity, which causes side effects due to global immunosuppression [1-5].

Ideally, treatment of autoimmune diseases, including MG, should specifically delete or suppress the function of the lymphocyte clones involved in the disease pathogenesis. High-dose tolerance to a given autoantigen has long been proposed as an effective means of treating autoimmune diseases. Cellular-mediated autoimmune diseases, including experimental autoimmune encephalomyelitis, collagen-induced arthritis, experimental autoimmune uveitis, and NOD type I diabetes, have been prevented by high-dose tolerance to specific autoantigen. These tolerance approaches are antigen-specific, which only suppress the antigen-specific immune responses and leave the rest of the immune responses intact. MG and EAMG are classical antibody-mediated autoimmune diseases. Pathogenesis of these diseases depends on T cell help for B cell production of pathogenic antibodies [6, 7]. Depletion of CD4 cells not only prevented EAMG development, but also reversed established clinical EAMG [7]. Moreover, CD4-deficient mice have a lower incidence of EAMG [8]. EAMG mimics MG in its clinical and immunopathological manifestations and is a prototypical model to study the cellular and molecular mechanisms of pathogenesis, and therapeutic effects of specific agents in antibody-mediated autoimmune diseases. MHC class II-restricted CD4+ cells and a dominant T cell epitope within the AChR α subunit region α146-162 have been implicated in EAMG pathogenesis in C57BL/6J (B6) mice [9-12]. It is suggested that α146-162 peptide-reactive CD4+ cells interact with AChR-specific B cells to produce pathogenic anti-AChR antibodies.

Thus suppression or deletion of AChR-specific CD4 cells should either prevent and/or induce clinical remission of EAMG. In this article we will provide an overview of studies performed in different laboratories on antigen-specific interventions of EAMG and the possible mechanisms which underlie each therapeutic approach.

Systemic Tolerance with AChR T Cell Epitope α146-162 Peptide

AChR α subunit peptide α146-162 is one of the dominant T cell epitopes involved in EAMG pathogenesis [11, 12]. Studies in our laboratory showed that neonatal injection of soluble α146-162 peptide could prevent adult mice from developing EAMG upon immunization with AChR in CFA [11]. To evaluate the effect of high-dose α146-162 peptide tolerance on EAMG, we performed a series of experiments. We first tested whether high-dose α146-162 peptide suppresses the AChR-specific T cell response. B6 mice were immunized with 20 μg of AChR in CFA. A week later 300 μg α146-162 peptide or PBS in incomplete Freund's adjuvant (IFA) was administered intraperitoneally (ip). Seven days after the induction of tolerance, draining lymph node cells (LNC) were exposed to AChR, its peptides α146-162 and α182-198, or PPD. T cell proliferation by ^{3}H-thymide incorporation and cytokine production in supernatant were measured. Tolerance induction with α146-162 peptide after primary immunization with AChR suppressed AChR and α146-162 peptide-specific lymphocyte proliferation. A similar suppression of α182-198 peptide-specific proliferation was also observed. However, there was no marked suppression of the PPD-specific response in these mice. Th1 cytokines IFN-γ and IL-2 and Th2 cytokine IL-10 produced by AChR, α146-162 and α182-198 peptide-specific T cells were suppressed. The α146-162 peptide-induced tolerance not only suppressed the response to α146-162 peptide itself, but also suppressed responses to the entire auto-antigen AChR and the other AChR subdominant peptide α182-198 due to a possible epitope spread (bystander effect), which is caused by reduction of IL-2, IFN-γ, or IL-10 production [13].

We also tested the effect of high-dose α146-162 peptide on the keyhole limpet hemocyanin (KLH)-specific T cell response. B6 mice were immunized with KLH in CFA. Seven days later the mice were injected ip with either 300 μg α146-162 peptide or PBS in IFA. After a week, draining LNC were collected to examine the T cell proliferative response to KLH. High-doses of peptide α146-162 failed to suppress the KLH-primed T cell response, implicating the antigen-specificity of α146-162 peptide-induced tolerance.

To study the effect of high-dose α146-162 peptide on the development of EAMG, we performed two *in vivo* experiments. B6 mice were immunized with 20 μg AChR in CFA on days 0 and 30. On days 10 and 18, 300 μg α146-162 peptide in IFA was injected subcutaneously (sc), the control mice were injected with either PBS or 300 μg ku peptide (control) in IFA. Clinical EAMG was evaluated, and its incidence was significantly lower in the high-dose α146-162-treated group compared to a control group (Table 1) [13]. The serum anti-AChR antibody response was lower in tolerance than that in the control group, even though there was no significant difference. However, anti-AChR IgG2b was significantly suppressed by high-dose α146-162 tolerance. Thus suppressing a fraction of pathogenic anti-AChR IgG2b antibody, rather than suppressing the overall antibody response could prevent EAMG [13]. The data also implicate for the first time the critical role played by anti-AChR IgG2b isotype in EAMG pathogenesis.

Table 1. Summary of clinical EAMG findings of systemic α146-162 peptide-tolerized and control mice [13]

Experiment	Treatment	Total number of mice	Muscle Weakness Grade 0	1+	2+	3+	Accumulated Clinical EAMG Incidence
1	PBS + IFA	20	3	3	6	8	85% (17/20)
	α146-162 + IFA	20	12	2	2	4	40% (8/20)
2	ku peptide + IFA	20	3	1	9	7	85% (17/20)
	α146-162 + IFA	20	10	2	4	4	50% (10/20)

In all of the above studies, we have used IFA as an adjuvant for peptide-specific tolerance induction. The main purpose is to slowly release the peptide *in vivo*. In humans, it is better to avoid the parenteral administration of IFA. Therefore, we tested the effect of intravenous injection of soluble α146-162 peptide on T cell response and clinical EAMG. The experimental procedure was the same as before. Results showed that AChR-specific T cell responses to AChR, peptide α146-162 and α182-198 were suppressed by IV injection of 300 μg α146-162 peptide. A high-dose of an irrelevant ovalbumin peptide 323-339 had little effect on the AChR-primed T cell response. However, soluble α146-162 peptide failed to prevent clinical EAMG development. To induce suppression of clinical EAMG, it may be necessary for the AChR immune cells to be in continuous contact with the peptide to suppress or delete (e.g. apoptosis) the pathogenic T cells. Because short fragments of peptides are rapidly removed *in vivo*, adjuvant may be required to maintain tolerance.

The effect of a high-dose of AChR in IFA given subcutaneously after the secondary immunization was also investigated. B6 mice were immunized with 20 μg AChR in CFA on days 0 and 30. Seven days after the second immunization, 500 μg AChR in IFA was injected sc, and PBS in IFA sc as control. The incidence and severity of EAMG were similar between the two groups. It is possible that a single dose of 500 μg of AChR in IFA may not be sufficient to induce tolerance once memory T and B cells specific for AChR have been established.

In our system, a high-dose α146-162 peptide in IFA ip suppressed AChR-primed T cell response and production of AChR, α146-162, and α182-198 peptide specific IFN-γ, IL-2 and IL-10. High-dose α146-162 in IFA sc prevented EAMG development. We could tolerize the T cell response and clinical EAMG after the primary immune response has been established. Whether this approach will be effective in reversing the established disease remains to be seen.

Oral Tolerance

Tolerance with the whole AChR molecule

Oral administration of antigen is one of the ideal methods of inducing tolerance. The drawback is that the peptic enzymes digest the majority of antigen, and therefore, a huge amount of antigen should be given to induce tolerance in EAMG. Either the entire AChR molecule or its fragments have been used to induce oral tolerance. Wang et al [14] fed Lewis rats with different doses of AChR prior to immunization, and consequently prevented EAMG development. The higher the dose, the more effective was the suppression. EAMG was believed to be suppressed through active suppression by endogenous cyokines, such as TGFβ, and suppression of both Th1 and Th2 cytokine production [15]. An oral high-dose of AChR failed to suppress both Con-A-induced cytokine production and the development of EAE in rats that were immunized with MBP in CFA [16]. Therefore, oral high-doses of AChR-induced tolerance is antigen-specific. Similar data were obtained by Okumura et al [17]. Either a low dose (0.25 μg × 5) or a high-dose (1 μg × 5) of purified AChR completely prevented EAMG. However, both low- and high-doses of unpurified AChR only partially prevented EAMG, while an oral high-dose of ovalbumin failed to prevent EAMG. The anti-AChR antibody response was initially increased, but later significantly suppressed by high-dose purified AChR tolerance. The AChR-specific T cell response to AChR and IL-2 production were partially suppressed by a low-dose of AChR tolerance, but significantly suppressed by a high-dose of AChR tolerance. A high-dose of ovalbumin feeding could not suppress cellular and humoral responses to AChR [17].

Drachman et al tested the effect of high-dose AChR tolerance on the ongoing immune response to AChR (18). They immunized Lewis rats with AChR. Two weeks later when the immune response was well established, but before the development of clinical EAMG, groups of rats were fed either pure AChR (1 μg every 3 days × 5) or control vehicle. The rats were examined for clinical EAMG. Oral high-dose AChR significantly reduced the clinical score. However, the antibody response to either *Torpedo* or rat AChR was enhanced in the AChR-fed rats. The cellular response to AChR and IL-2 production were not inhibited by oral high-dose of AChR. The authors concluded that the extra antibodies produced after oral tolerance were not pathogenic. Therefore, oral high doses of AChR in an ongoing immune response resulted in a paradoxical inverse relationship between the increased antibody response and clinical benefit.

Tolerance with α146-162 peptide

Recently oral tolerance with α146-162 peptide prevented EAMG and reduced anti-AChR antibody response (Baggi et al, this volume). Interesting, oral tolerance to α146-162 peptide suppressed AChR-specific lymphocyte response to peptides α146-162, α182-198 and whole AChR, as well as both Th1 (IL-2, IFN-γ) and Th2 (IL-10) cytokine production as observed for systemic tolerance with α146-162 peptide [13]. Control peptide failed to suppress the AChR-specific T cell response. Again studies are required to observe the effect of oral tolerance to

AChR or the peptides on established clinical EAMG, in order to apply this approach in the treatment of human MG.

Nasal Tolerance

Tolerance with the whole AChR molecule

An alternative administration of antigen by mucosal absorption for tolerance induction is nasal inhalation. Nasal administration of antigen requires very low doses without peptic proteolytic degradation of the antigen. Extensive studies using AChR or its fragments by nasal administration have been performed. Ma et al reported that nasal administration of micrograms of AChR could prevent EAMG, suppress serum anti-AChR antibodies, and decrease the delayed-type hypersensitivity response to AChR [19]. Nasal tolerance also suppressed the AChR-specific IgG-secreting cells, the AChR-reactive, IFN-γ secreting cells and T cell proliferation to AChR. Nasal tolerance not only prevented EAMG, but also induced protective tolerance in primed animals. Furthermore, nasal administration of higher doses of AChR to Lewis rats two weeks after immunization with AChR in CFA could ameliorate clinical EAMG [20]. Nasal tolerance reduced AChR-specific T cell proliferation, and IFN-γ secretion. The anti-AChR antibodies in the rats in which tolerance was induced had a lower affinity, and serum IgG2b and AChR degradation were reduced. The numbers of IFN-γ and TNF-α mRNA-expressing LNC cells were suppressed, while IL-4, IL-10 and TGFβ mRNA-expressing cells were unaffected. These data indicated that the prevention of EAMG by nasal administration of high-doses of AChR is associated with selective suppression of Th1 functions, without influencing Th2 cell functions. The impaired Thl functions may result in the production of fewer pathogenic anti-AChR antibodies and contribute to the amelioration of EAMG severity.

Tolerance with AChR peptide

In addition to nasal administration of the entire AChR to induce immune suppression of EAMG, other groups have tolerized EAMG by nasal administration of synthetic fragments of AChR. Karachunski et al observed the effect of nasal delivery of synthetic sequences of *Torpedo* AChR (TAChR) α chain epitopes recognized by anti-AChR CD4 T cells (α150-169, α181-200, and α360-378), given before and during immunization with TAChR, on clinical EAMG. Nasal administration of α150-169 alone or in combination with the above 3 peptides either before or during immunization induced lower CD4 responsiveness to those epitopes and to AChR, reduced synthesis of anti-AChR Ab, and prevented EAMG ([21], Karachunski et al, this volume). These effects were not induced by nasal administration of synthetic epitopes of diphtheria toxin. Studies on cytokine profiles by splenocytes showed that in sham-tolerized mice only Th1 (IL-2 only) cells responded to TAChR, while peptide-treated mice had AChR-specific Th2 (IL-4 and IL-10) responses. The AChR peptide treatment induced anergy *in vitro,* and IL-2 could reverse these anergized T cell responses.

However, Zhang et al showed that synthetic peptides of AChR α chain failed to induce nasal tolerance in EAMG [22]. Nasal administration of different doses

(25, 100, or 500 μg daily for 10 days) of AChR α subunit peptide α61-76, α100-116, α146-162, α261-277), or δ subunit δ345-367, or combination of these peptides to Lewis rats pre-immunized with AChR failed to prevent EAMG development [22]. This treatment also failed to affect the levels or affinities of anti-AChR antibodies in peptide(s)-treated rats when compared to control rats. Further studies are required to show effective suppression of ongoing clinical EAMG with nasal tolerance to AChR or its peptides.

Tolerance with AChR extracellular domain

A large portion of autoantibodies in MG is directed to the main immunogenic region (MIR) of the extracellular domain of AChR [23, 24]. Recombinant human AChR α chain fragments, Hα1-210 and Hα1-121, contain MIR. Fragment Hα122-210 has only ACh-binding site. Fragments Hα1-121 and Hα1-210 could prevent both passive transfer and actively induced EAMG. Myasthenic symptoms were prevented by one milligram of fragment Hα1-121 either preincubated with mAb 198 for 30 min, prior to the injection into rats, or injected into rats together with mAb 198, without preincubation. Similar results were obtained with the Hα1-210 recombinant fragment, but not with Hα122-210, and controls. Nasal administration of these fragments to rats over 10 consecutive days prior to immunization with AChR in CFA markedly prevented EAMG development. There were no significant differences between the groups that were pretreated with Hα1-210, Hα1-121, or Hα122-210. T cell responses to AChR and the production of IL-2 and IFN-γ were reduced in comparison to the controls [25].

Other Approaches of Antigen-Specific Suppression

Tolerance with AChR analog peptide

Single, substituted human AChR α chain peptides Hα195-212 and Hα259-271 analogs and dual analog, which contains the two single substituted analogs, could bind to MHC class II molecules on APC as effectively as the original peptides. These analogs significantly inhibited T cell responses induced by their respective myasthenogenic peptides [26]. Hα195-212 and Hα259-271 peptides are immunodominant T cell epitopes in SJL and BALB mice, respectively. The single, substituted analogs inhibited the proliferative response of T cell lines specific to relevant peptide and lymph node cells (LNC) of mice immunized to Hα195-212 and Hα159-271. The analog inhibited the *in vivo* priming of LNC of both SJL and BALB/c mice when administered iv, ip, or per os. The dual analog also suppressed the manifestation of EAMG induced by inoculation of a pathogenic T cell line. Therefore, a single peptide that is composed of analogs to two epitope specificity can be used to regulate T cell responses and diseases associated with each epitope ([26], Mozes et al, this volume).

Tolerance with AChR specific suppressor cells

Suppressor cells specific for AChR in EAMG were generated by McIntosh et al [27]. AChR-primed lymphocytes were cultured with the immunosuppressive drug cyclosporin A plus AChR for 7 days. These cells strongly suppressed anti-

AChR Ab production by lymphocytes from EAMG rats, but failed to suppress antibody response to an unrelated antigen. The authors suggested that this approach should be a potential way to induce specific suppressor cells from immunized populations of lymphocytes and could be used in the treatment of MG.

Tolerance by MHC class II competition peptide

Since MHC class II molecules play a crucial role in EAMG pathogenesis [10], blockage of MHC class II-peptide-TCR interaction through a competitive mechanism could prevent EAMG. Wauben et al [28] reported that MHC class II competitor peptides produced an altered immune response and suppressed EAMG. Co-immunizing Lewis rats with peptide OVA 323-339, which is a strong MHC class II-binding peptide, together with AChR resulted in complete disease inhibition. Not only was the total anti-AChR antibody response dramatically reduced, but also the IgG isotype was shifted from IgG2b to IgG1. However, this approach may not be antigen-specific. Any MHC class II-binding peptide could competitively block antigen presentation, and therefore inhibit any given immune response mediated by an MHC class II allele-specific response.

Tolerance with MHC class II: AChR peptide complex

T cell activation needs two signals. Delivering the first antigen-specific signal to the T cell in the absence of the second co-stimulatory signal induces T cell anergy. Nicolle et al [29] designed an approach to induce an AChR-specific T cell clone unresponsive to AChR. AChR-specific T cells were cloned from MG patients. One particular clone (PM-A1) with a known peptide epitope (α144-163) and MHC class II restriction (DR4 Dw14.2 or 4.2) was used. Soluble MHC-class II with AChR peptide complexes induced long-lasting tolerance in the PM-A1 clone. Preincubation of PM-A1 T cells with such a complex induced death by apoptosis in 40-50% of the AChR-specific cells. Surviving cells remained refractory to stimulation with AChR-derived synthetic peptides or recombinant polypeptides for 38 d after complex treatment. These effects were highly specific, dose-dependent and required more than 2 h preincubation. The T cells could be protected from the tolerizing effects of the complex by coincubation with DR-matched or -mismatched antigen-presenting cells.

MHC class II molecule derived from a rat was coupled with one of the AChR-dominant T cell epitope α100-116 peptides [30]. An irrelevant complex of MHC class II: HSP 180-188 or MHC class II alone was used as control. MHC class II: AChR α100-116 could bind to TCR with higher avidity and consequently initiate the early T cell signal events ordinarily induced by APC-associated MHC class II and peptide binding to TCR, but cannot activate T cells probably due to the lack of the second signal [30]. Preincubation of AChR-specific T cells with MHC class II:AChR α100-116 caused T cell unresponsiveness to AChR. *In vivo* treatment with soluble MHC class II: AChR α100-116 reduced the *ex vivo* proliferative response to AChR and peptide α100-116. *In vivo* MHC class II: AChR α100-116 treatment of rats co-immunized with peptides AChR α100-116 and MBP 69-88 inhibited the subsequent *in vitro* proliferative response to AChR α100-116, but not to MBP 69-88 peptide. The effect of MHC class II:α100-116

Table 2. Summary of experimental therapeutic approaches to prevent EAMG and possible mechanisms of tolerance

Tolerogen	Route	T cell response to AChR	Anti-AChR Antibody	Clinical EAMG	Mechanisms	Antigen Specific	References
α146–162 peptide + IFA	Systemic (S.C.)	Down regulated	Suppressed IgG2b	Suppressed	Decreased Th1 (IL-2 and IFN-γ) and Th2 (IL-10) cytokins	Yes	[13], This volume
α146–162 peptide	Oral	Down regulated	Suppressed	Suppressed	Decreased Th1 (IL-2 and IFN-γ) and Th2 (IL-10) cytokins	Yes	This volume
AChR	Oral	Down	Suppressed	Suppressed	Active suppression, Decreased IFN-γ IL-4, increased TGF-β	Yes	[14-18]
α chain recombinant fragment	Oral Nasal	Down regulated	Suppressed	Suppressed	Decreased Th1	Yes	[25], This volume
AChR or α chain peptides	Nasal	Down regulated	Suppressed	Suppressed	Decreased Th1; enhanced Th2 cytokines	Yes	[21]
MHC class II: AChR α100–116	I.V.	Down regulated	—	Suppressed	Anergy due to lack of costimulatory molecules	Yes	[30]
α chain analog	Oral	Down regulated	Suppressed	Suppressed	Decreased Th1, increased Th2 TGF-β	Yes	[26] This volume
MHC binding peptide	S.C.	Down regulated	Suppressed	Suppressed	Competitively bind MHC class II	No	[28]

on established EAMG was also tested. The EAMG rats were treated once a week for 5 weeks with 25 mg MHC II: AChR α100-116, 25 μg MHC II:HSP 180-188, 25 μg MHC II alone, respectively. The treatment of individual rats was started when net weight loss exceeded 10 g and clinical EAMG was reached. Four out of six (67%) rats in the MHC class II:AChR α100-116-treated group survived and showed clinical improvement, compared with 0-20% survival rate in all other treated groups. These data demonstrated that the MHC class II:AChR α110-116 complex not only specifically suppressed the T cell response to AChR, but also improved established clinical EAMG, which is more representative of the clinical situation encountered in human MG.

Conclusion

Ideally, treatment of autoimmune diseases should be antigen-specific. EAMG is an excellent model for developing antigen-specific therapeutic approaches because the auto-antigen, AChR, has been cloned, sequenced, and biochemically characterized. Thus far several approaches for intervention of EAMG have been investigated. Either the entire AChR molecule or its T cell epitopes and recombinant fragments administered through parenteral, nasal, or oral routes could suppress the AChR-specific T cell response and consequently prevent clinical EAMG (Table 2). However, the effect of these therapeutic approaches on ongoing clinical EAMG is not well established. Although few studies have been performed to study the mechanisms of the above tolerance (Table 2), further studies should be performed on the cellular and molecular mechanisms by which AChR- or peptide-specific tolerance is achieved.

Acknowledgements

Author's studies reported in this paper were partially supported by the Muscular Dystrophy Association and Francaise Centre Les Myopathis. Caishu Deng was a Myasthenia Gravis Foundation postdoctoral fellow and is now a James W. McLaughlin postdoctoral fellow.

References

1. Johns, J.R. 1987. Long term corticosteroid treatment of myasthenia gravis. *Ann. N. Y. Acad. Sci.* 505: 568–587.
2. Matell, G. 1987. Immunosuppressive drugs: Azathioprine in the treatment of myasthenia gravis. *Ann. N. Y. Acad. Sci. 505:588–594.*
3. Drachman, D.B. 1993. Myasthenia gravis. In: Current Therapy in Neurologic Disease. 4th ed. R.T. Johnson, J.W. Griffin, eds. St. Louis: Mosby-Year Book, p. 379–384.
4. Tindall, R.S., J.T. Phillips, J.A. Rollins, L. Wells and K. Hall. 1993. A clinical therapeutic trial of cyclosporine in myasthenia gravis. *Ann. N. Y. Acad. Sci.* 681: 539–551.
5. Wilensky, R., B. Dwyer and R.F. Mayer. 1993. Relapses in patients with myasthenia gravis treated with azathioprine. *Ann. N. Y. Acad. Sci.* 681: 591–593.
6. Christadoss, P., J. Lindstrom, R. Melvold and N. Talal. 1985. Mutation at I-A β

chain prevents experimental autoimmune myasthenia gravis. *Immunogenet.* 21: 33–38.

7. Christadoss, P. and M.J. Dauphinee. 1986. Immunotherapy for myasthenia gravis: A murine model. *J. Immunol.* 136: 2437–2440.
8. Zhang, G., B. Xiao, M. Bakhiet, P.V.D. Meide, H. Wigzell, H. Link and T. Olsson. 1996. Both CD4+ and CD8+ T cells are essential to induce experimental autoimmune myasthenia gravis. *J. Exp. Med.* 184: 349–356.
9. Hohlfeld, R., B. Conti-Tronconi., I. Kalies, J. Bertrams and K.V. Toyka. 1985 Genetic restriction of autoreactive acetylcholine receptor-specific T lymphocytes in myasthenia gravis. *J. Immunol.* 135: 2393.
10. Kaul, R., M. Shenoy, E. Goluszko and P. Christadoss. 1994. Major histocompatibility complex class II gene disruption prevents experimental autoimmune myasthenia gravis. *J. Immunol.* 152: 3152–3157.
11. Shenoy, M., M. Oshima, M.Z. Atassi, P. Christadoss. 1993. Suppression of experimental autoimmune myasthenia gravis by epitope–specific neonatal tolerance to synthetic region alpha 146–162 of acetylcholine receptor. *Clinical Immunology & Immunopathology.* 66(3): 230–8.
12. Shenoy, M., E. Goluszko and P. Christadoss. 1994. The pathogenic role of acetylcholine receptor α chain epitope within α146–162 in the development of experimental autoimmune myasthenia gravis in C57BL6 mice. *Clin. Immunol. Immunopathol.* 73: 338–343.
13. Wu, B., C. Deng, E. Goluszko and P. Christadoss. 1997. Tolerance to a dominant T cell epitope in the acetylcholine receptor molecule induces epitope spread and suppresses murine myasthenia gravis. *Journal of Immunology.* 159(6): 3016–23.
14. Wang, Z.Y., J. Qiao and H. Link. 1993. Suppression of experimental autoimmune myasthenia gravis by oral administration of acetylcholine receptor. *Journal of Neuroimmunology.* 44(2): 209–14.
15. Ma, C.G., G.X. Zhang, B.G. Xiao, Z.Y. Wang, J. Link, T. Olsson and H. Link. 1996. Mucosal tolerance to experimental autoimmune myasthenia gravis is associated with down-regulation of AChR-specific IFN-gamma-expressing Th1-like cells and up-regulation of TGF-beta mRNA in mononuclear cells. *Ann. N. Y. Acad. Sci.* 778: 273–87.
16. Wang, Z.Y., H. Link, A. Ljungdahl, B. Hojeberg, J. Link, B. He, J. Qiao, A. Melms and T. Olsson. 1994. Induction of interferon-γ, Interleukin-4, and transforming growth factor-β in rats orally tolerized against experimental autoimmune myasthenia gravis. *Cell. Immunol.* 157: 353–368.
17. Okumura, S., K. McIntosh and D.B. Drachman. 1994. Oral administration of acetylcholine receptor: effects on experimental myasthenia gravis. *Annals of Neurology.* 36(5): 704–13
18. Drachman, D.B., S. Okumura. R.N. Adams and K.R. McIntosh. 1996. Oral tolerance in myasthenia gravis. *Ann. N.Y. Acad. Sci.* 778: 258–72.
19. Ma, C.G., G.X. Zhang, B.G. Xiao, J. Link, T. Olsson, and H. Link. 1995. Suppression of experimental autoimmune myasthenia gravis by nasal administration of acetylcholine receptor. *J. Neuroimmunol.* 58: 51–60.
20. Shi, F.D., X.F. Bai, H.L. Li, Y.M. Huang, P.H. Van Der Meide and H. Link. 1998. Nasal tolerance in experimental autoimmune myasthenia gravis (EAMG): induction of protective tolerance in primed animals. *Clin Exp. Immunol.* 11: 506–512.
21. Karachunski, P.I., N.S. Ostlie, D.K. Okita and B.M. Conti-Fine. 1997. Prevention of experimental myasthenia gravis by nasal administration of synthetic acetylcholine receptor T epitope sequences. *Journal of Clinical Investigation.* 100(12): 3027–35.

22. Zhang, G.X., F.D. Shi , J. Zhu, B.G. Xiao, M. Levi, B. Wahren, L.Y. Yu and H. Link. 1998. Synthetic peptides fail to induce nasal tolerance to experimental autoimmune myasthenia gravis. *Journal of Neuroimmunology.* 85(1): 96–101.
23. Tzartos, S., L. Langeberg, S. Hochschwender and J. Lindstrom. 1983. Demonstration of a main immunogenic region on acetylcholine receptors from human muscle using monoclonal antibodies to human receptor. *FEBS Lett.* 158: 116–118.
24. Tzartos, S., A. Kokla, S.L. Walgrave and B.M. Conti-Tronconi. 1988. Localization of the main immunogenic region of human muscle acetylcholine receptor to residues 67–76 of alpha subunit. *Proc. Natl. Acad. Sci.* USA. 85: 2899–2903.
25. Barchan, D., O. Asher, S.J. Tzartos, S. Fuchs and M.C. Souroujon. 1998. Modulation of the anti-acetycholine receptor response and experimental autoimmune myasthenia gravis by recombinant fragments of the acetylcholine receptor. *Eur. J. Immunol.* 28: 616–624.
26. Katz-Levy, Y.M. Dayan, I. Wirguin, M. Fridkin, M. Sela and E. Mozes. 1998. Single amino acid analogs of a myasthenogenic peptide modulate specific T cell responses and prevent the induction of experimental autoimmune myasthenia gravis. *Journal of Neuroimmunology.* 85(1): 78–86.
27. McIntosh, K. and D.B. Drachman. 1986. Induction of suppressor cells specific for AChR in experimental myasthenia gravis. *Science.* 232: 401–403.
28. Wauben, M.H., A.C.W.E. Hoedemaekers, Y.M.E. Graus , J.P.A. Wagenaar, W. van Eden and M.H. Bates. 1996. Inhibition of experimental autoimmune mtasthenia gravis by major histocompatibility complex class II competitor peptides results not only in a suppressed but also in an altered immune response. *Eur. J. Immunol,* 26: 2866–2875.
29. Nicolle, M.W., B. Nag, S.D. Sharma, N. Willcox, A. Vincent, D.J. Ferguson and J. Newsom-Davis. 1994. Specific tolerance to an acetylcholine receptor epitope induced *in vitro* in myasthenia gravis CD4+ lymphocytes by soluble major histocompatibility complex class II-peptide complexes. *J. Clinical Investigation.* 93: 1361–1369.
30. Spack, E.G., M. McCutcheon, N. Corbelletta, B. Nag, D. Passmore and S.D. Sharma. 1995. Induction of tolerance in experimental autoimmune myasthenia gravis with solubilized MHC class II:acetylcholine receptor peptide complexes. *Journal of Autoimmunity.* 8(6): 787–807.

Index